ORDINARY FAMILIES, SPECIAL CHILDREN

Ordinary Families, Special Children

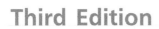

Third Edition

**A Systems Approach
to Childhood Disability**

Milton Seligman
Rosalyn Benjamin Darling

THE GUILFORD PRESS
New York   London

© 2007 The Guilford Press
A Division of Guilford Publications, Inc.
72 Spring Street, New York, NY 10012
www.guilford.com

Printed in the United States of America

This book is printed on acid-free paper.

Last digit is print number: 9 8 7 6 5 4 3 2 1

Library of Congress Cataloging-in-Publication Data
Seligman, Milton, 1937–
  Ordinary families, special children : a systems approach to childhood
disability / Milton Seligman and Rosalyn Benjamin Darling.—3rd ed.
    p. cm.
  Includes bibliographical references and index.
  ISBN-13: 978-1-59385-362-4 (hardcover: alk. paper)
  ISBN-10: 1-59385-362-9 (hardcover: alk. paper)
  1. Children with disabilities—Family relationships—United
States. 2. Parents of children with disabilities—United States. 3. Family
social work—United States. I. Darling, Rosalyn Benjamin. II. Title.
  HV888.5.S45 2007
  362.4′043083—dc22
                                                    2006033720

To the memory of my mother, Irma Seligman,
a woman of great warmth, social intelligence,
and remarkable culinary aptitude (1910–2004)
                                              –M. S.

To my extraordinary grandsons,
Elijah Wolf Darling and Isaac Olyn Darling
                                      –R. B. D.

About the Authors

Milton Seligman, PhD, is Professor Emeritus in the Department of Psychology in Education at the University of Pittsburgh. His chief academic interest is in the area of childhood disability and the family. Other areas of instruction and scholarship include individual and group psychotherapy and clinical supervision. Retired since 2004, Dr. Seligman maintains his private practice, serves on the editorial board for the *Journal for Specialists in Group Work,* and is currently writing a book for parents on childhood disability and the family. He lives in Pittsburgh with his wife.

Rosalyn Benjamin Darling, PhD, is Professor of Sociology at Indiana University of Pennsylvania, where she has taught since 1994. Prior to assuming her academic position, she served for 15 years as the executive director of an agency serving young children with disabilities and their families and was the founder and first president of the Early Intervention Providers Association of Pennsylvania. Dr. Darling has authored or coauthored eight books and numerous articles and chapters on disability and human services. She has played an active role in many state- and national-level disability-related organizations and committees and is currently engaged in research on orientations toward disability.

Preface

In this third edition of *Ordinary Families, Special Children*, we again want to share some thoughts about the title. Too often people have regarded families of children with disabilities as almost saintly. These parents' quotes from the Preface of the last edition describe this view:

> We parents of children with disabilities get a lot of "you are so wonderful as parents taking care of Scott/Heather (you supply the name). I don't see how you do it all . . . working, doing all the stuff for your child, and keeping a home. I know I could never do it."

> "You must be special people to get a child like that. . . . " Well, few people ask for a child "like that." You just look at what has to be done and do it. If the other person had a child with a disability, he/she would do what has to be done.

Children with disabilities are born into all sorts of families. Although such a birth is usually an unanticipated event, most families learn to accept, and sometimes even rejoice, in its occurrence. These parents do not begin their familial careers with any special gifts or skills; they simply "do what has to be done." Our title emphasizes this ordinariness in order to suggest the essential similarity of all families.

At the same time, ordinary families are usually poorly prepared to meet the special challenges posed by children with disabilities. They must confront a lack of specialized knowledge; often negative reactions from other family members, friends, and strangers; the limited accessibility of needed resources; and, often, professionals who provide insufficient or inappropriate assistance. As in the earlier editions of this book, we hope that the present volume will aid professionals in understanding the situation of ordinary families who happen to have children with out-of-the-ordinary needs and in helping these families to meet those needs.

As in the preceding editions, we examine the intertwined child, family, ecological, and sociocultural variables that are thought to contribute to the response of families to childhood disability. We want to illuminate those elements of family and community life that bear on the family's ability to achieve a satisfactory lifestyle. We also want to describe relevant intervention strategies and services for families when such help is being sought. Another task is to update our review of the research and to describe new programs and approaches that have emerged in recent years. We also include pioneering perspectives and approaches that have shed light on childhood disability and the family and that continue to maintain their relevance. In addition to research, we include clinical reports and personal observations from professionals and family members. The expansion of previously written chapters and the inclusion of new chapters reflect developments in the field since the last edition was published in 1997.

This edition is organized a little differently from previous editions. We have grouped the chapters into four sections to highlight our main themes. The first section provides the conceptual framework for the rest of the book and introduces the idea of family systems and social systems. The chapters in the second section use a sociological perspective and view the family over time, beginning in the prenatal period and ending with the child's future adulthood. The third section takes a psychological perspective in examining the impact of childhood disability on various members of the family system. Finally, the fourth section applies the material in previous sections to professional practice.

Since the publication of the second edition, the literature on the "partnership" model in human services has continued to grow. Although that model guided our thinking in the two earlier editions, we specifically discuss its importance in the present volume. Another kind of model that receives increased attention in this edition is the social or sociological model of disability, which has increasingly come to replace the medical or clinical model. Historical trends relating to the ascendance of the social model, such as the disability rights movement, are also addressed for the first time in this edition, as are some demographic trends in relation to children with disabilities.

There have been changes in counseling as well as other approaches to help families cope with childhood disability. Cognitive strategies, for example, have proven to be useful in helping families modify their thinking patterns and hone their coping abilities. Interest in group approaches has been an area of focus in helping families gain support, encouragement, and concrete information. Support groups and other types of group interventions are explored, including those for parents and separate ones for fathers, siblings, and grandparents.

Since the publication of the first edition in 1989, promising resources have been developed for families. For example, the Internet has become a wonderful resource. Subscribers to various lists can now get both information and support regarding children's disabilities and family issues. We have included material from such lists to illustrate the family experience and to highlight specific sites for information.

This edition reflects a shift in the language used to refer to persons with disabilities—a shift noted in the second edition. We embrace the perspective of Lyon, Knickelbaum, and Wolf (2005) who wrote:

> Disability is secondary to the person; it does not define who she or he is as a human being. The person is not a problem. Instead, attitudes and misconceptions about disability (and people with disabilities) can create barriers to their acceptance and participation as members of the adult community. (p. 831)

Although person-first language is occasionally awkward, this book uses it to acknowledge that a person who happens to have a disability is a person first. However, we want to acknowledge that not all people with disabilities prefer person-first language. Some in the disability rights community, for example, see the shared condition upon which their oppression is based as more salient than their identity as individuals. Members of this group have suggested that person-first language is euphemistic and individualistic. We agree with these arguments but do believe that language shapes thinking and that older constructions may perpetuate undesirable stereotypes about people with disabilities. We also have changed some other terminology to reflect newer preferences. For example, we use the term *intellectual disability* in place of *mental retardation*.

As suggested above, this edition reflects a number of new concepts. Concepts such as "putting the disability in its place," "family tra-jectory postdiagnosis," "disability identity," "disability pride," and "typology of adaptation" reflect conceptual lenses that provide fresh perspectives on family and disability. The concept of resilience in children and family members is discussed as well.

Moreover, this edition contains a new chapter that focuses on the "orientations" of adults with disabilities. After all, the desired outcome for children with disability is successful adulthood, however that may be defined by those individuals and their families. The newer orientation of disability pride, which derives from a social or sociological model of disability, is addressed in this new chapter, along with other orientations.

Information on fathers and grandparents occupied a single chapter in previous editions. We believe that separate chapters are warranted as the challenges and contributions of these family members have been brought into clearer focus. Recent conceptions of fathers' roles and scripts that contribute to major health problems and hinder their full participation in family life serve as a backdrop for a discussion of fathers and childhood disability. Recent research and commentary on grandparents sheds new light on their struggles and contributions.

For siblings, issues pertaining to a fear of contagion in very young children and caretaking in adulthood and in later life are presented along with emerging research and personal reflections of siblings of brothers or sisters with a major emotional or cognitive disability. This is an important topic that has not been given the attention it deserves.

The chapter on family diversity has been updated significantly in light of recent research on the impact of welfare reform and on the intersections between culture and disability. We also include information on single-parent and gay and lesbian families and on some ethnic groups, such as American Muslims, that was not included in earlier editions.

Our final chapter has been updated to include more information about the partnership model in human services and the relevance of that model to services for families of children with disabilities. In addition, we present a detailed discussion of areas to be considered in the identification of family resources, concerns, and priorities. We also address the development of outcomes and service activities, as these are conceptualized in the current evaluation literature.

As in previous editions, we have included the voices of family members themselves to explain and illustrate many of the concepts in the book. In this volume we have retained some older quotes that still ring true and added some newer ones that reflect more recent experiences.

M. S.:

I want to acknowledge the help and contributions of the following important people in my life:

My wife, Karen, who has considerable knowledge about disability issues from her academic background, her clinical and personal experience, and her point of view as a reader who gobbles up mysteries, biographies, and books written by those challenged by disability. She kept me from a dire fate as I wrestled with the vagaries of the computer world. She is my leaning post.

My daughter Lisa, who rescued me after my retirement from the University of Pittsburgh in September 2004. She graciously volunteered to type handwritten and often unreadable manuscript pages. There would not have been a third edition without her. I am blessed to have this lovely and accomplished lady as my daughter.

My daughter Lori, who provides me with many insights into what disability means to family life. Although she is challenged by disability, she forges ahead to be her own person, gaining independence, friends, and confidence—and winning a 2004 Jefferson Award in Pittsburgh, an award given to an individual who makes a difference in her community. I am proud of her and doubly blessed.

R. B. D.:

We both owe a great debt to several graduate assistants at Indiana University of Pennsylvania who made important contributions to this volume. Michelle Stagmer transferred all of the references from the last edition to EndNote format, and Patricia Heiple added many new references to the file. Debra Mason compiled information for an appendix, which we chose not to include because of limits on length. Debra and Julie Grant provided teaching support that allowed me time to work on this book. I am also indebted to Indiana University of Pennsylvania for providing me with a sabbatical semester, during which I completed most of my share of the writing.

As always, I want to thank my husband, Jon, for his unwavering support in all that I do. I am fortunate to have him as a partner.

Contents

IV. APPROACHES TO INTERVENTION

I.

CONCEPTUAL FRAMEWORK

■1■

Introduction and Conceptual Framework I

Social and Cultural Systems

To put the magnitude of extant disability in the U.S. population into perspective, the year 2000 disability status report from the U.S. Bureau of the Census counted 49.7 million people with a chronic illness or disability. This figure accounted for 19.3% of the U.S. noninstitutionalized population ages 5 and older—or nearly one person in five (U.S. Bureau of the Census, 2003a). These figures do not include infants and children from birth to 5 years of age. Among the population from 5 to 15, about 2.6 million, or 5.8%, had disabilities, with boys representing a larger proportion of the total than girls. Overall, 5.2 million children and teenagers—one out of every 12—have a physical or mental disability. These numbers represent an increase over those in data collected previously. In addition, in this population, disabilities are more common among Native Americans and African Americans than among European and Asian Americans. According to Schonberg and Tifft (2002) and Batshaw (2002), 3–5% of births result in a congenital disability or genetic disorder.

Childhood disabilities range from high-incidence impairments to those that are less frequent in the population. High-incidence impairments in persons 6–21 make up 92% of impairments overall, including specific learning disabilities, speech or language impairments, intellectual disability, and serious emotional disturbance (U.S. Department of Education, 1996; Hunt & Marshall, 1999). Lower-incidence impairments, which for each condition constitute less than 2%, include multiple disabilities, hearing impairments, orthopedic impairments, other health impairments, visual impairments, autism, deafness–blindness, and traumatic brain injury. Furthermore, more than 6.3 million children and youth, ages 3–21, received special education services during the school year (U.S. Department of Education, 2002).

We suspect that these statistics provide a meaningful yet incomplete picture of the portion of the U.S. population that has a disability. In accumulating data from various sources, one should be mindful that there are differences in definitions of what constitutes a disability, differences in how data on multiple conditions are determined and counted, sampling method differences, and decisions that are made about when certain age groups are included/excluded (Olkin, 1999; Shapiro, 1994). This concern does not diminish the validity of the reported figures, but it does suggest that there may be even more people with disabilities than the figures indicate. These numbers indicate that persons with disabilities constitute the largest minority group in the United States (Olkin, 1999), and one that anyone can join at any time as a consequence of illness or accident. Actually, less than 15% of people with disabilities were born with their disability (Shapiro, 1994).

Dramatic improvements in medicine have benefited the existing population of infants, children, youth, and adults with disabilities. Enhanced methods of assessment and diagnosis, along with a greater awareness of symptoms by informed family members have increased the early identification and remediation of disabling conditions. By keeping people alive, and by keeping them alive longer, medicine has contributed to a disability population explosion (Shapiro, 1994). Such medical discoveries as chemotherapy for cancer, insulin for diabetes, and the methods to sustain low-birth-weight infants have kept people with impairments alive and functioning, yet often with disabilities.

Social change has not kept pace with clinical progress. People with disabilities remain at a disadvantage in relation to those without them in virtually every area of life. These individuals are much more likely to be unemployed, to live in poverty, and to remain at home rather than attending social functions. In addition, only 34% of those with disabilities say they are very satisfied with their lives, compared with 61% of those without disabilities (*National Organization on*

Disability/Harris Survey of Americans with Disabilities, 2000). Children with disabilities also experience disadvantages in comparison with their nondisabled peers. For example, they are about twice or three times as likely as other children to be abused or neglected (National Clearinghouse on Child Abuse and Neglect [NCCAN], 2004). Eliminating such disadvantages requires societal-level changes to remove the structural and attitudinal barriers still faced by people with disabilities. Such interventions are often beyond the scope of professionals working with families on a one-to-one basis. Nevertheless, these professionals need to be aware of the effects of socially constructed barriers on the families they serve.

DEFINITIONS AND MODELS

The terms *impairment, disability*, and *handicap* have been used at various times to describe conditions that deviate from the norm. The most recent version of the International Classification of Functioning, Disability and Health—Second Edition (ICIDH-2; World Health Organization, 1999) no longer includes the term *handicap* because of its pejorative connotations. The document acknowledges that not all impairments limit or restrict participation in life activities; that is, they are not *disabilities*. Consequently, such limitations and restrictions are included as variables in the resulting classification scheme.

The ICIDH-2 still includes what is often called the *medical model* of disability. This model is based on an equation of, or analogy between, disability and illness. In short, disability is viewed as a negative condition requiring treatment, rehabilitation, or cure. A newer model that has become popular during the past few decades has been called the *social model* by Oliver (1996) and others. This model suggests that, although impairments may involve health-related conditions, disabilities are socially caused; that is, because society stigmatizes people with disabilities and creates physical and social barriers to their full participation in society, they are at a disadvantage in relation to more typical individuals.

Oliver and others have argued that disabilities are not inherently negative. In fact, many now speak of "disability pride" (see, e.g., Linton, 1998). Swain and French (2000) have suggested an "affirmation model" of disability, in which disability is viewed as a normal (and positive) form of human diversity. Russell (1994) and others have suggested an analogy between "black pride" (i.e., the positive identities of

African Americans) and disability pride. Many individuals with disabilities today recognize a vibrant disability culture of shared writings,
performances, meanings, and values that sets them apart from the
mainstream in a positive way.

Whereas the medical model is based on professional dominance
(Freidson, 1970), or control by physicians and other medical personnel, the social model places the locus of control in the hands of individuals with disabilities and inspires self-help movements based on
obtaining rights and choices. Expertise based on lived experience thus
replaces expertise based on education and training.

Finally, whereas the medical model views disability as a personal
tragedy, the social model views it as a social problem. The proposed
solution to the problem involves social change and social policy
change, such as the passage of the Americans with Disabilities Act,
rather than the treatment or rehabilitation of the individual.

Although the social model has been gaining adherents, not all
individuals with disabilities have rejected the medical model (see
Chapter 6 for a further discussion of the range of orientations toward
disability in today's population). Many parents of children with disabilities continue to focus on treatments or interventions that will improve
their children's ability to function in society. While recognizing the
diversity in orientations among families and individuals, in this book
we adopt the terminology of the ICIDH-2 and the social model by
using the term *impairment* to describe an anatomical or physiological
trait or condition, which sometimes may be ameliorated by appropriate professional intervention, and the term *disability* to describe conditions with social consequences.

We also adopt two perspectives that characterize recent trends in
human services by espousing a model that is both *family-centered* and
strengths-based (partnership). The family-centered care movement developed within the field of pediatrics (e.g., Hostler, 1991). Brewer,
McPherson, Magrab, and Hutchins (1989) wrote: "Within this philosophy is the idea that families should be supported in their natural
care-giving and decision-making roles by building on their unique
strengths as people and families" (p. 1055). This perspective also has
been adopted in special education legislation, such as the Individuals
with Disabilities Education Act and its amendments.

Like the family-centered model in the fields of medicine and education, the "strengths-based" approach in social work (e.g., Lee, 1994)
assumes that clients are capable of acting in their own best interest
and that they understand their own concerns and life situations better

than professionals. Unlike earlier deficit models, this approach focuses on family resources such as support from extended family member or from a church or other type of organization. In this book we reject the notion that the needs of families of children with disabilities can be met only by professionals. Similarly, we reject the notion, found in some of the early literature in this field, that all such families are pathological and in need of therapy. *All* families, whether or not they have children with disabilities, need a little help from time to time, and some need considerable assistance. This need is a normal aspect of family life and is met by most families in informal ways, with the help of family and friends. However, sometimes families' informal support systems are insufficient to address their concerns, and professional help is required. Although we focus on such instances in this book, we take the position that professionals need to work *in partnership* with the families they serve, rather than as powerful experts. The partnership approach is discussed in greater detail in Chapter 11.

RECENT CHANGES IN DISABILITY RIGHTS

The social model of disability shifts the focus away from treatment and care toward a demand for rights. This shift reflects changes that have come about as a result of a growing disability rights movement (DRM) as well as activism by parents of children with disabilities. Like other civil rights movements, the DRM has taken the position that people with disabilities are a minority group that is oppressed by the more powerful majority (e.g., Shapiro, 1994). Early disability legislation in the United States, such as workers' compensation insurance, created programs to support individuals with disabilities who were deemed unable to work. As a result of DRM activism, the more recent Americans with Disabilities Act (ADA), passed in 1990, promotes changes that enable individuals with disabilities to work and participate fully in other ways in society. Whereas earlier legislation resulted primarily from the efforts of nondisabled individuals, the ADA and similar laws in other countries resulted directly from the activism of people with disabilities. A DRM slogan that reflects this change is "Nothing about us without us" (Charlton, 1998).

Parents of children with disabilities also have engaged in activism, primarily in the area of education. Recent legislation, such as the Individuals with Disabilities Education Act (IDEA; 1997, originally enacted as the Education for All Handicapped Children Act in 1975) and its amendments, has reflected parent demands for education in "the least restrictive environment" and supports services that enable children to attend public schools with their nondisabled peers (Darling, 1988; Seligman, 2000). Parent activism is discussed further in Chapters 5 and 11.

Thanks to the efforts of the DRM and parent activism, changes in legislation, improved treatment, better educational alternatives and resources, along with more progressive social attitudes, the quality of life for many families of children with disabilities has improved. Community services and financial help, such as supplemental security income (SSI), have greatly contributed to the ability of some families to provide for their children at home.

However, along with these positive developments, many social and cultural obstacles remain, and the birth of a child with a disability still poses formidable challenges to the family: from the strain on available financial, time, and emotional resources to learning how to negotiate complex educational and medical systems, from dealing with dashed hopes and expectations to worries about what the future holds, these families face an uncertain journey. This edition of *Ordinary Families, Special Children* is dedicated to addressing this journey and to providing assistance to professionals who encounter these families along their way.

SOCIAL SYSTEMS AND FAMILY SYSTEMS

The concept of systems is a leading perspective in the social sciences. However, earlier conceptions of disability within the family contained scant reference to the family unit/system or to other social structures that surround the child and the family. In psychology, this approach has been marked primarily by the development of family systems theory and the social ecology model. In sociology, all theory relates to models of interacting individuals and groups or systems.

This edition of *Ordinary Families* focuses on systems models, as supported in both psychology and sociology, in relation to families of children with disabilities. Both disciplines have offered complementary theories to facilitate an understanding of the family in the context of childhood disability.

Conceptions of family systems theory are incorporated in the theoretical grounding of contemporary psychologists and other professionals who conduct research on, or provide services to, families containing a member with a disability. But this has not always been the case. Early theoretical formulations saw the child or the child and the mother as the central focus in both theory and practice. A drawback of this focus was that other implicated family members were neglected as important contributors and respondents to family events. The singular focus on the family member with a disability is also shortsighted in that it neglects the dynamic nature of family functioning. A problem experienced by one family member affects the entire system and, in turn, affects the family member with a disability.

In the past there was a grudging reluctance to embrace a broader, or ecological, perspective, which may have been partially a consequence of psychoanalytic theory and practice, which focuses on individual and intrapsychic rather than interpersonal processes. Early psychoanalytic theory focused on the mother, with a particular focus on the mother–child relationship. Fathers were discounted as nurturers because of the assumption that they were less important than mothers in influencing the developing child (Parke, 1981). Extant theories reflected the traditional conception of the remote, uninvolved father. Furthermore, the mother was seen as the first and most important object of infant attachment, and fathers were seen as playing a supporting role for the mother (Bowlby, 1951). Another contributing factor may be that, with few exceptions (Minuchin, Rosman, & Baker, 1978), family theorists and family therapists have not studied or shown a particular interest in childhood disability within the context of the family. Others implicate professionals who narrowly define the unit of care as the individual with a disability (McDaniel, Hepworth, & Doherty, 1992). Whatever the reasons for this narrow perspective, there is considerable interest in integrating theories of family systems with the available information on children with disabilities and their families (e.g., Elman, 1991; Ramsey, 1989; Rolland, 1994; Seligman, 1991b; Turnbull & Turnbull, 2001; Berry & Hardman, 1998; Marshak, Seligman, & Prezant, 1999; Marshak & Prezant, 2007). The marriage of family researchers and practitioners with professionals knowledgeable about childhood disability turned out to be a fortuitous merger in that it serves both parties. Chapter 2 provides an in-depth exploration of the value of family systems theory and related theories in the field of psychology for an understanding of families of children with disabilities.

Sociologists commonly classify theories into those that are "micro level" and those that are "macro level." Macro-level theories try to explain the workings and effects of larger social systems. These systems consist of *structures*, or forms of social organization, and *cultures*, or the operating principles of those organizations. Micro-level theories attempt to explain the workings and effects of interactions between and among individuals who reside in larger social systems. Family systems theory, as described above, is a micro-level theory. The remainder of this chapter (1) explores the sociocultural framework within which family systems operate and (2) describes two theoretical perspectives in sociology that are used in later chapters to further our understanding of families of children with disabilities. We begin with sociological systems theory because individuals and families operating at the micro level are affected by macro-level cultural factors (e.g., norms, values, beliefs, attitudes) and structural factors (e.g., social inequality) that are present in the larger society in which they live.

THE SOCIOLOGICAL PERSPECTIVE

Because we represent two different but not unrelated disciplines, namely psychology and sociology, we felt that it would be helpful to reflect on what each discipline brings to the field of disability and the family. In some ways sociological theory is similar to psychological theory. In other ways it is very different. In this section we provide a brief overview of two major sociological approaches that are applied in later chapters: structural–functionalism and symbolic interactionism. We will also suggest similarities and differences between these approaches and the systems perspective in psychology. Finally, we examine the differing foci of the psychological and sociological perspectives and suggest why both are valuable in understanding and working with families of children with disabilities.

Social Structure

The "structural–functional" school of thought in sociology is a macro-level body of theory that has been most closely identified with the systems concept. In the perspective of this school, which traces its American roots primarily to Talcott Parsons (1951), society is regarded as a network of interconnected groups. The structure is held together by shared values that shape the roles people play.

Each part of the system has a *function* that contributes toward the working of the whole. Functions may be *manifest*—generally acknowledged—or *latent*—not known or acknowledged. For example, the manifest function of a preschool program may be to provide an early educational experience for children; its latent function may be to provide a few hours of respite for parents.

In the structural–functional view, the actions of individuals are explained by their place in the social structure, and society has certain expectations about the behavior of people in different roles. Some of the determinants of these culturally based expectations include age, gender, ethnicity, and socioeconomic status (SES), among others. The values of the larger society, then, shape the ways in which parents relate to their children, husbands relate to their wives, and employers relate to their employees.

Much of the literature in the field on the sociology of the family looks very much like recent literature from the family systems perspective in psychology. Writings in both fields share a concern with family roles and functions, and with life-cycle stages and transitions between stages. A structural–functional perspective is used later in this book in discussions of "opportunity structures" and the socially structured barriers that limit individuals and families in the achievement of their goals (Chapters 5 and 6) and of the social expectations inherent in professional and parent roles and in the organization of services for families (Chapter 11).

Because individuals are shaped by the social structures in which they live, people from different societies or different groups within a society may view similar situations differently. Thus the perspective of parents of children with disabilities may not be shared by the professionals who provide services to them. Some (Mercer, 1965; Marshak et al., 1999; Naseef, 2001b; Seligman, 2000) have described conflicts between parents and professionals based on their differing life experiences. These conflicts are explored in greater detail in Chapter 11. Moreover, not even all parents view their life situations and their children's disabilities in the same way. For example, because of their beliefs and values, some Native American families may be less distressed by the birth of a child with a disability than families of other ethnic backgrounds. Family diversity with respect to reactions to childhood disability are discussed further in Chapter 3.

Social Process

Another important current of thought in sociology has suggested that structural–functionalism does not adequately account for the dynamic nature of society. These theorists suggest that social change is the norm and that social interaction is a process in which "reality" is constantly being renegotiated. In this view roles are not static sets of behaviors based on predefined values and expectations; rather, roles are continually recreated by those who play them, based on situational contingencies. All "fathers" do not always act in exactly the same way, nor do all "mothers," "teachers," "doctors," or "patients," and the same father may act differently at different times or in different places.

The sociological perspective that has been most concerned with the determinants of these social processes is *symbolic interactionism*, a micro-level perspective that focuses on individuals and small groups such as families, rather than on larger social structures. However, symbolic interactionism is a distinctly sociological form of social psychology, because it connects the thoughts and actions of individuals with the larger society in which they live. Mead (1934) and other early symbolic interactionists accepted the notion that individuals are shaped by society and attempted to explain the process through which social ideas are transmitted to them. The perspective suggests that individuals, in turn, continually reshape society through their interactions. This perspective is used (and elucidated further) in Chapters 4, 5, and 6 to explain the "career" path followed by families from the prenatal period, through the birth of a child with a disability, through the preschool and school years, and into adolescence and adulthood. The symbolic interactionist perspective is used again in Chapter 11 to describe the process of interaction between families and professionals.

A concept that derives from symbolic interaction theory is that of the *self* or *self-identity* and the related concept of *self-esteem*, which is used in both psychology and sociology to describe a positive attitude toward the self. Sociologists believe that a person's self-concept derives from interactions with other people. Cooley (1964) classically described the self as a "looking-glass self," to suggest this idea. Thus, if a person is always being told that he or she is a bad person, that person is likely to have low self-esteem. Obviously, the converse also is true: Positive evaluations produce high self-esteem. Because high self-esteem is usually one of the outcomes desired for children with disabilities (and, indeed, for all children), interventions are often directed toward achieving this goal. Chapter 6 explores the identities and orientations toward disability that are commonly found among adults with disabilities in society today and speculates as to the interactional paths that produce these differing outcomes.

The concept of stigma, used in several chapters, also has its roots in the symbolic interactionist literature. Stigma refers to the negative attitude held by others in society toward individuals with disabilities and other devalued statuses. Goffman (1963) classically described stigma as a perceived discrepancy between virtual and actual social identity, which prevents the nondisabled person from recognizing the positive attributes of a person with a disability. Although some early literature suggested that individuals with disabilities internalize the stigma they experience, resulting in low self-esteem, more recent literature has suggested and later chapters will show that, like members of other minority groups, people with disabilities can be "inoculated" against negative definitions through their interactions with supportive family members and friends.

Related Concepts

The concepts of stress and social support, which are discussed in Chapter 2, have received considerable attention in both the psychological and sociological literature. Sociological studies of disability, in particular, have typically regarded social support as a major mediating variable. These studies are discussed in Chapters 4 and 5.

How the Perspectives Complement Each Other

Although sociologists and psychologists have developed similar perspectives in trying to understand families of children with disabilities, their focus in practice tends to be different. For psychological practitioners, the object of intervention is usually the "client" (in this case, the family). Intervention, in the form of counseling, therapy, or treatment, is intended to bring about changes in the family system or its individual members. For the sociological practitioner, on the other hand, the object of intervention is often some aspect of the larger social structure. Sociologists generally focus on social change to create more opportunities for families.

Because of the difference in focus, both sociology and psychology (and other helping professions) are important in working with families. The helping professions that operate at the micro level (primarily psychology and social work) are important because family members need to learn to use existing resources and to adjust to, or *cope* with, situations that may be unchangeable. For example, the family that devotes all its time to finding a "cure" for a child's Down syndrome may need assistance in redirecting its efforts. Individual, family, or couple counseling can also be beneficial for families experiencing intolerable conflict and stress.

On the other hand, in many situations, the family would be able to cope very well without therapeutic assistance if enough supports or resources were available to them. The sociological perspective encourages the professional to assist families in creating new resources and expanding their "opportunity structures." For example, if no appropriate classroom for children with disabilities existed in a neighborhood school, the sociologically oriented practitioner might engage in advocacy for families by working with the school to develop the means to establish an appropriate classroom. Sometimes situational factors are so overwhelming that intervention at the family level is not at all helpful. Extreme poverty resulting from larger societal conditions, for example, cannot be eliminated by family counseling; much broader social change is needed in such a case. At other times, needed social structures are in place, yet the family continues to experience stress, marital disharmony, and major communication problems. Such feelings as guilt, shame, embarrassment, anxiety, and depression may be impossible to shake. Again, in such instances, psychotherapy or family therapy may be indicated.

Some families need both counseling and advocacy; some families need neither. What the family "needs" is increasingly defined by families themselves rather than by professionals. In the field of early intervention, for example, "family centered" is coming to mean "family driven." As one of us has described elsewhere (Darling & Darling, 1992), early intervention has shifted dramatically from a clinical or professionally directed field to one in which *parents* generally determine the desired outcomes of intervention for both the child and the family (see Chapter 13 for a further discussion of the process of outcome determination). Similarly, in the field of medical care for children with special health needs, legislation and policy have dictated a more family-directed approach (see Darling & Peter, 1994, for an indepth discussion of models using this approach in medical education). Social work, education, and other fields have also been moving toward family-centered models (e.g., Adams & Nelson, 1995).

Both psychology and sociology, therefore, are now using a family-centered perspective in relation to families of children with disabilities. Both fields have also moved beyond a simple family-centered approach to a consideration of the larger social system within which families live. Professionals working with families need to be aware of the various levels on which intervention can occur. Those counseling families need to be sure that the problem lies within the family itself, not in the family's larger (and perhaps changeable) social situation. Conversely, professionals who focus on social change and advocacy need to have the skills to help families cope with limited opportunities (or to refer them to professionals who do have these skills). In either case, successful intervention requires an understanding of the systems perspective and an ability to provide broadly based interventions.

OVERVIEW OF THE BOOK

This chapter has attempted to introduce the systems perspective on families of children with disabilities. The approach to be taken in the following chapters is a systems approach. Derived from both the psychological and sociological literature, this approach views the child as part of a family system of interacting units and a social system of interacting families, individuals, and social institutions.

This book has been organized into four sections. The first, encompassing Chapters 1–3, presents the conceptual framework for the remaining chapters. Chapter 1 has introduced the definitions and models that are used throughout the book and presented a brief overview of the sociological perspective. The relevant concepts from this perspective are explained in greater detail as they are used in later chapters. Chapter 2 presents an in-depth overview of the systems perspective in psychology. Chapter 3 completes the discussion of the book's conceptual framework by addressing family diversity. Although diversity is addressed primarily in a single chapter, readers should keep its importance in mind and think about its relevance for the ideas and situations explored throughout the book.

The second section of the book, consisting of Chapters 4–6, explores the "career paths" of families of children with disabilities. These chapters broaden the reader's understanding of the family experience by tracing it sequentially from the prenatal period through adulthood. Chapters 4 and 5 employ a sociological perspective to look at how family reactions to the birth and rearing of a child with a disability are socially shaped. Chapter 6 explores the possible outcomes of family careers by considering children as future adults.

The third section of the book, Chapters 7–10, based on the conceptual framework outlined in Chapter 2, presents an in-depth exploration of the family as a system. Using the principles of family systems theory, Chapters 7, 8, 9, and 10 explore the effects of childhood disability on various members of the family system and on the family as a whole.

The final section of the book consists of the last three chapters and focuses on applications of the material covered in the preceding theoretical and conceptual, chapters. Chapter 11 discusses the parent–professional relationship, beginning with a theoretical discussion of the sometimes opposing roles of parents and professionals. The chapter then presents the current strengths-based or "partnership" model of practice as the approach that guides the interventions suggested in the last two chapters of the book. Chapter 12 focuses on counseling as a family-based intervention practice rooted in family systems theory. Finally, Chapter 13 illustrates the application of a social systems perspective to assisting families in identifying their resources, concerns, and priorities and in using these family-defined elements in the development of a service plan to achieve the outcomes that they desire. By combining the systems literature from sociology and psychology, we hope to provide the reader with a broader and deeper understanding of families of children with special needs and to offer some tools to assist these families in achieving a higher quality of life.

■2■

Conceptual Framework II

Family Systems Theory and Childhood Disability

As we noted earlier but will mention here again because of its centrality, the family operates as an interactive unit, and what affects one member affects all members. With systems theory, the family is seen as a complex and interactive social system in which all member's needs and experiences affect the others (Friend & Cook, 2002). A family systems perspective rejects the view that linear relationships characterize family life and that the only important relationship is that between a mother and her child. Instead, families are viewed as interactive, interdependent, and reactive; that is, if something occurs to one member in the family, all members of the system are affected (Goldenberg & Goldenberg, 2003; Turnbull & Turnbull, 2001). As one family therapist observed, families can be likened to a baby's mobile that hangs over a crib (Elman, 1991). When one of the objects of the mobile is touched, all of the other objects are set in motion. General systems theory holds that each variable in any system interacts with the other variables so thoroughly that cause and effect cannot be separated. Writing about deafness in the family, Luterman (1991) notes, for example, "This notion implies that when a deaf child is born into a family, to some extent, everybody is deaf" (p. 2). All living systems are composed of interdependent parts, and the interaction of these parts creates characteristics not contained in the separate entities (von Bertalanffy, 1968; Goldenberg & Goldenberg, 2003). Others concur that the family is more than the sum of its parts. Indeed, Garbarino (1992) asserts that "a family is a little society of its own and in this sense every family has its own small-scale culture, government, language, foreign policy and even its own myths" (p. 77). Therefore, family life can best be understood by studying the relationship among its members. The family is the primary and most powerful system to which a person ever belongs.

Before examining the dynamic nature of family functioning, it is imperative to have an understanding of the characteristics, both static and dynamic, that comprise most family units. What follows, then, is an examination of these aspects of the family from authors who have merged family systems concepts with information from the disability studies area.

FAMILY STRUCTURE

Family structure refers to the variety of characteristics that serve to make families unique. These factors include membership characteristics, cultural style, ideological style, and family size.

Membership Characteristics

The early literature on families with members who have disabilities is based on the assumption of family homogeneity. Families, however, differ with regard to numerous membership characteristics: extended families with contributing grandparents who reside either in the household or elsewhere; single-parent families; families with an unemployed "breadwinner," a member with a major psychosocial disorder (e.g., substance abuse, mental illness), or a deceased family member whose influence continues to assert itself on the family's thinking and behavior. In addition, contemporary views of families must consider configurations that make room for other committed persons who may not be legally married (Goldenberg & Goldenberg, 2003). Families may be comprised of gay and lesbian partners, cohabitating or remarried heterosexual couples, or widows or widowers with children. (See Chapter 3 for a more detailed discussion of family diversity.)

Family membership changes over time. For example, the exiting of a family member will precipitate different communication and relationship patterns, just as an addition to the family increases the membership, the communication patterns, and the dynamics. Families are reduced in size through divorce and death and grow larger through remarriage and the inclusion of children and extended family members.

Cultural Style

The family's beliefs are the most static component of the family and can play an important role in shaping its ideological style, interactional patterns, and functional priorities. SES, ethnicity, race, and religious factors influence cultural style (Hanson & Lynch, 2004). Culturally based beliefs can affect the manner in which families adapt to a child with a disability, and these beliefs can also influence families' level of trust in caregivers and caregiving institutions. Cultural stereotypes account for many of the stigmatizing attitudes that continue to exist and add to evasion, exclusion, and limited opportunities for persons with disabilities.

Ideological Style

Ideological style is based on a family's history, beliefs handed down from generation to generation, values, and coping behaviors and is also influenced by culture. Cultural factors are generally considered unchanging, but according to Turnbull, Turnbull, Erwin, and Soodak (2006), cultural attributes can change over the lifespan. "One family may change its religion or choose atheism; another's economic status may improve or decline precipitously. Still another family may be influenced by racial or religious intermarriage" (p. 10).

Some Jewish families, for example, place a great deal of emphasis on intellectual achievement (McGoldrick, Giordano, & Pearce, 1996). Education is important in the Jewish culture because learning/education is portable; this value derives from the relocations Jews were forced to make (Rosen & Weltman, 1996). Intellectual achievement is sought because it reflects favorably on the family; in fact, education is viewed as an obligation. When their offspring do not achieve expected educational levels, Jewish families experience shame (Rosen & Weltman, 1996)—an ideological style that can be problematic for families who have a child with an intellectual disability.

Whereas a family's response to a child with a disability is influenced by ideological style, the reverse is also true: namely, that such a child may influence a family's values. For example, when a child with a disability is born, a family not only responds to the event itself but must also ultimately confront its beliefs about people who have disabilities. Because attitudes toward persons with disabilities continue to be influenced by negative stereotypes (Olkin, 1999; Fries, 1997; Marshak et al., 1999; Shapiro, 1994), confronting the birth of a child with a disability challenges most parents' belief system. Disability does not discriminate on racial, cultural, or socioeconomic grounds; a child with a disability may be born to a family that is very dogmatic and prejudiced. In such an instance, the family grapples with what the child's disability means to them psychologically and practically (Marshak & Seligman, 1993). There is a dissonance between what they believed about persons with disabilities and the existence of disability in their child. The disdain one may have for a stranger with a disability is impossible to harbor toward one's son or daughter. The birth of a child with a disability thus results in a double shock to the family.

As family members confront a childhood disability, they must also cope with their beliefs about what and who can influence the course of events (Rolland, 1994; Barnwell & Day, 1996). It is helpful to know if family members believe that the control of the disability is in their hands, in the hands of others, in the hands of God, or purely a matter of chance (Ariel & Naseef, 2006). Their views will influence their interpretation of events related to the disability, their help-seeking behavior, and their approach to care-giving. Rolland (1994) contends that professionals should assess the family's views about what caused a disability and what might influence the outcome. Strongly held opinions that someone is to blame or feelings of shame and guilt may negatively influence the family's ability to come to grips with disability.

Heritage, culture, beliefs, and values influence the coping mechanisms families employ. Coping behaviors can motivate the family to change the perceived meaning of the situation (Turnbull, Patterson, et al., 1993; Berry & Hardman, 1998).

Coping styles can be classified into internal and external strategies (McCubbin & Patterson, 1981; Houser & Seligman, 1991): *Internal* strategies include passive appraisal (e.g., problems will resolve themselves over time) and reframing (making attitudinal adjustments to live with the situation constructively), whereas *external* strategies include use of social support (family and extrafamilial resources), spiritual support (use of spiritual interpretations, advice from clergy), and formal support (use of community and professional resources).

FAMILY INTERACTION

We have established that children with disabilities do not function in isolation. Children live within a context—the family—and when something happens to one member, everyone is affected. However, the family is more than an assemblage of individuals who function in a dynamic interrelationship to each other; it is also comprised of subsystems, which we discuss below.

Subsystems

The composition of subsystems is affected by the structural characteristics of families (e.g., size of extrafamilial network, single mother or father, number of children) and by the current lifecycle stage (e.g., a couple with two children under 8 vs. a couple after they have "launched" their children; Goldenberg & Goldenberg, 2003).

Intervening in a subsystem can be problematic. An intervention designed to strengthen the bond between a mother and her child, for example, can have implications for the mother's relationship with her husband and other children. The other subsystems need to be considered so that the resolution of one problem doesn't bring about the emergence of others. Problems can be minimized by including (rather than excluding) family members and by communicating the purpose and expected outcome of a particular meeting or intervention.

Within the family there are many subsystems. However, there are three central subsystems in families that are constituent parts of the larger system (Goldenberg & Goldenberg, 2003); the spousal, parental, and sibling subsystems. Turnbull et al. (2006) add the extended family subsystem, which we address in Chapter 10.

Spousal Subsystem

This subsystem is basic. Chronic conflict between the parents reverberates throughout the family and contributes to the children's stress and worry. Children can be scapegoated or brought into alliances with one parent against the other. For example, we can predict discord when the mother feels insecure about her nurturing and child-care responsibilities after her first child is born with Down syndrome and her husband reacts to his son's birth by avoidance and withdrawal.

The spousal subsystem models for the children how to deal with differences, how to make decisions and negotiate conflicts, and how to interact in an intimate relationship. A sound spousal dyad is one in which both partners experience a fulfilling relationship with one another and where intimacy, support, and growth opportunities are present (Goldenberg & Goldenberg, 2003).

In the above illustration, a well functioning spousal subsystem would be one in which the mother could rely on her husband to be supportive and understanding. If he were able to be supportive, understand his own fears regarding his son, and cope with those fears without escaping, the couple would stand a good chance of becoming an effective spousal team. Without such changes in thinking, however, the spousal subsystem is in jeopardy and the family's future compromised.

The presence of childhood disability prompts questions about the effects it might have on the parents' relationship (Turnbull & Turnbull, 2001; Turnbull et al., 2006). Is the couple negatively or positively impacted by the presence of a child with a disability, or is the evidence inconclusive? Do divorce rates hover around the national average, or are they significantly greater than those of parents of nondisabled children? Is marital satisfaction compromised or enhanced in these families? Is the prebirth relationship of the couple a critical variable during postbirth adjustment, or is the impact of childhood disability such a shattering event that the couple's emotional health is compromised?

We consider these questions to be pertinent to the discussion of the spousal subsystem (and to a subsystem of cohabitating partners as well), yet the responses to these questions are fairly complex.

Parental Subsystem

This subsystem consists of interactions between parents and their children; its tasks include discipline, nurturing, limit setting and guidance (Goldenberg & Goldenberg, 2003). Through modeling it also offers children important opportunities to learn how to deal with authority and to indulge in independent decision making and self-direction. The extended family can be included in the parental subsystem, as well as other kin or even older children who may assume parental roles for a limited period of time. An example of the latter is an older son assigned to take care of a younger brother while the parents are at the hospital tending to their other son, who has hemophilia.

According to Kliman and Madsen (1999), parental authority in working-class families is often shared with grandparents, relatives, neighbors, or other kin. Parental caretakers can be biological, step, adoptive, or foster parents (Turnbull & Turnbull, 2001). Certain family configurations can present challenges to the parental subsystem. An illustration of a potential problematic situation is a child with a disability whose parents have both remarried. It is fairly well established that blended families need to negotiate roles, caretaking responsibilities, and discipline, and determine lines of authority (Visher & Visher, 1996). When a child with a disability is introduced into a blended family, issues of responsibility, discipline, and caretaking become paramount to the survival of the family. This is not only an issue for the parental subsystem, but it is also a concern for the "blended" children, namely, the sibling subsystem.

Sibling Subsystem

Sibling relationships are lifelong and constitute a child's first peer group (Powell & Gallagher, 1993; Bank & Kahn, 1997; Cicirelli, 1995). Through this subsystem children learn how to provide mutual support, compete, negotiate with each other, and develop social skills. Generally speaking, the quality of the sibling subsystem depends on how the other subsystems function (Goldenberg & Goldenberg, 2003). The sibling relationship is culturally rooted; different cultures have unique expectations for siblings in response to birth order, age, and gender (Harry, Day, & Quist, 1998). As siblings grow older, they assume greater responsibility within the family, but the distribution of responsibility is not always seen as fair by siblings and can thus become grounds for negotiation or conflict (Orsmond & Seltzer, 2000). Caretaking responsibility is a major issue when a sibling has a disability, especially when the sibling is female (Harris & Glasberg, 2003; McHugh, 2003; Turnbull et al., 2006). Furthermore, parents can place future caretaking responsibilities and expectations on their non-disabled children, which can also become problematic, though not always. The assignment of responsibility for a child with a disability is taken with aplomb by some children and deeply resented by others. Issues pertaining to sibling relationships are discussed in Chapter 9.

The spousal, parental, and sibling subsystems constitute the most important systems in the family, yet they are not the only ones. Alliances between mother–son, father–oldest son, and father–daughter suggest more transitional relationships that exist within families (Goldenberg & Goldenberg, 2003). Thus, there are numerous active subgroupings within the family. Central to the understanding of subsystem functioning is the concept of boundaries. The next section addresses boundary issues in family functioning.

Boundaries

Boundaries exist between subsystems. They are invisible, yet a keen observer can detect them within a family system. One can sense who in the family is the chief disciplinarian and who is the main nurturer. There are boundaries between the parents and the children and between the children. There are boundaries too between the family unit and outside forces, such as educators or medical personnel. Within the family, boundaries help to define its members' roles in relation to one another (Turnbull & Turnbull, 2001). In contemporary society role reversals occur with some frequency; in traditional families, however, it would be rare for a father to become the chief caretaker of the children and the mother to assume the breadwinner role. In such a family the father is aware that the family caretaking role has a boundary placed around it.

Nuclear and extended family boundaries tend to be permeable, but not always. Boundary violations can emerge when grandparents want to help or offer advice to parents in regard to their grandchild with a disability (see Chapter 10). The parents may interpret the help or advice as intrusive and as an indication that they are not competent caretakers. They may feel that the grandparents violated an unspoken rule (boundary). In contrast, in some poor, African American families, grandparent participation in an expanding family is more likely to be the norm, as they provide care and support for grandchildren, adult children, and other kin (Hines, 1999). Perhaps the most heinous boundary violations occur when children are abused, a concern of considerable relevance to children with disabilities (Garbarino, 1989; Matich-Maroney, 2003).

The clarity of the subsystem boundaries is important. Family members tend to know who does the parenting and the breadwinning, who assumes responsibility for limit setting and discipline. When these boundaries are ambiguous and crossed, there can be confusion and tension. Thus, within families, the boundaries should be clear to everyone.

An *open* system has continuous information flow to and from the outside. *Closed* systems perpetuate rigid boundaries that are not easily crossed; in other words, they have impermeable boundaries. Examples of closed systems are religious cults that close off the outside world and totalitarian countries that do not permit information from other sources that can threaten their reign (Goldenberg & Goldenberg, 2003).

Closed families coping with childhood disability are at risk of isolation, whereas an open family with permeable boundaries may become overloaded with information, both good and bad, and perhaps even susceptible to quack treatments or supposed cures. In childhood disability, closed boundaries tend to be more frequent and more of a problem than open ones. The family that believes it can solve all of its problems without outside help (or, as perceived by the family, interference) can become isolated from the community, from needed resources (e.g., early intervention) and from other families of children with similar disabilities (e.g., through support groups). Little or no contact with external systems can result in fearful, confused, and inadequate responses during crises. Closed families run the risk of regressing because of insufficient input, and they are susceptible to disorganization and dysfunction (Goldenberg & Goldenberg, 2003). Such families may be suspicious of outsiders and depend exclusively on the family, which can put considerable strain on the system because the family is seen as its own resource. However, in some cultural groups, the family is sometimes able to provide all the resources a family needs or wants, and insistence on professional intervention or support group involvement is inappropriate.

Effective families develop a balance between openness and rigid self-containment: open enough to take advantage of available resources, and discriminating enough to discern legitimate programs or treatments from those that are unproven, not beneficial, or even harmful. In addition to being open and closed, families have other properties, such as the ability (or lack thereof) to form a cohesive bond and to adapt to change and crises.

Cohesion

The concepts of enmeshment and disengagement are components of cohesion. Cohesion refers to close emotional bonding *and* independence among family members (Turnbull et al., 2006). The dilemma faced by family members is how to be close yet separate. Some families have weak boundaries between subsystems and can be characterized as overinvolved and overprotective, in other words, enmeshed (Minuchin & Fishman, 1981; Goldenberg & Goldenberg, 2003). A considerable amount of emotional closeness and demands for loyalty and consensus (Olson, 1993), extreme proximity and intensity in family interactions, and overconcern in each other' lives (Goldenberg & Goldenberg, 2003) are additional characteristics. The family feels betrayed when a member makes any move toward separation. Such families have difficulty allowing for member individuality. Overly protective families can have deleterious effects on children with disabilities. These families experience considerable anxiety in allowing their children to become independent and, hence, may keep them from participating in growth-promoting activities that can contribute to future independent functioning. It is important to remember that what may be overly close in one culture may be the opposite in another. According to Zuniga (2004), in Latino families, preteens and even adolescents are allowed to sit on their mother's lap, and preschoolers are allowed to drink from a baby bottle, behaviors deemed unacceptable by European American parents.

Disengaged families have rigid subsystem boundaries (Minuchin, 1974) and tend to be underinvolved. A familiar pattern in middle-class families is one in which the father is disengaged and preoccupied with work and the mother is overinvolved with the children (Minuchin & Nichols, 1993). The mother's closeness to the children may be a substitute for the lack of closeness from her husband. In families in which there is a child with a disability, this distance (from each other) and enmeshment with work or the children can be a recipe for family problems. The partners have not coalesced in terms of the challenges that confront them; the father will feel left out of the parental subsystem, and the mother will fail to get the needed emotional and instrumental support she needs.

Becoming involved creates anxiety, and disengaged families tend to avoid anxiety. As a result, someone with a disability can initiate independent activity but fails to receive support for these endeavors. Families that function optimally are characterized by a balance between enmeshment and disengagement. Boundaries between subsystems are clearly defined, and family members feel both a close bonding and a sense of autonomy.

Adaptability

The family's ability to change in response to a stressful situation—to negotiate differences and make decisions during times of crisis and change—is called *adaptability* (Olson, Russell, & Sprenkle, 1980). Rigid families do not change in response to stress, and chaotic families are characterized by instability and inconsistent change. A rigid family would have difficulty adjusting to the demands of caring for a child with a significant impairment (Turnbull & Turnbull, 2001).

A father's steadfast "head of household" role, for example, would not allow him to help with domestic chores or to assist with the child ("woman's work"), thereby placing an inordinate burden on the mother. The mother must put all of her energies into care-giving responsibilities, leaving little time for the other children in the family or for interacting with other people. This family is in jeopardy of becoming isolated and dysfunctional. One study showed that the adjustment of parents of adult sons and daughters with an intellectual disability was related to the family's adaptability (Lustig & Akey, 1999a).

In determining a family's adaptability, one needs to be constantly aware of culturally determined values and behavior (Kalyanpur & Harry, 1999). For example, teachers need to be sensitive to the degree of student decision making that the family believes is appropriate (Turnbull & Turnbull, 2001). The teachers' Western values may be the opposite of those of the parents. Nevertheless, both teachers and practitioners must be respectful of parents' choices, always remembering that although differences in values can make a professional feel uncomfortable, those different values should not be cast into right or wrong judgments.

Chaotic families have few rules by which to live, and those that do exist are changed frequently. Commitments and promises are rarely kept, making it difficult for family members to depend on each other (Turnbull et al., 2006). Although chaos is expected during a crisis, it is problematic when it becomes way of life and especially troublesome when parents are coping with childhood disability. There is often no family leader, and there may be endless negotiations and frequent role changes (Turnbull & Turnbull, 2001). Chaotic families can move quickly from enmeshment to distance and disengagement. Although it is normal for family members to experience chaos during a crisis, chronic chaos in families of a child with a disability can lead to confusion regarding routines, treatments, and medication management, not to mention emotional reactions. Family members who interact in a functional way maintain a balance between emotional unity and autonomy, between reacting to change and maintaining a sense of stability, and between closed and random communication.

Problematic Family Systems

Communication breakdowns generally reflect a problematic family system rather than faulty people. Communication problems reside in the interactions between people, not within people (Turnbull & Turnbull, 1986). In the family therapy literature and in practice, there has been a shift from blaming and pathologizing individuals to examining interactional patterns, adopting a no-fault outlook, and exploring recurring behavioral patterns (Goldenberg & Goldenberg, 2003; Elman, 1991). When working with families from a systems point of view, the emphasis is on changing patterns of interaction and not on changing individuals. When families believe that a particular member is responsible for the problems they are experiencing, they usually discover that difficulties often reside in faulty communication that leads, in turn, to misunderstanding, confusion, and conflict. It is not uncommon to blame a child with a disability for the family's financial woes rather than the family's excessive, impulsive spending patterns.

FAMILY FUNCTIONS

Family functions are tasks that help the family achieve certain outcomes and meet established needs. Considerable interdependence between the nuclear family and its extrafamilial network is required to successfully carry out essential tasks. Families differ with regard to the priorities they attach to different functions, and they differ with regard to who is designated to carry out certain functions. For example, the Goldmans place considerable emphasis on coordinating and assigning roles relative to home tasks (who takes out the garbage, who does the dishes, who dusts, who generally drives). The Tolands are less concerned about these issues and prioritize financial concerns such as who is the main breadwinner, who balances the checkbook. The Tolands' financial worries are related to their care for their adolescent daughter, who has spina bifida and requires expensive adaptive equipment.

Typical family functions can be categorized into eight domains:

1. Economic (e.g., generating income, paying bills, banking)
2. Daily care/health care (e.g., transportation, purchasing and preparing food, medical visits)
3. Recreation (e.g., hobbies, recreation for family and individual)
4. Socialization (e.g., developing social skills, interpersonal relationships)
5. Self-identity (e.g., recognizing strengths and weaknesses, sense of belonging)
6. Affection (e.g., intimacy, nurturing)
7. Educational/vocational (e.g., homework, career choice, development of work ethic)
8. Spiritual (e.g., religious community, understanding child's exceptionality; Turnbull & Turnbull, 2001; Turnbull et al., 2006).

According to Turnbull et al. (2006), spirituality generally refers to how family members "find meaning in their lives, how they respond to the sacred, and how they perceive the connections between themselves, others, and the universe" (p. 55). In terms of spirituality, some parents regard their child's disability as a blessing in that such a child would only be bestowed on those who are strong emotionally. In a survey study of grandparent responses to their grandchild with a disability, a majority of the respondents endorsed religion and belief in God as the reason acceptance came so easily to them (Frisco, 2002). Furthermore, having a child with disabilities can be a catalyst for families to seek out a spiritual connection (Poston & Turnbull, 2004). There are other instances where a child's condition is considered to be a sign of God's blessing or good luck because the family was considered especially worthy or because God was challenging them to be better people (Skinner, Correa, Skinner, & Bailey, 2001). However, some spiritual interpretations propose that disability is a punishment for one's sins (Chan, 1998; Rolland, 2003; Chan & Lee, 2004). Families may have difficulty finding a religious community that is responsive to their child's needs—locating and becoming integrated into such a community poses another challenge to the family (Poston & Turnbull, 2004). Yet families derive considerable support from their religious communities. It is important to keep in mind that different religions, cultures, and individuals bring their own interpretation of what constitutes spirituality.

A child with a disability can change the family's self-identity by reducing its earning capacity, constricting its recreational and social activities, and affecting career decisions. These negative consequences reflect how a child with a disability can affect the family by reflecting on the family functions noted above. This discussion also asserts that well-functioning families need to be flexible, open to change, and resilient (Singer & Powers, 1993; Walsh, 2003a). Family members who can assume the functions of other family members enhance the family's coping ability. For example, when parents first learn that their child has a disability, it is important, during this period of crisis, that family members abandon rigid, long-held roles and be open to input from others whom the family now needs.

Children with disabilities can have a positive or negative effect on family functions (Featherstone, 1980; Turnbull & Turnbull, 2001; Lambie, 2000; Hornby, 2000; Friend & Cook, 2002). In the past there has been more emphasis on negative outcomes, but that has changed as research reports and personal observations provide a more balanced perspective (Trainer, 1991; Turnbull et al., 1993; Klein & Schive, 2001; Ariel & Naseef, 2006; Meyer, 1995; Klein & Kemp, 2004) For example, in one study, Turnbull, Brotherson, and Summers (1985) report that parents and siblings described positive attitudinal and values changes that they attributed to the family member with retardation.

In terms of an educational function, some question the emphasis placed on the role of parents as teachers of their children (e.g., Seligman, 2000; Turnbull & Turnbull, 2001), although Turnbull et al. (2006) believe that fathers rarely assume this role. It is important to remember that the educational function is only one of several functions. Parents have many roles to play and many functions to perform, and as the various functions interact with each other, one needs to be concerned about how the overemphasis of one role or function affects the others.

In asking parents to assume an educational function the professional should first inquire about the parents' wish to take on that role, whether they are comfortable with it or feel prepared to assume it. Parents are sometimes asked to do more at home with their child than the family system can tolerate. Too much stress may be placed on the family when professionals fail to coordinate the activities they ask the family to assume (Laborde & Seligman, 1991). If the family or one of the professionals fails to assume a leadership/coordinator role, the family can assume too much responsibility, leading to stress, confusion, tension, conflicts, and possibly even depression. With certain types of childhood impairments, a family may be given "homework" by the teacher, speech therapist, and physical therapist, among others. Again, there needs to be careful monitoring of the functions professionals ask a family to assume and a recognition that overburdening one aspect of a family function can negatively impact the successful functioning of the other ones.

FAMILY LIFE CYCLE

Cultural and ethnic factors, along with childhood disability in the family, suggest that family movement along its life cycle may not necessarily coincide with conventional theories of what families face over time (Turnbull et al., 2006). Others note that the family's movement through the life cycle is influenced by their developmental past and the historical era in which they are living (Walsh, 2003b; Goldenberg

& Goldenberg, 2003), such as whether they lived through the Great Depression, the baby boomer period, or came of age during the Vietnam War. Each of these periods offers a different orientation to life (Walsh, 2003b; Goldenberg & Goldenberg, 2003).

The family life cycle is a series of developmental stages in which, during a particular stage, the family's lifestyle is relatively stable and each member is engaged in developmental tasks related to that period of life (Duvall, 1957; Carter & McGoldrick, 2003). According to Friend and Cook (2002), "transitions are the periods between stages when family members are readjusting their roles and interactions in order to meet the next set of expectations and tasks, and they are characterized by confusion and often by increased stress" (p. 335). For example, a family with two late adolescent children is coping with the usual intensity and ambivalence of adolescent life in addition to the concerns that characterize adult (the parents') midlife. Change occurs for this family when one of the children leaves home, which affects the family structure (e.g., changing from four to three persons at home) and may affect other aspects of family life, such as family interaction and communication.

We could hypothesize that certain family dynamics will change if the adolescent who left home is a nondisabled child. The parents can become more focused on the child with a disability, restricting their own activity and blocking efforts toward independence. Once the nondisabled child is gone, the burden of caretaking may become more intensified for the parents. This can motivate grandparents to become more involved. Another scenario would be one in which the parents become more active consumers of community services and recreational opportunities for their child, thus freeing them to engage in other pursuits. Furthermore, if the nondisabled child has played a major caregiving role in the family, he or she may experience guilt and loss in leaving. This life cycle change has the potential of setting in motion a series of family responses. For most families these changes result in some initial turmoil, followed by the achievement of an equilibrium characteristic of that stage.

Olson and colleagues (1984) identified seven stages of the life cycle: couple, childbearing, school age, adolescence, "launching," postparental, and aging. The main task that the family must negotiate is the contraction, expansion, and realignment of family relationships to support the exit, entry, and ongoing development of the system (Carter & McGoldrick, 1999).

Each stage has its own developmental tasks; for example, parenting tasks are salient during the childrearing stage and largely nonexistent during the postparental stage. If launching fails to occur when it normally does (and it may not with children with severe impairments), parents may need to extend their parenting beyond the usual period. The failure to launch can result in challenges for family members if the parents resent remaining in a parental role and the youth with disabilities is unable to achieve independence. The nondisabled children may feel burdened by their sibling's disability (Harris & Glasberg, 2003). They may have to assume caregiving roles for their brothers or sisters. These children may feel that life is passing them by and that they are unable to achieve goals and dreams or perhaps even engage in fulfilling relationships. Other siblings seem not to resent caregiving but need to be monitored so that they don't assume an overly responsible life role of caregiving, while abandoning other goals.

Developmental transitions (moving from one stage to another) can be a major source of stress and possibly even family dysfunction for any family (Carter & McGoldrick, 2003). Launching a child creates stress in the family. It should not be assumed that all families negotiate life cycle changes and transitions successfully. We have noted that some families of children with disabilities may not be able to move beyond the parental stage. Likewise, lower SES families may experience numerous blocks to a fulfilling family life because "their life cycle constitutes a virtually endless series of crises and their adaptive capacities are often pushed beyond human limits" (Hines, 1989, p. 514). Families of children who are deaf encounter increased amounts of stress during the process that leads to the identification of hearing loss (Moores, 2006).

According to Carter and McGoldrick (2003), the family at midlife may be the most troublesome of all phases. The most significant aspect of this phase is that it is marked by the greatest number of exits and entries of family members. It begins with the launching of grown children and proceeds with the entry of their spouses and children. It is a time when grandparents often become ill or die. Parents must deal with the change in their own status as they make room for the next generation and prepare to move up the position of grandparents. They must also forge a different type of relationship with their own parents, who may become dependent, giving them (particularly women) considerable caretaking responsibilities (Carter & McGoldrick, 2003).

The developmental stages derived from systems theory can be related to the stress that families of children with disabilities experience, as Turnbull, Summers, and Brotherson (1986) have done:

1. *Childbearing:* Getting an accurate diagnosis, making emotional adjustments, informing other family members.
2. *School age:* Clarifying personal views regarding inclusive versus segregated placements, dealing with reactions of child's peer group, arranging for child care and extracurricular activities.
3. *Adolescence:* Coping with the chronicity of the child's disability, dealing with issues of sexuality, coping with peer isolation and rejection, planning for the child's vocational future.
4. *Launching:* Adjusting to the family's continuing responsibility, deciding on appropriate residential placement, dealing with the lack of socialization opportunities.
5. *Postparental:* Reestablishing relationship with spouse (i.e., if child has been successfully launched), interacting with disabled member's residential service providers, planning for the future.

THE SOCIAL ECOLOGY MODEL

In the early studies of families with children who have disabilities, researchers defined the unit of study or intervention in very specific terms. They accomplished this specificity by focusing exclusively on the child and neglecting the family as a legitimate unit of study. Later studies focused on the mother, with a particular emphasis on mother–child bonding. The consideration of the family as a dynamic, interdependent unit was a major step forward, yet there continued to be something missing in the conceptualization of the family. We know that young children with disabilities do not live in isolation. Likewise, the family lives in a broader context of their immediate community and beyond. The formulation of the family within a social ecological framework has been discussed extensively by Bronfenbrenner (1979, 1990), and more recently has been discussed in relation to families of children with disabilities (Bubolz & Whiren, 1984; Hornby, 1994a; Mitchell, 1983; Hanson & Lynch, 2004).

The ecological paradigm suggests that a change in any part of the system affects subparts of the system, creating the need for system adaptation. The ecological environments of a family furnish the resources necessary for life—and make up the life support and social support systems.

The ecological model is concerned with the permeability of the family in interacting with environmental systems. This model would ask whether a family with a child with a disability is, or is not, open to the supportive influences of other similarly situated families (e.g., support groups or parent-to-parent programs) or whether they are amenable to being assisted by social agencies or other sources of help.

The social ecological view asserts that a child or family can be affected by events occurring in settings in which the person is not even present. For example, a young child can be affected by the conditions of parental employment, and the parents' employment status can be the consequence of the health of the local economy. In turn, the health of a local economy can be affected by events occurring on a national (e.g., a severe economic downturn) or even international (e.g., a war) scale. Thus the behavior of a child and family unit can be influenced by a variety of external, even remote events. This view encourages a broad conceptualization of the forces that impinge on the family. Such a framework incorporates contributions to the literature that focus on the social policies that affect families of children with disabilities.

It simply is not sufficient to study only the child, the child and his or her mother, or the dynamics occurring within the family. It is becoming increasingly important to examine the family within the context of larger social, economic, and political realities.

OTHER CONCEPTS RELATED TO CHILDHOOD DISABILITY AND THE FAMILY

A number of important dimensions of family life are discussed in the following pages. These dimensions reflect aspects of life that can contribute to either family adaptation or family challenges. This discussion centers on several key concepts that are often cited in the literature and relate directly to families of children with disabilities.

Resilience

Most families adapt and cope effectively with childhood disability. Although most, if not all, parents experience disappointment, stress, and worry when they first learn about their child's disability, it should not be assumed that parents are chronically traumatized by this unsettling event. As Turnbull et al. (2006) have noted, professionals themselves may focus only on the weaknesses of the family or child, not their strengths: "sadly, many families are accustomed to getting bad news about their child or getting a litany of problems. That emphasis on weaknesses can cause families to feel sad, frustrated, and defensive" (Turnbull et al., 2006, p. 87).

Parents may be anxious, and some mild and transitional depression is expected, but most are able to come to terms with their circumstances with support and attention to potential problems. However, not all families emerge from the experience of childhood disability unscathed, and some undergo significant struggles in their efforts to cope (Power, DuPaul, Shapiro, & Kazak, 2003). The marital relationship may experience chronic stress and dissension, which can end in divorce and/or other serious problems due to the perceived demands of raising a child with a disability (Marshak & Prezant, 2007). Furthermore, there are some reports of the deleterious effect an impaired child might have on nondisabled siblings (Safer, 2002; Ufner, 2004; Simon, 1997; Moorman, 1992b).

In considering the impact of factors that contribute to risk in children, it is important to include poverty and discrimination, lack of parenting skills, work-related stress, alcoholism and drug abuse, as well as physical, emotional, and sexual abuse (Marshak et al., 1999). Evans (2004), in his extensive review of the effects of childhood poverty, puts this major social concern into proper perspective as he delineates its many contributors:

> Compared to their economically advantaged counterparts, they are exposed to more family turmoil, violence, separation from their families, instability, and chaotic households. . . . Low-income neighborhoods are more dangerous, offer poorer municipal services, and suffer greater physical deterioration. Predominantly low-income schools and day care are inferior. The accumulation of multiple environmental risks rather than singular risk exposure may be an especially pathogenic aspect of childhood poverty. (p. 71)

Although not all poor children experience these risks, this sobering description suggests that the care of children with disabilities who are born into such an environment may be a major unmet challenge to families, service providers, and to policy makers. These factors pose significant obstacles to the development of resilience in children. Another risk factor for some children can be residing in a single-parent home where the stress of work and caretaking, especially if there is childhood disability, can become overwhelming. A more detailed discussion of such situations appears in Chapter 3.

Thus some families do well in the face of adversity whereas others struggle and succumb. The study of resilience in individuals and in families should provide clues to which families can overcome risk factors when confronting problems and which cannot. The following discussion pertains to the factors and characteristics of resilient and nonresilient families.

The concept of resilience acknowledges that not all people are destroyed by negative events (Butler, Rosenbaum, & Palfrey, 1987; 1997; Alvard & Grados, 2005). In colloquial terms, it refers to "bouncing back" after an adverse event. Resilience shows that the event itself does not predict one's reaction to it (Wolin & Wolin, 1993)—although the accumulation of risk factors, such as those mentioned by Evans (2004), presents compelling challenges to resilience in children.

Research shows that resilient children have an active approach to problem solving, an ability to gain others' positive attention, an optimistic view of their experiences even in the face of stressful aspects, and a tendency to seek novel experiences (Rak & Patterson, 1996). These children also tend to be firstborn, recover more quickly from illness than nonresilient children, and are described as active and good-natured by their mothers (Werner & Smith, 1992). Success at making friends, intelligence, and an ability to regulate behavior are examples of internal strengths that contribute to resilience (Alvard & Grados, 2005).

In the aftermath of trauma, illness, disability, and dysfunction, children and their families can come to new insights and develop new abilities. As reflected in the writings of parents, grandparents, and siblings, the initial shock of childhood disability is a wake-up call and a challenge, an event that ultimately changes family members' outlook and perspective, alters goals, strengthens family ties, and changes roles in the family (Frisco, 2002; McHugh, 1999; Meyer, 1995; Simon, 1997; Harris & Glasberg, 2003; Hornby, 1995b; Naseef, 2001b). It can marshal resources and promote growth out of adversity, so that future crises are met with improved emotional and instrumental resources. Some family members write about how the shock of childhood disability can eventually become an opportunity for the reappraisal of priorities leading to more fulfilling lives and compelling relationships. It can also lead to involvement in issues and causes that contribute to a person's sense of altruism, achievement, and meaning.

Specific to the situation of childhood disability, Patterson (1991) offers the following advice to help families develop resilience:

1. The family should make active efforts to stay together, sharing responsibility and tasks and maintaining a positive outlook.
2. Learn to balance the special needs of the children with the needs of the other family members. This shift promotes inde-

pendence for the child and helps the family shift from the exclusive focus on the child to a broader consideration of all family members.

3. Maintain normal family routines and embrace shared family values and priorities.
4. Resilient families tend to find meaning in the face of challenges. The family should avoid blaming a member for having caused or contributed to the disability.
5. Flexibility in setting rules, establishing roles, and promoting expectations contributes to resilience.
6. Be proactive in learning about the disability and in locating needed services and formats for support (e.g., support groups, church, counseling).
7. Recognize that the family–professional relationship is a two-way street and attempt to maintain good relationships with teachers, physicians, and other providers. Poor relationships can lead to added stress and promote withdrawal from needed medical, educational, and social services.
8. Communication is vitally important for any family, but especially when there is a child with a disability.
9. The perspective of family members is enhanced when they are able to attribute a positive meaning to the situation.
10. Resilient families rarely approach challenges with an attitude of passive resignation. The family is enhanced when its members actively seek out resources and opportunities.

Stress in family life is inevitable and can be harmful when it is severe and chronic. The study of resilience provides hope because we learn that most children and adults do not crumble in the presence of stress and that there are ways to enhance resistance to negative events (Alvard & Grados, 2005). In the following section we address the concept of stress, how to recognize it, and how to decrease its negative effects.

Stress

Someone once opined that, "If you ain't got stress, you ain't living." These words suggest that stress is ubiquitous. Not only is it a common phenomenon but it also varies in intensity. Stress and its partner, anxiety, can fuel great performances and motivate people to attain unexpected achievements, it can also be the curse that cuts short ambition, demoralizes, saps energy, and lead to depression, withdrawal, and iso-

lation. Mild, time-limited, intermittent stress can energize and motivate, whereas excessive, unremitting stress can debilitate. Stress has
been implicated in illness, family dysfunction, concentration difficulties, and depression. Due to its pervasiveness, scientific journals and
popular magazines and books trumpet the newest, innovative stress
reducing techniques. Some claims may reflect innovative strategies,
whereas others promote techniques that have been around for some
time, camouflaged as something new.

Hill (1949, 1958) developed a theoretical model of stress that is
still cited in the family literature (McCubbin & Patterson, 1983;
Wikler, 1981; Walsh, 2003b; Hanson & Lynch, 2004) and has been designated as the *ABCX* family crisis mode, where *A* (the stressor event),
interacting with *B* (the family's crisis-meeting resources), interacting
with *C* (the definition the family makes of the event) produces *X* (the
crisis).

The *A* factor, the stressor, is any life event or transition that produces change in the family system. It can include a *normative* stressor
that is expected (e.g., the family losing an elderly parent or adding a
new member through birth) or a *nonnormative* event (e.g., the birth of
a child with a disability) (Hanson & Lynch, 2004). The family's boundaries, goals, patterns of interaction, roles, or values may be threatened
by the change caused by a stressor (McCubbin & Patterson, 1983).

The *B* factor (family resources) is the family's capacity to meet
challenges and obstacles and shift its course of action to counter the
stressor. This factor relates directly to the notion that the family's flexibility and quality of relationship prior to the presence of the child
with a disability may be an important predictor of its ability to adapt.
Resources can also be acquired outside of the family by initiating contact with community services.

The *C* factor is the definition the family attributes to the experienced stressor. This factor reflects the family's values and previous
experience in dealing with change and meeting crises. In other words,
it is not the event itself that is disturbing but the meaning attributed to
the event that constitutes the source of anxiety. Research has shown
that cognitive strategies are helpful in gaining more positive perspectives on a situation. Cognitive strategies are explored in Chapter 12.

These three factors all influence the family's ability to prevent the
stressor event from creating a crisis (the *X* factor). A crisis reflects the
family's inability to restore balance and stability. It is important to note
*that stress may never become a crisis if the family is able to use existing
resources and defines the situation as a manageable event.*

Psychosocial Stresses Associated with Childhood Illness or Disability

Although illness and disability are different phenomena, some researchers have looked at factors common to both and noted five areas of stress commonly experienced by families as a consequence of either chronic illness or disability. These areas are intellectual, instrumental, emotional, interpersonal, and existential (Brinthaupt, 1991; Chesler & Barbarin, 1987).

Intellectual Stress

Intellectual stress is chiefly associated with the process of first information—that is, when determining an accurate diagnosis occupies the parents' attention. It is not uncommon for parents of children with certain impairments to engage in the frustrating process of consulting a number of specialists. With some impairments, there can be several misdiagnoses before a correct one is given. As noted in Chapter 4, once the diagnosis is made, parents usually experience a compelling need for information (Darling, 1979; Hobbs, Perrin, & Ireys, 1986; Hornby, 2000; Marshak et al., 1999).

The quest for information regarding etiology, prognosis, and treatment may be very anxiety provoking. Parents may engage in "doctor shopping," which may make them susceptible to "quack" treatments, although some shopping may be necessary to reach a professional who is empathic, responsive to the parents, has had experience with disability, and can make a definitive diagnosis. Unproven money-making schemes and supposed cures constitute heinous acts toward children with disabilities and their caretakers, taking advantage of vulnerable families and distracting them from seeking appropriate treatment for their children. "To my mind, promoters of such treatments are up there with televangelists who oversell religious retirement communities and keep the change, and used car salesmen who set back odometers 50,000 miles" (Siegel, 1996, p. 323).

A 5-year-old child was given a controversial treatment, chelation therapy, to cure or reduce the effects of autism (Linn, 2005). The goal of the treatment is to rid the body of lead and mercury (apparently there is a mercury preservative in childhood vaccinations). The child died during the treatment. A physician quoted in the article said, "I wish there was more outrage with his death. The boy was sacrificed on the altar of bad science and that was unconscionable" (p. 2).

Various intellectual stresses are imposed as parents attempt to comprehend their child's disability (Brinthaupt, 1991). Parents may be required to integrate vast amounts of information about physiology, timing and type of treatments and the rationale for them, symptoms of decline or improvement, and complications and side effects of treatment (Rolland, 2003). In writing about childhood cancer, Chesler and Barbarin (1987) observed: "The stress of wondering if they are handling treatments and side effects properly is escalated by the stakes involved—the child's comfort and even life may hang in the balance" (p. 42). Brinthaupt (1991) noted: "The overriding task of learning the skills necessary to effectively operate within a medical subculture is an intellectual stress not to be underestimated for its difficulty as well as importance" (p. 301).

Instrumental Stress

Instrumental stress involves tasks that are necessary to incorporate the child's care and treatment into the lifestyle of the family. The goal is to achieve as much equilibrium as possible in the family system. Parents become frontline caregivers of their child and, as a result, become proficient in treatment management. While simultaneously attending to their child's needs and their own needs, they must also attend to the needs of other family members, such as other children or their spouses (Turnbull & Turnbull, 2001; Marshak et al., 1999). Brinthaupt (1991) noted the following instrumental challenges:

1. Managing finances.
2. Determining the division of labor in the family so that adequate care is provided for the child with a disability.
3. Accomplishing necessary household chores in addition to caretaking.
4. Becoming aware of signs that indicate a negative impact of the illness or disability on family members.
5. Knowing when and how to seek assistance.
6. Fostering a sense of normalcy despite the demands of the illness or disability.

The financial demands on a family are often given short shrift in the professional literature. As noted in Chapter 5, both direct medical care and in-home and self-care expenses, as well as expenses for special diets, special schools, time lost from work, home modifications, and the like, constitute significant sources of stress. "Disability is expensive. Medical and therapy services, special equipment, and adapted toys and clothing are examples of the financial impact of disability" (Berry & Hardman, 1998, p. 54). These financial demands can interfere with potentially restorative and interpersonally rewarding family activities, such as vacations (Brinthaupt, 1991).

Emotional Stress

Emotional stress is a response to the demands of caregiving that might include lack of sleep, loss of energy, and excessive worry and anxiety (Chesler & Barbarin, 1987). A factor contributing to the emotional response to illness or disability is uncertainty regarding prognosis and responses to periodic exacerbations (Jessop & Stein, 1985; Perrin & MacLean, 1988; Rolland, 2003). Furthermore, the uncertainty and ambiguity that can accompany illness or disability can compromise one's sense of perceived control (Pollin, 1995; Wright, 1983).

Parents of children with rare disorders may feel particularly isolated, which increases emotional stress, because it is unlikely that they will encounter another family with a child who has the same condition. A useful resource for parents of infants who have rare disorders is the "Reader's Forum" in the magazine *Exceptional Parent*. Letter writers often offer to correspond with other parents who have an infant or child with the same uncommon disorder as their child. Another contributor to emotional stress is the heart-wrenching experience of watching a child suffer and not being able to relieve that suffering. Also, in the case of medical illness, heightened vigilance for signs of relapse or disease exacerbation can add to stress and anxiety (Rolland, 2003).

Interpersonal Stress

Interpersonal stress can follow on the heels of childhood disability or illness and may involve family members, friends, and medical or educational personnel. Although divorce rates among these families tend to be roughly equivalent to rates in families in which there is no illness or disability (Brinthaupt, 1991; Kalins, 1983; Sabbeth & Leventhal, 1984), there does appear to be evidence of marital distress. Siegel (1996) claimed that about one-third of American marriages end in divorce and that in families of children with disabilities the rate is 20% higher. She also stated that it is difficult to obtain accurate figures on divorce rates (Marshak & Prezant, 2007). In their review of studies of marital adjustment in families of children with congenital impairments, Benson and Gross (1989) noted that the influence of stress was negative in some cases and positive in others (increased cohesiveness). These researchers were critical of the studies they reviewed in terms of methodology. Another older review of studies that used control groups of parents who had children without disabilities indicated that parents of children with disabilities were not more likely to divorce but did experience marital dissatisfaction and stress (Sabbeth & Leventhal, 1984).

The available research suggests that having a child with a disability does not necessarily lead to divorce or major marital problems, although some families are challenged by this situation and others seem to grow stronger (Berry & Hardman, 1998; Hunt & Marshall, 1999). More research is needed to clarify the role of marital distress in these families in comparison to families with nondisabled children.

In terms of family dysfunction and divorce, one of us noted previously (Seligman, 1995):

> One needs to be careful about attributing marital conflict or divorce to the presence of a child with special needs. The decision to dissolve a marriage is a complex one, made up of personal styles and values, family of origin issues, external factors, and the like. We suspect that the general public believes that a child with a disability creates enormous tensions within the family, eventually culminating in divorce. However, parents who speak and write about their experiences with their child project the notion that a child with a disability marshals constructive forces within the family system and eventually brings family members together. Our guess is that the truth probably falls somewhere between what the general public seems to believe and what some parents have projected in their public utterances and in their writings. We need to openly address this issue so that the public is better informed and that parents who have experienced divorce are not filled with guilt and shame because of the perception that most other families are actually brought closer. (pp. 178–179)

As noted throughout this book, interpersonal distress exists in other family members because nondisabled children and extended family members are also affected by childhood disability (Marshak et al., 1999). Finally, interpersonal stress can emerge from potentially stressful encounters with the public (Siegal, 1996; Wikler, 1981;

Heatherton, Kleck, Hebl, & Hull, 2000). Depending on the extent to which parents "go public" with their child's disability, they must negotiate the sometimes stressful and awkward transactions with strangers (discussed further in Chapter 4).

Existential Stress

The term *existential stress* is used to discuss the family's ability to construct an explanatory meaning framework for its experience (Rolland, 2003). Childhood disability is an affront to an assumed developmental order of the family life cycle. "Childhood is supposed to be a time of well-being, or, at worst, a period of self-limited, transitory illness, and not a time of threats to viability or function" (Stein & Jessop, 1984, p. 194). Parents grapple with such existential issues as "Why me?" or "Why my family?" (Kushner, 1981). B. Gill (1997) believes:

> For those of us with a strong sense of personal God, acceptance of this can be very difficult. We may feel betrayed, even abandoned by God, or question God's love for us. All of us must struggle in our own way to square what has happened with our idea of God and of the universe. Our challenge is to accept randomness. Why did this happen? Because it did. Why me? Why not? Maybe "why" is not a useful question. Maybe the real question is "what now?" (p. 20).

Existential questions regarding "Why me" or "Why us" are salient concerns to children with disabilities and their parents. Dinsmore (2004) quoted the observations of a 30-year-old man with spina bifida:

> As a boy, I often felt angry about why I ended up with my disability. I questioned God and throughout my life have battled with my faith. Why would a just and fair God give this disability to an innocent baby? I never asked for it.
>
> I later learned the reason why I was chosen. God picked me because he knew I could handle it. In this way, it was a gift from Him. More times than not though, it seemed like a curve.

Cherished notions about God, fate, and a just world are challenged (Chesler & Barbarin, 1987). "If the child is seen as a divine gift, the unexpressed question, 'why did this happen to me?' has the corollary 'why did He do this to me?' and raises the age-old philosophical question, 'If God is good He would not have done this.' " (Ross, 1964, p. 62).

A child with a disability may be perceived as a reflection of the mother's inadequacy (Featherstone, 1980). In situations where a child is viewed as salvaging an unstable marriage, the birth of a child with a disability may be another indication that the marriage is doomed to failure. On the other hand, as noted by Ross, the infant may be seen as a divine gift, a sign of grace.

Some parents appear to be able to explain their child's disability within the framework of a particular life philosophy, whereas others alter or abandon their prior religious or spiritual commitments. It is apparent that existential stresses are a formidable challenge for parents of children with chronic illness or developmental disabilities (Brinthaupt, 1991).

Social Support

Social support is viewed as a mediating or buffering factor in meeting the demands of a stressful event (Cobb, 1976; Crnic, Greenberg, et al., 1983). According to Biegel, Sales, and Schulz (1991), social support can intervene between a stressor and a stress reaction (i.e., an appraisal of the event) by preventing the reaction, or it can intervene after the stress is experienced and prevent the onset of a problematic response. As described by Freund and McGuire (1999):

> Social ties can serve as nets that hold us up or keep us from falling when we are threatened. They function as sources of information and financial or other kinds of aid and as mirrors that help reflect messages of self-affirmation back to us. Just as a fetus needs a womb to receive nourishment, shelter, warmth, and life support, human beings do not function effectively as isolated individuals. (p. 101)

Thus social support increases one's sense of well-being, resilience, and feeling of competence, whereas its absence in a time of crisis contributes to a diminished network of social relationships, isolation, depression, doubt, and less positive outcomes.

The forms of social support can include a variety of formats, including group and one-to-one support. The nourishing effects of one-to-one support (e.g., spouse, trusted friend) are poignantly reflected in Naseef's (2001b, p. 195) quote of an Arab proverb:

A friend is one to
whom one may pour out
all the contents of one's
heart, chaff and grain
together, knowing that the gentlest of hands
will take and sift it,
keep what is worth keeping
    and
with the breath of kindness
blow the rest away.

As we know, the birth of a child with a disability is considered a stressful event (Crnic, Greenberg, Ragozin, Robinson, & Basham, 1983; Marshak et al., 1999; Beckman, 2002), and one that is chronic in nature. The use of social support is an external coping strategy that has been shown to reduce family stress (Beckman & Porkorni, 1988; Berry & Hardman, 1998). Indeed, results from research indicate that supportive social networks are linked to increased well-being, positive caregiving, positive parental attitudes, improved child behavior, and better parent–child relationships (Dunst, Trivette, & Cross, 1986).

As we have noted, childhood disability can have an isolating effect on families. A disability can serve as a familial "membrane" that separates the family from mainstream society (Marsh, 1992). Some of the reasons for this isolation include the emotional and physical exhaustion of family members, the stigma experienced by the family, social exclusion coming from a lack of acceptance and understanding, the support needs of extended family members, and the specialized needs of children with disabilities (Marsh, 1992; Marshak et al., 1999; Turnbull & Turnbull, 2001; Heatherton et al., 2000; Berry & Hardman, 1998). The availability of social support helps to buffer some of the more arduous effects of childhood disability.

When informal support in the form of family, friends, neighbors, or coworkers is insufficient, formal support from professionals may be needed. It is important to recognize the degree (e.g., from considerable help to modest assistance) and type (e.g., information, counseling) of support needed in relation to the disability or illness (Marsh, 1992; Goodheart & Lansing, 1997). Families of children with disabilities tend to have smaller networks of support than other families (Herman & Thompson, 1995; Kazak & Marvin, 1984). Most of the support comes from the nuclear family and from extended family members. However, when family members gain access to supportive professionals, groups, and organizations, they tend to experience improved functioning (Turnbull & Turnbull, 2001).

Both formal (e.g., social service agencies) and informal (e.g., family, kin, friends) support can contribute to coping, adaptation, and a reduction in stress (Boyd, 2002; Turnbull et al., 2006; Lyon, Knickelbaum, & Wolf, 2005). By the same token, certain forms of support can add more stress to the family unit. Rejecting grandparents (informal) or cold, distant, uncommunicative professionals (formal) are likely to strain the family with their lack of sympathetic attitudes. From the reported positive effects of social support, it is easy to assume that it is always easily available and accepted gratefully. This is not always the case. Poverty can limit access to needed support due to limited funds for respite, recreation, or transportation or dues or other expenses for clubs and similar groups (Pilisuk & Parks, 1986; Evans, 2004). Furthermore, it can be stressful and counterproductive at times to have family and friends around (Freund & McGuire, 1999). An ill person, for example, may experience pressure to quickly improve beyond his or her capacity to do so (Horton, 1985). Additionally, overreliance on social support can undermine family members' sense of competence by making them feel that they cannot function on their own or that they will be unable to reciprocate the help they received (Pilisuk & Parks, 1986).

It is usually assumed that social support should come primarily from close friends and family, but, as Chapter 3 suggests, "people from various cultural backgrounds differ in what they see as social support and where they are apt to turn for support. In some cases, it is one's spouse or one's children; in other cases, friends and neighbors" (Freund & McGuire, 1999, p. 105). Thus, in attempting to facilitate support for families, it is important to take multicultural and ethnic factors into account as well as the expressed preferences of family members. In this respect, it is helpful to be aware of the support preferences of individuals within the family. For example, a father/husband may be willing to discuss pressing feelings with an old, trusted friend, whereas his wife expresses the need to be involved in a support group of women who have children with similar disabilities. A nondisabled child may be receptive to joining a sibling support group of like-aged children, whereas the grandparents are satisfied by confiding only in family members. Generally speaking, the provision of unwanted support can be problematic, and the provision of support over the long haul can be difficult to achieve as well (Goodheart & Lansing, 1997). Unfortunately, there are fewer programs and activities available and families receive less support as children grow into adolescence and adulthood than they do during their childhood years (Marshak et al., 1999).

To sum up, social support reduces the subjective distress of families, encourages positive personal, family, and child functioning, and enables parents to maintain a sense of normalcy and coping effectiveness (Schilling, Gilchrist, & Schinke, 1984; Turnbull & Turnbull, 2001; Berry & Hardman, 1998). In addition, peer or professionally led self-help groups are a powerful resource for some family members (Santelli, Turnbull, Sergeant, Lerner, & Marquis, 1996; Katz, 1993; Seligman & Marshak, 2003). As noted, these groups provide a forum for catharsis, information, emotional support, mutual aid, and advocacy. Such groups are discussed further in Chapter 12.

Developmental Transitions

Because of the nature and severity of a child's impairment and the family's response to it, families of children with disabilities negotiate a series of stages that, at least to some extent, are unique to them. Because of plateaus, exacerbations, setbacks, and achievements that continue to occur throughout the child's lifetime, typical developmental stages may not apply. Consider, for example, a family with a child with hemophilia, for whom periodic "bleeds" cause considerable ongoing stress. Such events trigger a new cycle of upset, changing demands, and new adaptations. Similarly, the families of children with cancer or mental illness need to adjust to unanticipated events such as a recurrence or side effects from medication (Moores, 2006).

Children with developmental disabilities are generally slower in accomplishing certain life cycle or developmental milestones, and some may never achieve them. As the child approaches critical periods, parents may experience renewed anxiety or sadness. Fewell (1991) describes several periods that are particularly stressful to parents of children with disabilities.

Encountering the Disability

The nature of a child's disability generally determines when the parents learn about it. Genetic disabilities, such as Down syndrome, are usually apparent soon after birth. Conditions such as deafness, chronic illness, and language and learning disabilities may not be discovered until the child is older. In the case of mild to moderate disability, Fewell (1991) observes that "When there is a problem, knowledge comes slowly, bit by bit, until the parent acts to seek an answer" (p. 224). After parents realize that there are problems, they must then obtain a diagnosis so that proper remediation procedures can begin. The path of obtaining a diagnosis can be a convoluted one as professionals differ in their opinions and because a diagnosis is not always able to be determined. Families are apt to seek a favorable diagnosis, which can have the paradoxizal effect of prolonging treatment (Fewell, 1991). The diagnostic phase is considered one of the most stressful times for parents (Berry & Hardman, 1998). Contributing to this stress is the dissatisfaction that parents feel when they were told about their child's disability in a negative way (e.g., cold, dispassionate, condescending; Quine & Rutter, 1994; Sloper & Turner, 1991). More is said about the initial diagnostic phase in Chapter 4.

Families may be confronted with impairment that is caused by an accident or develops when their child is older. The confirmation of a serious and chronic problem often precipitates a crisis and affects the entire family. Immediate reactions may include shock, great disappointment, anxiety, and depression (Hornby, 1994a). As we have noted, the loss experienced because of having a child who is different than expected may precipitate a mourning period much like the death of a family member (Marshak & Seligman, 1993). Contact with physicians and health care workers is particularly intense at this stage. It is also during this time of considerable stress that the family needs to inform other family members, friends, and work acquaintances of their situation. A minority of parents consider disclosure so difficult that they hide or delay telling others, which can lead to isolation during a stressful period when social support might be helpful.

Parental adjustment is complicated by the fact that a child's disability is an unanticipated event. Generally speaking, adults have expectations of proceeding through the life cycle in a fairly predictable sequence. An unanticipated life event (e.g., the birth of a child with a disability; death of a young parent) is likely to be experienced as traumatic. Major stressors tend to be "off time" events that fall outside of the family's expectations (Marsh, 1992; Rolland, 2003).

Early Childhood

The early childhood years can be difficult ones for parents, as they anxiously watch for their child to achieve certain developmental milestones. The chronicity of a child's disabilities and what it means to the family is a major issue during this stage of the child's development

(Hunt & Marshall, 2005). All families expand in membership when a child is born. But for families of children with disabilities, the family expands because of the addition of the child *and* of professionals who populate the services families need (Berry & Hardman, 1998). The inclusion of professionals is not a welcome addition, yet in time they generally prove to be beneficial and provide a supportive alliance. The nature and severity of the impairment play a key role in the family's perception and behavior (Fewell, 1991; Lyon et al., 2005). In regard to a child's developmental delay, Fewell (1986) observe that

> the task of diapering a three-year-old is simply not as easy as it was when the child was one year old. The larger and heavier child requires more energy to lift and carry. The emotional burden is also great: parents anticipate the end of diapers and two o'clock bottles, and when these things don't end, it can shatter dreams and invite questions about the future. (pp. 16–17)

Helen Featherstone, in her classic book, *A Difference in the Family* (1980), poignantly speaks to her anxieties about the future:

> I remember, during the early months of Jody's life, the anguish with which I contemplated the distant future. Jody cried constantly, not irritable, hungry cries, but heartrending shrieks of pain. Vain efforts to comfort him filled my nights and days. One evening when nothing seemed to help, I went outside, intending to escape his misery for a moment, hoping that without me he might finally fall asleep. Walking in summer darkness, I imagined myself at seventy, bent and wrinkled, hobbling up the stairs to minister to Jody, now over forty, but still crying and helpless. (p. 19)

Early intervention programs that provide services typically beginning at birth or shortly afterward are generally applauded (Hornby, 2000; McWilliam et al., 1995; Erickson & Kurz-Riemer, 1999; Bauer & Shea, 2003). One overview of the literature in this area concludes that a significant number of families are helped to gain more confidence in their parental roles, to work with professionals, and to help their child learn (Turnbull et al., 2006). These authors also report that some families from culturally and linguistically diverse backgrounds tend to be less satisfied with early intervention programs.

Fewell (1986) noted that a crisis can develop when a child enters an early intervention program and families encounter one or more of the following:

1. Families see older children with a similar condition and wonder whether their child will resemble them as he or she develops.
2. Families who share their experiences with other families realize that they may need to "fight" for the services their child needs, further draining the family's emotional resources.
3. Families learn that they are expected to be their child's primary caregivers and teachers.

Parents come into increasing contact with professionals following the diagnosis of their child, who may treat parents more like patients who need treatment rather than as experts on their children (Seligman, 2000; Alper, Schloss, & Schloss, 1994). Parents may be traumatized by their experiences with professionals and "the system" and avoid further contact, if possible (Erickson & Kurz-Riemer, 1999). Perhaps most discouraging at this stage is the realization of the chronic burden a child might constitute for family members as they view the future with some degree of apprehension. However, early intervention programs help to prepare the family for the marathon ahead. The infancy and preschool periods are discussed further in Chapter 4.

School Entry

Another period of adjustment comes when parents realize that their child fails to fit into the mainstream of the traditional educational system. A child may require special education classes and a separate transportation system or extra help from the school nurse to assist with medical problems and regimens. This can be a particularly difficult period for siblings as more of their schoolmates learn that they have a brother or sister who has a disability. This stage can be characterized as the period when the family "goes public," as they venture beyond their own boundaries (Marshak et al., 1999). If they have not done so already, parents must also adjust the educational and career goals they had envisioned for their child.

The challenges parents face depend on both the nature of the child's impairment (e.g., there may be relatively few adjustments if the child has a mild physical impairment) and the preparedness of the school system to provide adequate educational and adjunct services for children with special needs. Another issue is the difficulty of finding playmates during the school years. Parents look on with dismay as they see their child fail at making friendships:

There is a helpless feeling that you get when you pick up your child at 3:00 in the school parking lot and watch her going from child to child inviting each one over only to be refused. If you only had the power to create a friend, you would do it. How many times can you tell her that they must have other things to do today and maybe they'll be free another day before she catches on they just don't want to play with her? And then what do you do? (anonymous personal communication, September 1997; Marshak et al., 1999, p. 73)

One of us had the following reaction after watching his daughter and her sister being rejected by neighborhood kids:

My heart ached to see either Lisa or Lori hurt. I felt impotent to help either one avoid the pain, although, on occasion, I would call the kids in so that they could escape the conflicts. Although I'm sure that they were suffering from the rejection they felt, I now know that I called them into the house because of my own anguish. (Seligman, 1995, p. 176)

Issues faced by families during the school years are discussed further in Chapter 5.

Adolescence

Lidz (1983) described adolescence as "a time of seeking: seeking inward to find who one is; a searching outward to locate one's place in life; a longing for another with whom to satisfy cravings for intimacy and fulfillment" (p. 306). Another author added that adolescents are preoccupied with what others think about them. They crave attention yet complain about being "on stage." They move toward independence but are anxious about losing the protection and nurturance from parents (Mondimore, 2002). Adolescence marks the period of separation from parents, increasing independence, and searching for one's individuality or uniqueness. It also commences a period of anxiety as maturing children experience considerable change, turmoil, and ambivalence. For families of children with disabilities, this stage can be a painful reminder of their offspring's failure to negotiate this life-cycle stage successfully, of their child's continuing dependence. Furthermore, children with disabilities and their families may face a prolonged period of adolescence (Strax, 1991). Citing a national study of more than 1,000 families, Turnbull et al. (2006) reported that adolescence and young adulthood are the two most stressful life stages. These authors fur-

ther noted that adolescence can exacerbate or mitigate typical adolescent issues. In terms of adolescents with disabilities:

> Parents might experience only minor rebellion and conflict because
> their children might have fewer peers after whom to model such behav-
> iors, fewer opportunities to try alcohol or drugs, or decreased mobility
> and, therefore, fewer changes to take dangerous risks. In other cases,
> adolescence may bring greater isolation, a growing sense of difference,
> and confusion and fear about emerging sexuality. (p. 82).

Peer acceptance is particularly painful for the entire family during
the adolescent years, even though it does occur during the school
years and in adulthood as well. Peer acceptance may determine the
extent to which the child feels rejected and isolated, which in turn may
contribute to the stress other family members experience.

Adolescence is a particularly difficult phase of life for many with
disabilities. Nondisabled adolescents can be cruel in their comments
and behavior toward their peers with disabilities. The value placed on
conformity during adolescence typically causes considerable distress
because of the difference inherent in having a disability. Being different and distinct becomes bad. "To be different when every adolescent
instinct begs for sameness, is to be denied the protective coloration
that helps other kids endure the teen years, the mean years" (Leslie
Milk, quoted in Kriegsman, Zaslow, & D'Zmura-Rechsteiner, 1992). An
additional source of distress is the heightened importance placed on
dating. Issues of independence and emancipation also become pronounced and a source of considerable turmoil (Marshak & Seligman,
1993). Additionally, how do adolescents establish a positive identity in
a society that generally views them in negative ways? (Olkin, 1991).
How are individuation and separation achieved if the adolescent has
limited access to peers? Is a level of separation possible for the adolescent, even if he or she is unable to attain full separation, as do nondisabled peers?

Acknowledging the challenge of coping with the ups and downs
of adolescence with the additional challenge of having a disability,
Milk wrote: "Adolescence is the ultimate disability. All teenagers hate
their hands or their hair, feel stupid or awkward, and are certain that
their tiny flaws and foibles are the only things that others see about
them. So to be a teenager coping with a disability is to be doubly disabled" (quoted in Kriegsman et al., 1992, p. v).

Beginning Adult Life

Public education offers both children and parents several benefits: It helps the child gain important educational and vocational skills and independence, and it provides respite for the parents. The transitions from school to community and work are major challenges for families (Bauer & Shea, 2003). These authors noted that the successful adjustment to work and community for those with disabilities is significantly below that of their nondisabled peers. As a child's education draws to an end, parents must make some difficult choices. Limited vocational possibilities and inadequate community living arrangements and social programs leave families with few choices. This is a stressful period in that the specter of the child's future looms and causes considerable concern and anxiety, especially in the area of severe disability (Lyon et al., 2005).

Maintaining Adult Life

As the family prepares for their child's adult years, one of the more significant threats is the failure of the child to achieve independence and self-sufficiency. Although there have been efforts to establish transitioning programs, mostly driven by parent outcry and legislation, "the longitudinal, developmental bases of transition and the implications for individuals, families, and professionals are frequently ignored in the bureaucratic hodgepodge of guidelines and mandates that currently exist" (Marshak et al., 1999, p. 153).

Where an adult with a disability will live and the level of care he or she will need constitute the family's concerns at this stage (Bauer & Shea, 2003). A major source of worry is the future care of their adult child as parents look to the ensuing years when they may not be able to function as active overseers or when they are deceased.

Competent professionals are particularly important to help families plan for their children's future in terms of living arrangements, vocation, and leisure-time activities. Adult siblings as well as extended family members may be useful adjunct resources and should be considered potential helpers during this period. Although mental health and community support services are always needed, their availability and accessibility may be particularly acute at this point.

When formal schooling is over, late adolescents and young adults are not protected by entitlement systems of educational services but are thrust into an adult service system governed by different guidelines and funding streams. Those with disabilities and their families may become lost in attempting to access training and employment, community participation, and independent living. There is a great need for a coordinator to ferret out available services—a person who knows the needs of the family, the resources in the community, and can actively act as an advocate and source of information and support (Laborde & Seligman, 1991). Adulthood ushers in a period of concern as new rules and guidelines need to be learned and new services need to be negotiated in the context of fewer resources and supports.

Employment is a particularly difficult issue because attitudes continue to be negative regarding job applicants with disabilities. It is especially problematic for women with disabilities in that there are higher unemployment rates for them, as opposed to men with disabilities. Women of color and gay and bisexual women with disabilities are multiple victims of discrimination (Banks & Kaschak, 2003). African American women with disabilities are triply victimized due to prejudice based on gender, ethnicity, *and* disability (Beatty, 2003; Feldman & Tegart, 2003). All of these factors combine to make job opportunities problematic. Issues of adulthood are addressed further in Chapter 6.

Rolland's Model of Family Adjustment to Chronic Illness

Chronic illness in children, with its steady, declining, or episodic course, can be compared to developmental disabilities in some ways. Some children with developmental disabilities also have a chronic illness (Goodheart & Lansing, 1997). It is for these reasons that we have included Rolland's (1994, 2003) theory of adjustment to chronic illness in children. By doing so we acknowledge the unique circumstances that illness can present for the family and the fact that the medical model is not always an appropriate framework for the understanding of disability.

Rolland's (1994, 2003) model of family adaptation to chronic illness relies on an understanding of a series of life-cycle and illness-related variables. An illness can have an *acute* or *gradual* onset. For acute-onset problems (e.g., stroke, accident), families are forced to cope with the situation in a short period of time. There is a need to mobilize resources quickly to cope with the situation, whereas a gradual-onset illness develops more slowly and requires patience and a tolerance for ambiguity as symptoms are experienced. In addition, the patient and family may have to endure rounds of medical tests and examinations before a diagnosis is known.

The *course* of an illness is another disease variable that must be considered. For example, illnesses can be progressive, constant, or relapsing/episodic. In a constant-course illness, family members face a fairly stable and predictable situation, whereas in an episodic-course illness, family members may find it stressful to cope with the transitions between crisis and noncrisis and the uncertainty of when an episode will occur.

Outcome and *incapacitation* are two other factors. In terms of outcome, a condition can be fatal (e.g., AIDS, cancer) or chronic and nonfatal (e.g., arthritis). The key difference between these outcomes is the degree to which family members anticipate loss (Rolland, 2003). In terms of incapacitation, an illness or impairment can affect one's cognitive abilities (e.g., Alzheimer's disease), mobility (e.g., stroke, auto accident), or sensation (e.g., blindness, deafness), or can result in stigma (e.g., AIDS) or disfigurement (e.g., burns). The timing, extent, and type of incapacitation imply differences in the degree of family response (Rolland, 2003).

Illnesses also have *time phases*, such as crisis, chronic, and terminal. During periods of *crisis*, families are particularly vulnerable. Professionals have enormous influence over a family's sense of competence during this phase. Rolland (1994) views the initial meetings with professionals (diagnosis and advice) as a "framing event." This can be a period of considerable anxiety, misunderstanding and miscommunication (Seligman, 1995). Rolland (2003) advises professionals to be very sensitive in their interactions with family members at this stage. For example, who is included during these early meetings can influence family communication patterns about the illness. Family members tend to have vivid memories around their initial professional contacts, especially those with physicians as they attempt to establish a diagnosis.

The *chronic* phase may be marked by constancy or by periods of episodic change or even death. This phase challenges the family to maintain a semblance of a normal life while living with uncertainty. Chronic illnesses can strain family relations as expectations and personal life/career goals may need to be altered. This phase resembles the period when families realize that their child has a lifelong developmental disability.

Families that adapt well to the *terminal* phase are those that are able to shift from trying to control the illness to "letting go" (Rolland,

2003). Being open to experience and dealing with the numerous practical tasks that need to be done characterize a family that is coping well. A family with a track record of coping during crises will negotiate this phase well, though certainly not without the grieving period common to loss.

Rolland (2003) noted that there are other implications of disease onset, course, incapacitation, and so forth, as they interact with individual and family life-cycle phases. In the face of chronic illness, professionals need to be mindful that the demands presented by an illness can seriously interfere with the personal life goals of family members. This is the case for families who have a child with a developmental disability as well. A balance between meeting the requirements of the disease and achieving dreamed-of personal goals would be an optimal situation. To help achieve such a balance, Rolland (1994) suggested that

> it is vital to ask what life plans the family or individual members had to cancel, postpone, or alter as a result of the diagnosis. It is useful to know whose plans are most and least affected. By asking a family where and under what conditions they will resume plans put on hold or address future developmental tasks, a clinician can anticipate developmental crises related to "independence from" versus "subjugation to" the chronic illness. (p. 454)

SUMMARY

In this chapter we have reviewed some of the literature related to the effects of childhood disability on the family system. Most of this literature has involved families of European ancestry, and much of it has been based on families of middle and upper SES. In the next chapter we consider the important variable of family diversity—both cultural and structural diversity. As we will see, professionals need to use caution in applying general principles of family functioning to the diverse families they may encounter.

∎3

All Families Are Not Alike

Social and Cultural Diversity
in Reaction to Childhood Disability

The birth of a child with a disability has different meanings in various societies throughout the world. Even within a single complex society, this event can have a variety of meanings that are shaped by subcultural values and beliefs. In addition, family reactions and lifestyles are structured by a family's place in the social order, which includes economic opportunities, neighborhood characteristics, and other factors. In this chapter, we briefly review some of the cross-cultural diversity in reactions to childhood disability and look more closely at the variety of meanings and adaptations that may be attached to childhood disability in U.S. society.

Understanding social and cultural diversity is essential in a systems perspective. A family's definition of its situation and of the roles that various family members should play will vary considerably depending on the family's background. Although individual differences certainly exist, cultural values and meanings and social opportunities shape reactions to children with disabilities. Professionals need to know as much as possible about the potential differences they might encounter in the families with whom they interact. Moreover, as

Jezewski and Sotnik (2005) suggested, service providers can be "culture brokers" who provide bridges, links, and mediation between groups to reduce conflict.

CROSS-CULTURAL DIVERSITY

As Groce (2005, p. 6) wrote: "In all societies, individuals with disability are not only recognized as distinct from the general population, but value and meaning also are attached to their condition." Values attached to disability have varied both geographically and historically. In ancient Sparta, malformed babies were thrown over a precipice; in contrast, in some Native American societies people with disabilities were believed to have supernatural powers and are held in high esteem. Safilios-Rothschild (1970) suggested that prejudice toward people with disabilities varies from one country to another by (1) level of economic development and rate of unemployment; (2) beliefs about the role of government in alleviating social problems; (3) beliefs about individual "responsibility" (sin) for disability; (4) cultural values attached to different physical conditions; (5) disability-connected factors, including visibility, contagiousness, part of the body affected, physical versus mental nature of the disability, and severity of functional impairment; (6) effectiveness of public relations efforts; and (7) importance of activities that carry a high risk of disability—for example, war.

A sampling of varying reactions to disability in different cultures throughout the world illustrates the role of cultural values in shaping attitudes. Obesity in women is greatly admired in most African tribes (Chesler, 1965) yet stigmatized in the U.S. middle class. Among Middle Eastern Muslims, the term *saint* is applied to people with intellectual disability, and they are given benevolent and protective treatment (Edgerton, 1970). According to Wright (1983), among the Wogeo, a New Guinea tribe, children with obvious deformities are buried alive at birth, but children disabled in later life are cared for lovingly. Groce (1987) has suggested that disability issues in developing countries are different from those in the Western world: "High tech, hospital-based, rehabilitative approaches to care, urban-based educational facilities, and even support groups, do little to reach the majority of the Developing World's disabled people, the vast majority of whom are poor and an estimated 80% of whom live in rural areas" (p. 2). Many of the impairments found in these areas are preventable, and those that are not preventable only worsen because of lack of early intervention and rehabilitative services. The difficulties faced by families as a result of a lack of resources, which are noted throughout this book, are likely to be grossly magnified in the developing world.

MODERN AMERICAN SOCIETY

As noted in earlier chapters, the most pervasive attitude toward disability in modern American society is stigma. As Goffman (1963) classically noted, individuals with disabilities have commonly been discredited and relegated to a morally inferior status in American society. Safilios-Rothschild (1970) classically suggested that people with disabilities are a minority group in U.S. society and share the following characteristics with other minority groups:

1. They are relegated to a separate place in society (encouraged to interact with their "own kind").
2. They are considered by the majority to be inferior.
3. Their segregation is rationalized as being "better for them."
4. They are evaluated on the basis of their categorical membership rather than their individual characteristics.

Although stigma continues to shape much of the interaction between people with and without disabilities in U.S. society, attitudes may be slowly changing. The DRM has had an impact in reducing some stereotypical thinking, and legislation such as the IDEA and the ADA has placed more individuals with disabilities in the societal mainstream. In the remainder of this chapter, we consider variations in attitude toward childhood disability that exist within this larger, still negative but evolving framework of American society as a whole.

As we have just indicated, attitudes toward children with disabilities vary considerably from one culture to another. In a pluralistic society, various groups *within* a culture may also hold divergent views of these children. Although sharing some of the aspects of the culture of the larger society, these subcultures also have their own beliefs, values, attitudes, and norms, which are learned through interaction with their members. Until recent decades, most of the literature on families of children with disabilities ignored subcultural variation. Theories of stages of parental adaptation (described in Chapter 2), for example, seemed to imply that all parents pass through similar stages regardless of SES, race, or ethnicity. In the following pages, we examine the idea that families' views are, in fact, shaped by the segment of society within which they live.

Societies are stratified along a number of different dimensions that are not mutually exclusive. Probably the most important dimension is SES, or social class. Although SES has a number of components, the most important are occupation, education, and income. Socioeconomic levels have been grouped in various ways, but a five-class system has been commonly used (e.g., Hollingshead & Redlich, 1958). Social classes are not separate subcultures in the same sense as some ethnic groups. Socioeconomic diversity is more a matter of differential access to opportunity than of different beliefs and values; this fact is discussed further in the section on social class. In addition to SES, differences based on race, ethnicity, and religion also exist.

FAMILY DIVERSITY

What is a family? Certainly, what has sometimes been regarded as the white, middle-class, heterosexual ideal—the nuclear family, consisting of a married couple and their unmarried children—is not universal in modern society. Most children in the United States today will spend at least part of their lives with a single parent. In addition, many receive out-of-home care while their parents work.

Although diversity is not new, our families today are more diverse than at any time in U.S. history. This diversity can be attributed to both cultural and structural factors (Zinn & Eitzen, 1993). Cultural factors have become more important as the United States has become more ethnically diverse; structural conditions have recently been rooted in economic changes that have had a major impact on the labor market.

In 1980 fewer than one in five Americans was a member of a racial or ethnic minority. In 1990 the ratio had changed to one in four, and demographic projections suggest that by 2030, the ratio will be one in three. As we show later in this chapter, different racial and ethnic groups have different values, norms, and beliefs regarding children and disabilities. Furthermore, in some ethnic groups, the nuclear family was never the norm. Rather, households typically included various extended family members or even "fictive kin" not related by blood or marriage to the nuclear family. In some U.S. communities today, parents and children still live in close proximity to grandparents, aunts, uncles, and cousins. In others, homelessness and isolation from relatives are common.

Structural factors affecting families today result largely from a decrease in high-paying blue collar jobs since the 1970s. Consequently, more married women with children are in the labor force, and mother-only households have become more common as a result of the postponement of marriage and increase in lifetime levels of divorce. Although many partners today postpone having children until they are in their 30s or 40s, teen pregnancy also occurs. Often, grandparents are involved in the care of their teenage children's children. Parents also have varying educational levels. In some communities, few have finished high school; in others, most have graduated from college or have advanced degrees. Some parents have intellectual or physical disabilities. Different family structures are also sometimes found in urban and rural areas. Professionals who work with families need to take this diversity into account.

DIVERSE FAMILY FORMS

Single-Parent Families and Stepfamilies

At any one time, approximately 27% of U.S. children live with just one parent (Moore, Jekielek, & Emig, 2002). However, not all of the others live with a married couple. Cohabitation involving unmarried partners has been increasing, and many children of unmarried parents live in two-parent households. Approximately 40% of cohabitating households in the United States include children (Bumpass, Sweet, & Cherlin, 1998).

A number of studies has suggested that children in single-parent households do not fare as well as children in two-parent households. McLanahan and Sandefur (1994) found, for example, that children from single-parent homes are less likely to graduate from high school and college and are more likely to become teen parents. However, they found that most of the disadvantage could be explained by the fact that economic resources are scarcer in single-parent than in two-parent homes. As we note in other chapters, childhood disability is expensive. Thus, single parents are likely to have an especially difficult time making ends meet when their children have disabilities. In addition, child care issues become magnified when only one parent is available to provide care.

Other issues emerge when single parents marry or remarry, creating step- or blended families. Hetherington and Stanley-Hagan (2000) suggested that children with difficult temperaments are more likely to have problems with their parents' marital transitions, resulting in negative parental reactions. Given that difficult temperaments are sometimes associated with disability, the presence of a child with a disability could be a risk factor for the success of such unions.

Gay and Lesbian Families

Although virtually no research has focused on gay or lesbian unions that include children with disabilities, the literature suggests that these families do not pose any particular risks for such children. Laird (as quoted in Stacey, 1998, pp. 130–131) wrote:

> A substantial number of studies on the psychological and social development of children of gay and lesbian parents have failed to produce any evidence that children of lesbian or gay parents are harmed or compromised or even differ from, in any significant ways along a host of psychosocial developmental measures, children raised in heterosexual families.

In fact, such families may be able to provide additional resources for children with disabilities. For example, Gavin-Williams and Esterberg (2000) mentioned a number of studies showing that lesbian communities typically are important sources of support for lesbian parents.

THE INFLUENCE OF SOCIAL CLASS

Families do not become poor in the same way that they become African American or Latino American. Social class is not so much a matter of cultural diversity as of structural constraints. SES can be attributed to the differential allocation of opportunities in society. Given a choice, most people would want to be rich. However, economic changes resulting in a decreased need for semiskilled labor and low wages for unskilled jobs have led, during the past few decades, to an increase in young families living in poverty. Poverty severely limits the lifestyle choices available to families; most of the attitudes and behaviors attributed to lower-class families in the literature are best explained by limited opportunities rather than differences in basic values. As Rank (2000) and others noted, some of the major consequences of poverty include "doing without," stress, and marital breakdown. The added stress of a child with disabilities suggests a strong need for support in such families.

Park, Turnbull, and Turnbull (2002) reported that 28% of children with disabilities ages 3–21 live in families whose incomes fall below the federal poverty line. Poverty is associated with disability in two ways. First, because of poor nutrition and health care, poor parents are more likely to give birth to children with impairments. Second, as noted in Chapter 5, a child with a disability tends to reduce family income because parents often must work less or at less lucrative jobs in order to stay home and provide the specialized care their children need and because specialized health care and other services are expensive.

Since the passage of welfare reform legislation in 1996, the poor have been under increased pressure to work. Especially in families of children with disabilities, the new work requirements create added strains related to the lack of affordable, appropriate child care options. Working parents also have less time to spend with their children and to attend to their special needs. In some cases, working poor families lose their medical assistance benefits, resulting in difficulties in obtaining needed health care for their children. Parents caring for children with disabilities may be exempted from work requirements; however, exemptions vary widely among states (Shields & Behrman, 2002).

Attitudes toward Disability

Families of children with disabilities come from all social classes. Professionals, on the other hand, are more likely to come from middle- and upper-class backgrounds. As a result, professionals and the families they serve may have highly divergent views of disability and its treatment. Perhaps the greatest conflict in this area has occurred in the field of intellectual disability, especially in the mild ranges. Although parents and professionals from middle- and upper-class backgrounds may regard mild intellectual disability as a devastating condition, lower-class parents may not even define it as a disability.

In a classic study of institutionalized children, Mercer (1965) found that the children who were discharged generally came from low-status families. High-status families were more likely to concur with official definitions of intellectual disability and the need for institutionalization. The low-status families, who were not as achievement oriented, were able to envision their children playing normal adult roles. In another older study, Downey (1963) found, similarly, that more educated families tended to show less interest in their institutionalized children, because the children were unable to conform to the family's career expectations.

As Hess (1970), Kohn (1969), and others have noted, middle-class parents expect independent behavior and achievement from their children. They have higher educational and occupational aspirations for their children and higher expectations that those aspirations will be attained. Socially appropriate behavior is also likely to be viewed by these parents as necessary for achievement.

This class-based pattern does not seem to occur as clearly in the case of physical disability. Dow (1966) found no correlation between social class and parental acceptance of their children with physical disabilities and noted that parents of all classes tend to have optimistic attitudes. These favorable attitudes are maintained by depreciating the importance of physique.

Recent studies of the influence of social class on attitudes toward disability are lacking. Recent literature on SES and childhood disability has been epidemiological, reaffirming the link between labeling and SES, especially in the case of mild intellectual disability (see, e.g., Stromme, 2000), or has looked at the relationship between labeling and service delivery (see, e.g., Harris, 1996). Typically in current studies, SES is used as a control variable, based on an *assumption* of a link with attitudes toward disability; however, recent research has not focused on the link itself. Much recent literature (see, e.g., Duvdevany & Vudinsky, 2005; Horton & Wallender, 2001; also, Chapter 7, this volume) has demonstrated an association between social support and favorable outcomes for families of children with disabilities. Other research (see, e.g., Gallo, Bogart, Vranceanu, & Matthews, 2005) has shown that those of higher SES tend to receive more social support, leading to the conclusion that lower SES families would have less favorable outcomes. However, none of this research has addressed differences in preexisting attitudes toward disability in families of varying SES levels.

Intervention Issues

In working with families of different social classes, professionals should be aware of differences in lifestyle or in parent–child interaction that may affect acceptance of professional recommendations or reactions to the professional. Professionals working in home-based programs that use parents as teachers need to be especially aware of the varying teaching strategies employed by parents of different social-class backgrounds. Laosa (1978) found, for example, that in a group of Chicano families, mothers with more formal education tended to use inquiry and praise in teaching their children, whereas mothers with less education were more likely to use modeling as a teaching strategy. Another study of low-SES mothers of preschoolers with mild intellectual disability (Wilton & Barbour, 1978) found that they showed less encouragement of their children's activities than comparison mothers. Attempting to get such parents to use more "middle-class" techniques could result in lack of compliance with a treatment program.

Lower-class parents are also likely to have less time and money to spend on their children's disabilities than their middle-class counterparts. Resources such as transportation, employment opportunities, adequate or appropriate housing, and access to good medical care are limited in the lower classes. When the necessities of life are scarce, a child's disability may not be a family's number-one priority. The disability may be only one of the many problems faced by the family. Professionals who judge such families by middle-class standards are often unwittingly creating a situation of noncompliance by their unrealistic expectations.

As noted earlier, SES and social support are linked. Dunst, Trivette, and Cross (1988) found that low-SES families of children with disabilities had less family support and more physical, emotional, and financial problems than a higher-SES group. Without a strong support network to share the burden, such families are likely to experience considerable stress in managing their children's disabilities, regardless of their level of acceptance. A number of studies has used the concept of *social capital* to explore the interpersonal networks of families in different population groups. Social capital can be as important as economic capital in linking families to resources. One study of low-income African American and Latin American mothers (Dominguez & Watkins, 2003) found that immersion in dense, localized, family- and neighbor-based networks sometimes prevented mothers from gaining access to societal resources. However, they also found that some of the African American women they studied had turned from informal support to the more formal support of social service agencies, which tended to be more reliable. Acceptance of formal support was less common among the Latin American women. As later sections of this chapter suggest, agencies have commonly been unsuccessful in winning the trust of this population.

At one time, researchers believed that a "culture of poverty" existed (e.g., Lewis, 1959). However, studies have generally indicated that poor people share most of the values of the larger society. Nevertheless, the conditions imposed by a chronic shortage of cash affect lifestyles and can restructure the priorities of a group. "Getting ahead" is not a major concern when survival is uppermost in people's minds. In a review of the literature on poverty and families of children with disabilities, Park et al. (2002) found that poverty had an impact on five domains of the quality of life: health, productivity, physical environment, emotional well-being, and family interaction. Professionals working with such families need to be sensitive to their priorities, especially in terms of the lack of material resources. As one of us (Darling, 2000) noted elsewhere, families that lack food, clothing, or shelter may regard participation in early intervention, therapeutic, or educational programs as an extra imposition on time needed to address survival concerns. For example, she discusses the case of a family without a working refrigerator in which the mother needed to walk to the store several times a day to buy fresh milk; this mother was not especially receptive to working on exercises with her child until the in-home teacher had helped her procure a refrigerator.

ETHNIC VARIATION

An ethnic group has been defined as "those who conceive of themselves as alike by virtue of their common ancestry, real or fictitious, and who are so regarded by others" (Shibutani & Kwan, as quoted in McGoldrick, 1982, p. 3). Ethnic identification may be based on race, culture, or national origin. Census data from 2002 indicated that the population of the United States was composed of ethnic groups in the following proportions (U.S. Bureau of the Census, 2003b):

Group	Percentage of population, July 1, 2002
African American	12.7
Hispanic/Latino (of any race)	13.4
Asian, Pacific Islander	4.2
Native American	1.0
Two or more races	1.5
White	80.7

(Note: Hispanics may be of any race and are therefore counted under more than one category.)

These data indicate a decrease in the European American population in proportion to the other groups, compared with data from the last census. Among the European Americans are people with various ethnic identifications, including Irish, Italian, Jewish, and German. Some members of ethnic groups may identify very strongly with the group, whereas others may think of themselves more as Americans. Attitudes toward disability and toward children, in general, vary by ethnicity to some extent. For example, in a study of families in an early intervention program, McDowell, Saylor, Taylor, and Boyce (1995) found that the stress level in European American families changed in response to changes in family resources, social support, and children's developmental progress, whereas stress level change was correlated only with income change among other ethnic families.

The following discussion is not intended to be an exhaustive review of the literature on various ethnic groups, but rather to suggest the kinds of ethnic differences that may be relevant to professionals working with families of children who have disabilities. More detailed reviews can be found in many of the works cited in the remainder of this chapter.

African American Subculture

Until a few years ago when their numbers were surpassed by Latino Americans, African Americans were the largest ethnic minority in the United States. Because African Americans are overrepresented in the lower classes, much of the literature on these families has focused on issues related to social class rather than ethnicity. Consequently, many of the patterns that have been uncovered have been socioeconomic. However, Tolson and Wilson (1990) and others have shown that African American families are not homogeneous and that considerable diversity exists among two- and three-generational families of varying socioeconomic levels. Moreover, considerable diversity exists within the African American community as a result of immigration; African American families today include immigrants from the West Indies, Latin America, and Africa, in addition to those who have been in the United States for many generations. Willie and Reddick (2003) have noted that 28% of African American families have incomes above $50,000 a year and that middle-class African Americans conform in most ways to the norms and values common to middle-class Americans of other ethnic backgrounds. In one study, Heiss (1981) found that no major difference exists between African American and European American women on attitudes toward marriage and family. Similarly, Scanzoni (1985) found that SES is a more important determinant than race in shaping parental values. African American parents were found to have the same values as European Americans of the same social class. Thus an African American family might be just as devastated as a European American family by the birth of a child with intellectual disability.

However, an African American subculture, based on the background and history of this ethnic group, does appear to exist apart from SES, and aspects of this subculture can be found in African American middle-class families as well as in the lower classes. We need to be careful to distinguish these ethnic patterns from characteristics associated with poverty. We consider the effects of poverty first and then describe some aspects of a distinctive African American subculture.

Because so many African American families are poor, the incidence of poverty-based impairment resulting from poor nutrition and poor prenatal care is disproportionately high in these families. Edelman (1985) noted that almost one in two African American children is poor compared to a general poverty rate for U.S. children of one in five. Infant mortality and low birth weight, a leading cause of childhood disability, are twice as high for African Americans as for European Americans. Franklin, Franklin, and Draper (2002) and others noted that African American children are much more likely than European American children to be placed in special education classes in school—a consequence of labeling, racism, and SES. Poverty also contributes to stress, and Korn, Chess, and Fernandez (1978) found, in one sample of children with physical disabilities, that African American families were more vulnerable to stress than European Americans.

Family patterns among poor African Americans often reflect macro-level structural factors, such as high levels of unemployment. In such an environment, marriage may be less advantageous—and, in fact, many African American children live in female-headed, single-parent households (e.g., Taylor, 2002). Hill (1999) and others noted that African American families have a history of destabilization as a result of social forces and social policies, including racism, sexism (because many African American families are headed by women), urban renewal, and the suburbanization of employment. Some of these forces have affected poor European American families as well. Yet, even in the face of adversity, African American families have been shown to exhibit many strengths, including family unity and a strong religious orientation. Hill notes as well a strong achievement orientation, as evidenced by a greater emphasis on educational achievement among African American mothers than European American mothers of all income levels in his study. Similarly, Ho, Rasheed, and Rasheed (2004) noted that African Americans value education as a form of social mobility. Denby (as quoted in Willie & Reddick, 2003) noted a high value placed on children in African American families. With respect to the strengths of these families, Wilkinson (1997) wrote: "Although its structure has been modified dramatically since its beginnings in the United States, the African American family has thrived as an essential communal network of sharing, support, protection, emotional reinforcement, and adaptation to the regularity of change" (p. 41).

Studies of poor African American families indicate that teenage pregnancies are fairly common and women tend to start families at early ages (e.g., Franklin & Boyd-Franklin, 1985). These young mothers may be poorly prepared to care for a child with a disability. However, as Dodson (1981), Franklin and Boyd-Franklin (1985), Harrison, Serafica, and McAdoo (1984), and others have suggested, childrearing in African American families has historically been a communal process, with a high level of involvement by the extended family, including fictive kin. Mutual-help patterns are usually strong. Hill (1999) cited a study showing that 85% of African American families had a relative living in the same city. A system of informal adoption also exists (Hines & Boyd-Franklin, 1982; Hill, 1999), along with an emphasis on group responsibility for the individual (Willie & Reddick, 2003). However, financial aid from relatives may be less available among African Americans than among European Americans because of higher levels of poverty (Edin & Harris, 1997).

An additional family strength that could be valuable to families with a child who has a disability is the flexibility of family roles. Willie and Reddick (2003) and others noted that black families tend to be more egalitarian than European American families, with more power sharing and role interchangeability between partners, both married and unmarried. Although traditionally, in poor, urban African American families the mother was usually the person responsible for providing care for a family member with a disability (Jackson, 1981), in two-thirds of African American couples today, the women are employed (Hill, 1999). The pattern is even stronger in middle-class families, where African American women are more likely to be in the labor force than European American women (Willie & Reddick, 2003).

Thus, role flexibility among other family members is especially important.

Some writers have argued that human service models developed
with European American populations are not appropriate for African
Americans. Schiele (2000) argued that elements of African culture
continue to exist in the United States and that Eurocentric human service models are not appropriate for people with African roots. Contrary to the Eurocentric social work model based on individualism
and conflict, an Afrocentric model would emphasize interdependency,
collectivity, spirituality, and affect. Traditionally, human service professionals have been trained to be affectively neutral, avoiding emotional involvement with their clients. However, Parham (2002) suggested that "many African American clients . . . may respond to a style
that seeks to access their affective and spiritual core" (p. 104). Martin
and Martin (1995) argued that social workers need to view the African
American experience as a unique historical and cultural entity marked
by African roots and survival in a hostile environment. They suggested that professionals use three concepts in working with African
American populations: *moaning* (reflecting African American pain
and suffering), *mourning* (a collective effort to overcome grief), and
morning (an ideal state of health and happiness). This model recognizes the tendency in the African American community (at all SES levels) to solve problems informally, with the assistance of the group
rather than with the aid of professionals.

As in the study reported by Hill above, Hatchett and Jackson
(1999) found a high level of geographic propinquity to relatives among
African Americans, especially among single parents, those of higher
SES, and those living in urban areas. Their respondents reported frequent contact with kin, and two-thirds reported receiving some help
from family members. Thus, African American families with children
who have disabilities may potentially receive more family support than
those in some other ethnic groups.

In naming significant others who are not relatives, half of the
African American respondents in Manns's (1981) study mentioned a
minister. Other studies (Franklin & Boyd-Franklin, 1985; Hines &
Boyd-Franklin, 1982; Rogers-Dulan & Blacher, 1995) have also mentioned the importance of religion in African American family life at
all social levels. In the African American community, the church often
provides food, clothing, shelter, counseling, economic aid, child care,
social activities, and youth programs. The willingness of the religious
community to provide emotional support and help in caring for a
child with a disability can greatly ease the burden on a family.

Variations in childrearing patterns among African American families have been reported. For example, some studies (Bartz & Levine, 1978; Polk, 1994; Young, 1970) found that African American parents encourage earlier independence training in their children than parents of other ethnicities. African American parents who expect accelerated development and early assumption of responsibility by their children may be disappointed by a child with a disability, whose development is considerably slower than the norm.

Latino Subculture

Latino Americans constitute the largest ethnic minority in the United States. Although the U.S. Bureau of the Census has used the term *Hispanic*, many members of this population group prefer the term *Latino*, which we adopt here. As Baca Zinn and Pok (2002) noted, although the census defines Hispanic as an ethnic category, Latinos often are treated as a racial group by others in society. As in the case of African Americans, socioeconomically based lifestyle characteristics among Latinos are sometimes incorrectly attributed to cultural differences. Like other groups with high levels of poverty, Latinos may not have a regular source of health care and may experience barriers to service use, such as lack of child care, lack of transportation, lack of knowledge, lack of insurance, or inability to pay. Zambrana, Dorrington, and Hayes-Bautista (1995) noted that Latinos are even more likely to be uninsured than other groups in poverty. They cite evidence, however, to suggest that the problem is structural (based on social barriers), not cultural (a matter of different values).

Harry (1992a) suggested that, although intragroup diversity exists, Latino Americans share a common language (Spanish) and worldview based on Roman Catholic ideology, familism, and values of personalism, respect, and status. She further suggested that a strong sense of family pride sometimes makes acceptance of a severe disability difficult in these groups. Mild disability, on the other hand, may not be recognized by the family.

Other studies suggested that some Latino cultural characteristics may assist families in adapting to children with disabilities. One study (Mary, 1990) found that, in comparison with African American and European American mothers, Latino mothers were more resigned and less angry about having a child with intellectual disability. Similarly, Zepeda and Espinosa (as quoted in Santiago-Rivera, Arredondo, & Gallardo-Cooper, 2002) noted that lower-SES Latinos tend to have lower expectations for developmental milestones in children, which could promote acceptance of those with developmental disabilities. Another group characteristic that would facilitate adaptation in the case of children unable to achieve independence during adolescence and adulthood is continuing interdependence between parents and their adult children (Santiago-Rivera et al., 2002).

Although similarities exist among various groups of Latino origin, Mexicans, Puerto Ricans, and other Latino Americans have separate identities and subcultures. Structures of economic opportunity also have been different for different groups, and Cuban Americans generally have fared better economically than other Latino groups (Baca Zinn & Wells, 2000). Recent immigrants also tend to have higher poverty rates than those who have lived in the United States for a longer period of time (Beinart, 1997). Most of the human service-related literature on Latinos has focused on Mexican Americans and Puerto Ricans, who together have had the highest levels of poverty in the Latino community and have constituted the largest Latino groups in some areas of the country.

Mexican Americans

The Mexican American population is the most youthful and rapidly growing ethnic minority in the United States (Martinez, 1999). Mexican Americans tend to be geographically concentrated in the Southwestern states, and many maintain strong ties to family in Mexico. However, recent immigrants may have different characteristics from those who are American-born (Baca Zinn & Pok, 2002).

As in the case of African American families, a significant proportion of Mexican Americans live in poverty. As a result, they are prone to labeling by professionals, and Mexican American children are much more likely than European American children to be placed in educable mentally retarded (EMR) classes. Such placements are attributable in part to assessment techniques that discriminate against non-English-speaking children and those whose culture differs from that of the majority. The poor Mexican American family may also lack access to treatment facilities and consistent care for a child with a disability.

In addition to high levels of poverty, Mexican culture is also marked by language and lifestyle differences from the mainstream. As a result, Mexican American parents may find interactions with professionals difficult and may be uncomfortable in institutional settings. Stein (1983) reported that Latino parents do not participate as actively in the development of their children's Individual Education Plans

(IEP) as do European American parents or parents in general. Both schools and medical settings tend to be intimidating to these parents. Azziz (1981) noted that, to Latinos, hospitals are places where the sick go to die. Hospital visiting rules, which exclude some family members, are also foreign to them. In addition, the Spanish-speaking patient may have difficulty distinguishing among various hospital personnel and may pay more attention to a technician who speaks Spanish than to a physician who speaks only English. Romaine (1982) noted, too, that time has a different meaning in Mexican culture, and some Mexican Americans may not keep appointments, creating scheduling problems for professionals. Differences in acculturation are related to SES, and middle-class Mexican Americans are more likely to speak English and have familiarity with the mainstream culture. On the other hand, undocumented immigrants are especially unlikely to turn to professionals for help because of fear of deportation (Bonilla-Santiago, 1996).

The traditional Mexican family has been characterized as marked by values of familism, male dominance and gender-specific division of labor, subordination of young to old, and person orientation rather than goal orientation (Alvirez & Bean, 1976; Baca Zinn & Pok, 2002). However, Baca Zinn and Pok (2002) and Vega (1995) have noted that the entry of women into the labor force has resulted in family patterns that are becoming more egalitarian than those in traditional families. Coltrane (1998) reported shared decision making and participation in housework in a sample of dual-earner Chicano couples, and Powell (1995) reported that Latino fathers willingly participated with their wives in a parent education and support program. Thus professionals need to be careful when making assumptions about cultural differences as more groups become acculturated to mainstream norms and values.

Guinn (as quoted in Williams & Williams, 1979) noted a number of additional differences between traditional Mexican American and European American values: Mexicans stress *being*, whereas European Americans stress *doing*; European Americans value material well-being more than Mexicans; Mexicans have a present-time orientation, whereas European Americans have a future orientation; European Americans value individual action, and Mexicans value group cooperation; Mexicans are fatalistic, whereas European Americans value mastery of the universe. All these values may cause more traditional Mexican American parents to be more accepting of a child's disability than European American parents.

The importance of the extended family in Mexican culture has been noted by many writers. Heller (as quoted in Williams & Williams, 1979) stated that the web of kinship ties imposes obligations of mutual aid, respect, and affection. Santana-Martin and Santana (2005) suggested that in Mexican culture the family is expected to care for members with disabilities. Falicov (1982) noted that the family protects the individual and that extended family members may perform many parental functions. Cousins may be as close as siblings. In addition, *compadres*, or godparents, play an important role. Sanchez (1997) noted that godparents commonly provide financial assistance in times of need. Lieberman (1990) also mentioned the *madrina*, who is selected by the parents to share responsibility for the child. In a study of the extended family as an emotional support system, Keefe, Padilla, and Carlos (1979) found that Mexican Americans consistently relied on relatives more than friends, regardless of geographical proximity. Children are more likely to have close relationships with siblings and cousins than with extrafamilial peers. Both Falicov and Karrer (1980) and Keefe and colleagues (1979) noted that Mexican women have a strong tendency to confide in female relatives. The young Mexican mother is likely to rely on her mother for advice and support. The support network provided by the family can be very helpful to parents of children with disabilities. However, Baca Zinn and Wells (2000) noted that extended kinship networks have been declining among Mexican Americans and that recent immigrants tend to have smaller kin networks than second-generation Mexican Americans.

The proximity of the extended family can also create problems for parents. Falicov and Karrer (1980) explained, for example, that the presence of the extended family puts pressure on members to compare themselves to their relatives. The mother of a child with a disability who is surrounded by sisters, sisters-in-law, and cousins whose children do not have disabilities may be upset by the constant reminder of her child's "differentness." Keefe and colleagues (1979) also noted that their Mexican American respondents sometimes resented their relatives' intrusion into their personal affairs. Friends who react negatively to a child with a disability can be avoided by parents; avoidance of close family is more difficult.

Traditional Mexican American attitudes toward childrearing also sometimes differ from those of the cultural mainstream. Falicov (1982) and Falicov and Karrer (1980) noted a relaxed attitude toward the achievement of developmental milestones and self-reliance, along with a basic acceptance of the child's individuality. Such an attitude would certainly be favorable for a child whose development proceeded much more slowly than the norm or who was not able to achieve independence from the family.

Mexican Americans and other Latinos tend to value modesty. One study ("Adapting Research to Cultures and Countries," 1995–1996) found that Mexican American adults with disabilities were reluctant to use personal assistant services because they view the body as private. These adults preferred family providers. Professionals working with children with disabilities might find that Mexican American families prefer the training of family members in therapeutic techniques rather than direct professional intervention.

Like other ethnic groups, Mexican Americans, depending on their degree of identification with the traditional culture, may have folk beliefs about the nature of disease and disability. Spector (1979) and Santana-Martin and Santana (2005) noted, for example, that Mexicans may regard illness as a punishment for wrongdoing. Such beliefs could result in guilt—and, in fact, Wendeborn (1982) has noted the presence of—guilt feelings in Mexican parents of children with intellectual disability and cerebral palsy. Santana-Martin and Santana (2005) noted that Mexican parents are more likely to blame themselves in the case of mental disability; physical disability, on the other hand, is viewed as "normal."

A social worker in a birth defects evaluation center serving a large number of Mexican American families described a case illustrating the influence of folk beliefs (H. Montalvo, personal communication, 1982):

> A young couple, legal residents of the United States, arrived at our clinic with their 4-year-old son. He was diagnosed as having classical Schwartz–Jampel (Pinto–DeSouza) syndrome. This very intelligent couple followed our counseling session well and understood the autosomal recessive transmission and the subsequent one-in-four risk of recurrence for each pregnancy. However, it was not until the mother was alone with the social worker that she intimated she'd had a severe *susto* (fright) during her pregnancy. She noted that her husband, an activist in their native Mexico, had been jailed over several days with no word available on his release. Mrs. G. was concerned and afraid for her husband's well-being, and she felt that this fright and anxiety may have infiltrated the fetus and caused a gene mutation. Interestingly, then, an articulate woman who capably followed our concise and detailed session on autosomal recessive transmission nevertheless felt a *susto* could also contribute to such a birth defect.

Schreiber and Homiak (1981) also noted the belief that children are susceptible to *susto*, even in utero.

Those who believe in folk medicine may employ the services of a *curandero(a)* (folk healer) in addition to, or instead of, those of a health care professional. The *curandero/curandera* derives his or her ability to cure from the supernatural (Spector, 1979). Because these healers maintain a close, warm, personalized relationship with the family, they may be preferred over the impersonal medical professional who works in a clinic or hospital setting. Keefe and colleagues (1979) found, however, that among urban Mexican Americans in one sample, the use of the *curandero* as a means of emotional support was negligible. Similarly, in a large sample of Latino (Mexican American and Puerto Rican) parents of children receiving early intervention services, Bailey, Skinner, Rodriguez, Gut, and Correa (1999) found little use of alternative practices.

Physicians, in particular, may be less likely than folk healers to become significant others for parents. Schreiber and Homiak (1981) noted that any diagnosis or treatment is likely to be evaluated and accepted or rejected by the patient's family, and that Mexican women usually prefer to go home and discuss any proposed treatment with their entire family. When the professional recommendations are not highly valued, the family may seek other consultations. Wendeborn (1982) noted that Latino families of children with cerebral palsy have difficulty accepting the fact that the condition cannot be healed completely and may consult with numerous practitioners, at considerable expense, before accepting the approach of any professional or facility.

Although many Mexican American families may behave in the ways suggested above when they have children with disabilities, many others exhibit attitudes and behavior that do not differ significantly from those of European American or other non-Mexican families. One study of poor Mexican mothers (Shapiro & Tittle, 1986) found, for example, that, like their European American counterparts, their subjects experienced difficulties in the areas of social support, child adjustment, perceived stress, and family functioning as a result of their children's disabilities. Similarly, a study of decisions related to amniocentesis by Mexican-origin women (Browner, Preloran, & Cox, 1999) found that health care providers incorrectly assumed that decisions would be governed by "deep-rooted, cultural givens," such as opposition to abortion. In fact, these women's decisions were related more to such variables as their understanding of risks and their faith in their doctors.

Puerto Ricans

Ortiz (1995) reported that Puerto Ricans have been more affected than other Latino groups by deindustrialization and showed a decline in SES during the 1980s. She noted that Puerto Ricans also have more female-headed households than other Latinos. Perhaps even more than other ethnic groups, the Puerto Rican community relies very heavily on the family as a source of strength and support. García-Preto (1982) wrote:

> In times of stress Puerto Ricans turn to their families for help. Their cultural expectation is that when a family member is experiencing a crisis or has a problem, others in the family are obligated to help, especially those who are in stable positions. Because Puerto Ricans rely on the family and their extended network of personal relationships, they will make use of social services only as a last resort. (p. 164)

The structure of the traditional Puerto Rican family also differs from the nuclear family model of the larger society. The basic family unit is commonly extended among Puerto Ricans and may consist of *compadres* (godparents) and *hijos de crianza* (children of upbringing) in addition to blood relatives (Mizio, 1974).

Although the extended family is the primary source of help and social support, members of the Puerto Rican community may also approach friends, neighbors, or a neighborhood spiritualist. Secondarily, they may approach professionals whom they know well. Ghali (1977) suggested that Puerto Ricans will not confide in anyone until *confianza*, or a familial-type of trusting relationship, is established. Professionals working with such families must, therefore, work toward establishing a personal bond with them. Another frequently noted aspect of the Puerto Rican subculture is fatalism (e.g., Fitzpatrick, 1976; García-Preto, 1982; Ghali, 1977). Submissiveness and acceptance of fate are encouraged, in contrast with the American values of achievement and aggressiveness. As in the Mexican American subculture, such fatalism may help parents cope with a child's disabilities.

Harry (1992c) noted that the low-income Puerto Rican families in her study did not accept professional definitions of their children's disabilities because of different meanings they attached to terms such as *handicapped* or *retarded*. One parent said, "They say the word 'handicap' means a lot of things. . . . But for us, Puerto Ricans, we still understand this word as 'crazy' " (p. 31). Similarly, Gannotti, Handwerker, Groce, and Cruz (2001) found that attitudes toward child development and disability were different from American norms in a sample of Puerto Rican parents. In particular, these parents valued interdependence and *sobre protectiva* (overprotectiveness) and did not define their children's continuing dependence in negative terms.

As in the case of other ethnic groups, Puerto Rican values tend to change with increasing acculturation. Carrasquillo (2002) noted that, although familism is still an important value among second-, third-, and fourth-generation Puerto Ricans, it is not as strong as among first-generation immigrants.

Implications for Professionals

Santiago-Rivera et al. (2002, p. 17) noted the following competencies as needed in professionals working with Latino families:

1. Understand these concepts and their meaning for relationship building: *personalismo, familismo, respeto, dignidad, orgullo*.
2. Recognize the role of spirituality and formalized religion in the family's life.
3. Determine the approach most suitable for the family based on SES and other considerations.
4. Understand one's own identity as a facilitator or impediment to a relationship with the family.
5. Identify and modify approaches in order to be culturally effective.

They noted further the importance of recognizing diversity among Latino families based on both SES and level of acculturation.

Santiago-Rivera et al. (2002) suggested further that for Latinos, family–professional matching by language may be more important than ethnic matching, as 90% of Latinos in the United States continue to use Spanish. They noted studies showing that language barriers can result in underutilization of services, diagnostic errors, and inappropriate interventions. In addition to language, interactional style can be important with Latinos. Some recommendations include:

1. Begin formally, then move to a more informal style.
2. Address adults with formal titles, that is, Mr. and Mrs.
3. Allow proximity in seating arrangements.
4. Address adults before children.

5. Maintain a flexible time frame.
6. Start with small talk.
7. Make a telephone call before the first in-person meeting to establish rapport and determine language preferences.
8. Assure family members that the church can be included in intervention planning, if they so desire.
9. Do not suggest interventions that may conflict with preferred gender roles.
10. Present sensitive issues with an apology or recognition that questions may be offensive.
11. Provide some concrete suggestions for action during the first session.
12. Conduct informed consent procedures carefully; some Latinos may sign forms they do not understand because of *respeto* for the professional. (Adapted from Paniagua, 1998, p. 94, and Santiago-Rivera et al., 2002, p. 115.)

Newer family-centered partnership approaches may be difficult with Latino families, because their culture traditionally mandates deference to the professional. Perry, Bedell, and Paniagua (as quoted in Santiago-Rivera et al., 2002) noted that "Latinos generally approach [services] with the expectation that the professional will be direct, give advice, and know what is best" (p. 127). Partnership issues are addressed further in Chapter 11.

Asian American Subculture

Asian Americans are the third largest ethnic minority group in the United States. The income levels of Asian Americans are high relative to other ethnic minorities; however, those from Southeast Asia tend to be relatively disadvantaged (Paniagua, 1998). Just as one should not necessarily generalize from one Latino group to another, one must be careful in assuming that all Asian subcultures are alike. Yet, similarities do exist. Segal (1998) noted that traditional Asian families in the United States share a set of characteristics, including (1) group, rather than individual orientation; (2) valuing of males more than females; (3) expecting children to be docile and obedient and to bring honor to the family; (4) expecting difficulties to be handled within the family rather than through formal support; (5) relationships based on obligation and shame.

Like other ethnic groups, Asian Americans value the family very highly. Any problems are likely to be solved within the family. Family problems are regarded as private, and bringing them to the attention of outsiders is considered shameful (Shon & Ja, 1982). Professionals might have a difficult time attempting to provide counseling services to such families. On the other hand, reticence in revealing coping difficulties does not necessarily mean that a family will not accept more "technical" medical or therapeutic services. For example, Vietnamese parents in the early intervention program directed by one of us (R. B. D.) were very receptive to physical therapy and other services offered to their daughter, who has cerebral palsy.

Harry (1992a) noted that the essence of Eastern cultures is collectivism and harmony, and that modesty is important. She noted that major disabilities are traditionally interpreted in one of four ways: (1) as retribution for sins of the parents or ancestors; (2) as possession by evil spirits; (3) as resulting from the mother's behavior during pregnancy; or (4) as an imbalance in physiological function. Such disorders are therefore seen as bringing shame to the family and may be met with fatalism or folk healing. She noted, too, that Asian parents are protective of young children and may be reluctant to seek help for them.

Japanese Americans

In the traditional Japanese family, the *ie*, or household unit, is the most important frame of reference (Kitano & Kikumura, 1976). Although the family is residentially nuclear, close ties to relatives are maintained. Children are expected to be respectful and considerate toward their parents and to have a high degree of self-control. Obligation to the family is also important (Harrison et al., 1984). However, like other ethnic groups, Japanese Americans are becoming increasingly acculturated to American patterns. Glenn (as quoted in Ishii-Kuntz, 1997) noted that although older families retain traditional elements of family life such as gender hierarchy, younger families are more egalitarian. As a result, Takagi (as quoted in Ishii-Kuntz, 1997) stated, "it is now difficult to speak of a singular Japanese American family experience" (p. 145).

Kitano and Kikumura (1976) noted that the Japanese are taught to defer to those of higher status, and that open confrontation is avoided. As a result, members of this group are unlikely to challenge the professional, even when they do not agree with a recommended course of treatment. Shon and Ja (1982) noted, too, that communication tends to be indirect.

Chinese Americans

Among Chinese Americans as well, the family—not the individual—is the major unit of society. Huang (1976) noted that, traditionally, Chinese children usually grow up in the midst of adults and are not left with babysitters.

Like Japanese parents, Chinese parents may not show their feelings for fear of "losing face," making interaction with a counselor difficult. Other group values, however, may encourage acceptance of a child with a disability. For example, traditionally the Chinese tend to be fatalistic and to believe in collective responsibility among kin (Gould-Martin & Ngin, 1981; Lee, 1982). Although the past is more valued than the future, Chinese parents do have high educational aspirations for their children (Harrison et al., 1984; Huang, 1976). Acceptance of a child with an intellectual disability could be problematic within such a value orientation; Yee (1988) has, in fact, noted that denial of a child's disability is common in Asian families. Wang, Chan, Thomas, Lin, and Larson (as quoted in Liu, 2005) suggested that the Chinese are more positive toward people with physical disabilities than toward people with developmental or mental disabilities. Liu (2005) noted, further, that Chinese people are generally more accepting of acquired than congenital disability.

Professionals working with Chinese families should also note that they may not adopt the "ideology of normalization" common among Western families of children with disabilities (Anderton, Elfert, & Lai, 1989). In the area of education, Chan (as quoted in Harry & Kalyanpur, 1994) suggested that the mandate that parents participate in their child's educational planning may be "both alien and threatening" to those with a traditional Asian background. Similarly, both Fong (1994) and Liu (2005) suggested that the client empowerment or partnership model (see Chapter 11), in general, may be inappropriate for some Asian families, because they prefer to defer to the expertise of professionals. As in the case of other ethnic groups, however, considerable intragroup variability is likely to be present among Asian American families, especially those with long exposure to mainstream American culture. Glenn and Yap (2002) noted, for example, that Chinese American professional families resemble other families of similar SES, regardless of ethnicity.

Indian Americans

Traditional Indian American families tend to be characterized by interdependence, conformity, and group solidarity (Pais, 1997). Like other Asian families, Indian Americans are strongly influenced by the extended family, and the family serves as an important source of information and support (Pais, 1997; Purkayastha, 2002). Segal (1998) noted, however, that the extended family may not provide long-term help. She noted further that most Indian families are loathe to utilize formal human services, especially mental health services, and that the most effective services are those that use the family resource network. Academic success and obedience to parental authority are valued (Pais, 1997). Like other groups that emphasize high achievement for their children, Indian Americans might be more disappointed than some other groups upon learning of a diagnosis of intellectual disability.

Vietnamese Americans

Traditional Vietnamese American families are male-focused, hierarchical by age, and extended (Gold, 1999), and modes of childrearing encourage dependence rather than independence (Kibria, 2002). The traditional Vietnamese view attributes disability to the sins of one's ancestors; however, the Vietnamese war and the effects of Agent Orange have "modernized" this view (Hunt, 2005). In addition, these families have rapidly adopted American patterns, in part because of a lack of elders in the United States. Another traditional pattern involving the responsibility of siblings for one another (Tran, 1998) may disappear more slowly, raising some of the issues discussed in Chapter 8.

Korean Americans

Korean American families also have adapted their traditional patterns to the American environment. Min (2002) reported, for example, that patterns such as authoritarian child socialization practices may be declining. Cho, Singer, and Brenner (2000) found important differences between a group of Korean American families of young children with disabilities and a group of similar families in Korea. In the United States, parents' adaptations to their children's disabilities were facilitated by early intervention programs and greater public acceptance. In Korea, parents tended to blame themselves for their children's disabilities, whereas the Korean American parents, who were strongly influenced by the local ethnic church, favored religious explanations.

Although much intragroup diversity exists, professionals working with Asian American families should initially adopt the following guidelines (adapted from Paniagua, 1998, p. 94):

1. Use a formal, professional mode of interaction; avoid personalism.
2. Do not pressure or encourage family members to reveal problems.
3. Do not emphasize the independence of children from the family.
4. Offer concrete assistance rather than counseling or psychotherapy.
5. Be cautious about using family-centered, partnership approaches (see Chapter 11), because the family is likely to be passive and respectful toward the professional.

Native American Subculture

The appropriate terminology for this group is a subject of some controversy. Some Native Americans, especially in Canada, prefer the term *First Nations* because it does not include any suggestion of European oppression. On the other hand, some have advocated a return to the previously rejected *American Indians*. Because preferred terminology is in flux at the time of this writing, we use the generally accepted term *Native Americans* in our discussion of this group.

As Altman and Rasch (2003) noted, Native Americans report the highest levels of disability of all race/ethnic groups in the United States, with 32% of adults reporting some type of activity limitation. Thus Native Americans may be more likely than other groups to be acquainted, or to have family members, with disabilities.

Because of much intertribal variation, Native Americans cannot be regarded as constituting a single subculture. Trimble and Thurman (2002) noted that the Native American population is more diverse than populations of European origin. In some ways, however, various tribes seem to be more like one another than like the cultural mainstream. Attneave (1982) and others have noted, for example, that Native Americans tend to be stoic and to accept fate. Attneave (1982), Harrison and colleagues (1984), Pepper (1976), and Price (1976), among others, have listed the following differences in values between Native Americans and the American middle class:

Native American	American middle class
Cooperation	Competition
Harmony with nature	Control over nature
Adult centered	Child centered
Present time orientation	Future time orientation
Expression through action	Verbal expression
Short childhood	Extended childhood
Education for knowledge	Education for grades

Ho et al. (2004) wrote: "The Native way teaches one to expect life's unpleasant events, and to gain honor from being able to survive the inevitable trials and tribulations of life" (p. 81). Because these families are more accepting of fate and less achievement oriented than others in society, they are likely to have less difficulty coping with a child with a disability. Attneave (1982) noted: "Since children are considered precious and are accepted for themselves, a handicapped child is usually given all the support needed to reach his or her own level of fulfillment" (p. 81). Red Horse (as quoted in Devore & London, 1999) related the story of a family trip to a wild rice festival. A three-year-old child who was unable to walk was carried around by many different individuals, and "as the evening wore on, a circle of care surrounded him; friends, family, elders, and teenagers joined together to meet his needs" (p. 314).

Locust (1988) has noted that among the Hopi, some of the gods, in fact, have disabilities and that the Native American belief system stresses the strengths of individuals rather than their disabilities. Harry (1992a) observed that most Native American languages do not have words for *disability*.

In addition, Native American families are likely to receive help and support in rearing a child with a disability. Traditionally among Native Americans, the extended family shares in childrearing duties (Yellowbird & Snipp, 2002). Williams and Williams (1979) also noted that Native American children tend to be loved by everyone in the family. Anderson (1988) suggested that grandparents may be even more important than parents in childrearing among Native Americans.

Joe and Malach (1992) noted that developmental milestones are perceived differently by some Native Americans, citing the example of a family that did not know when their child sat or walked but knew exactly when the child first laughed. The day a child laughs or is named is regarded as a major milestone.

Lewis (as quoted in Ho et al., 2004) noted that Native Americans seek help from others in the following order: (1) extended family; (2) religious leader; (3) tribal elders; and (4) outsiders. Formal support may not be sought at all, even when informal supports are not helpful. A history of oppression and inappropriate labeling by "helping" professionals such as missionaries, teachers, and social workers has left a legacy of mistrust of outsiders (White, 1995).

Professionals involved with these families should be aware of a tendency toward reticence. Spector (1979) also noted that Native Americans may be offended by direct questions or note taking by professionals. Interactions may be marked by long silences and little self-disclosure or show of emotion (Attneave, 1982; Ho et al., 2004), and some Native Americans react to stress with passivity, rather than by "doing something" (Trimble & Thurman, 2002). In addition, some Native American families still make use of traditional healers, such as medicine men and shamans. The professional who desires to win the trust of these families should not belittle the efforts of these healers. However, French (1997) noted that in recent times some imposters have posed as native healers and have exploited their "clients"; consequently, the professional should consult with the family's tribe or a Native American church to verify the authenticity of a healer.

French (1997) suggested that professionals try traditional means of problem solving when working with Native American groups. Such means include the use of "talking circles" led by a tribal elder and storytelling that involves books about disability. One report ("Developing Systems of Support," 1998) described a culturally appropriate service delivery model being used with Native American families in Wisconsin. This model reverses the Western system of "one serving many" (e.g., one counselor treating many clients) by using a principle of "many serving one" (e.g., many women "baby-showering" one pregnant woman). In this model, the entire community is mobilized to provide the services needed by an individual or family.

Native Americans, like other ethnic groups, may hold folk beliefs about various childhood disabilities. Kunitz and Levy (1981) have written that, among the Navajo, a child's illness is believed to be caused by a taboo broken by the mother during pregnancy. Seizures are called "moth sickness," which is believed to result from a broken incest taboo. Whereas seizures result in stigma, other impairments, such as blindness, may be ignored.

Native Americans range from those adhering to traditional beliefs, values, and practices to those who do not differ significantly from families in the cultural mainstream. John (1998) noted, however, that most Native American families are characterized by a greater degree of interdependence than other families.

Professionals should adhere to the following guidelines in initial interactions with Native American families (adapted from Herring, as quoted in Trimble & Thurman, 2002; and Paniagua, 1998):

1. Emphasize listening rather than talking and respect periods of silence.
2. Allow for flexibility in the ending time of a session and do not chide families for being late.
3. Be open to allowing extended family participation.
4. Avoid the use of control and authority; stress cooperation.
5. Avoid personalism.
6. Maintain the highest level of confidentiality.
7. Avoid taking notes.

Other Ethnic Subcultures

African Americans, Latino Americans, Asian Americans, and Native Americans are all generally regarded as minority groups in American society. Harry (1992a) noted that, in general, (lower-class) minority parents are likely to exhibit a pattern of "passivity" in relation to their children's special education programs. Similarly, Sontag and Schacht (1994) found that minority (Latino and Native American) parents reported less participation than European American parents in their children's early intervention programs. The special education system and other mainstream systems are typically not structured to recognize the strengths of families whose behavior differs from normative expectations.

Although ethnic variation is also present among the European American majority, value differences from the cultural mainstream may not be as pronounced—especially among the third, fourth, fifth, and later generations. However, some ethnic differences relevant to childhood disability have been noted by various writers. For example, Femminella and Quadagno (1976) noted that strong family ties continue to be important even among third-generation Italian Americans. Squires and Quadagno (1998) also noted a high degree of sibling solidarity. Italian parents of children with disabilities are thus likely to have a strong family support system. The extended family may be a source of support for some Jewish families as well. In contrast with the Italian family, which encourages dependence in children, the Jewish family encourages children to be independent and achieve personal success. Herz and Rosen (1982) wrote: "Through the child's success, parents are validated; through their defects and wrong-doings parents are disgraced and ashamed" (p. 380). The high value that Jewish parents place on achievement may create difficulties when a child has a disability.

RELIGIOUS VARIATION

Some early studies (see, e.g., Boles, 1959; Zuk, 1959; Zuk, Miller, Batrum, & Kling, 1962) considered the effect of Protestant, Catholic, or Jewish religious affiliation on parental acceptance of children with disabilities. However, more recent research has not focused on affiliation with these mainstream religions at all. Some more recent studies have considered the role of religiosity in general rather than religious affiliation in particular. For example, Rogers-Dulan and Blacher (1995) have suggested that more religious families might be more accepting of children with disabilities than less religious families, because religious participation is often associated with social support from fellow church members.

Muslim American Families

A growing religious group in the United States is the Islamic or Muslim community. This community consists of families of diverse national backgrounds, including those from Asia and the Middle East, as well as those born in the United States. Yet some common characteristics are of relevance for professionals working with families of children with disabilities.

In most Muslim families, women are primarily responsible for childrearing (Sherif, 1999), and family systems approaches that insist on the inclusion of fathers may not be appropriate. In the early intervention program directed by one of us (R. B. D.), attempts to include the father in home visits with one such family met with repeated failure, and the mother (a highly educated professional) finally told the interventionists that "in our culture, men don't get involved in these things."

As in many other ethnic groups, the extended family is more important than the nuclear family or the individual and is a central source of emotional support (Carolan, 1999; Sherif, 1999). Aswad (1997) noted that in many Arab families one son emigrates to the United States, and other family members follow. As a result, many relatives may live in close proximity. Families generally try to solve problems without the assistance of professionals, although technical support, such as physical therapy, may be welcomed. Carolan (1999) noted that, because of the value placed on modesty, professionals should be of the same gender as the client.

Amish Families

A European American family type for which religion plays an important role is the Amish. Such families are common in rural areas in some geographic regions. They tend to be self-reliant and do not seek outside help. The Amish receive strong support from the extended family, neighbors, and the church (Huntington, 1998). MacNeal and Leach (1997) suggested the following strategies for health care professionals who provide services in an Amish community:

1. Don't be afraid to give them literature, but ask whether anatomically explicit literature would be offensive.
2. Seek out trusted "English" people, such as a community friend, a driver with whom they contract for transportation, or a shopkeeper. These people can introduce you to community leaders, such as bishops and schoolteachers.
3. Dress conservatively; women should not wear jeans or slacks.

IMPLICATIONS FOR PROFESSIONALS

Professionals who work with families of children with disabilities should be aware of structural and subcultural differences. At the same time, professionals must be careful not to stereotype families on the basis of social class or ethnic, or religious identification. Within most subcultures, a considerable amount of intragroup variation exists. Professionals should not assume that individual members of a group will share all of the values and beliefs commonly held by the group as a whole.

Intragroup variation was found in a study of lower-class European American, African American, and Latino couples (Cromwell & Cromwell, 1978). No ethnic differences were found among the groups in styles of conflict resolution. Stereotypical characterizations of African American matriarchy and Latino patriarchy were thus not supported. The authors concluded that "categorical labeling of family structure based on ethnic group membership is unwarranted and inappropriate" (p. 757). Similarly, several studies (as quoted in Martinez, 1999) have shown little difference in parenting styles among Mexican American, European American, and African American families when SES is held constant. The value of subcultural studies, then, is in making professionals more aware of *possible* characteristics they may encounter.

The need for a better understanding of subcultural differences is demonstrated by a number of studies that reveal misunderstandings between professionals and clients of a different cultural background. One study of therapists and their Spanish-speaking patients (Kline, Acosta, Austin, & Johnson, 1980) found that the therapists did not accurately perceive patients' wants and feelings and instead projected their own wishes onto the patients. Such misperceptions may persist even when interpreters are used. Marcos (1979) found, for example, that clinicians evaluating non-English-speaking patients through an interpreter were faced with "consistent, clinically relevant, interpreter-related distortions, which may give rise to important misconceptions about the patient's mental status" (p. 173).

Studies with Mexican American groups (Delgado-Gaitan; Ada; as quoted in Harry, 1992a) have shown that passivity can be overcome by professional techniques that are inclusive rather than exclusive. The parents in these studies were empowered by the realization that their social (nonacademic) skills were valuable. Thus the process of encouraging families to share their concerns may require special techniques. A number of recommendations emerge to guide professionals who work with culturally and socially diverse families:

1. *Do not overlook resources or overemphasize concerns.* Particularly in the case of families of lower SES, professionals may tend to focus on their clients' deficits rather than their strengths. All families have strengths, but professionals may have to work harder to discover them when families feel as though they have no power. VanDenBerg and

Grealish (1997, p. 2) suggested some questions that are useful in eliciting strengths:

- If you could say one good thing about yourself, what would it be?
- I like your (hair, makeup, clothes, etc.). Did you come up with that yourself?
- What do you do for fun?
- Who has been the biggest influence on your life?
- What are the best things about your family? Your community?

Additional information on identifying family strengths can be found in Chapter 13.

2. *If at all possible, the professional should speak the family's native language.* As Laosa (1974) has suggested, abandonment of one's native language may imply abandonment of one's entire culture. Also, as indicated earlier, much misunderstanding occurs when professionals and families do not speak the same language, even when an interpreter is used. Hanson (1981) also noted the importance of providing written materials in the family's native language. Fracasso (1994) suggested the technique of "back translation," whereby materials that have been translated be translated back to English by an independent translator, to assure that meanings have not been changed. Harry (1992a) suggested that when interpreters must be used, they should always be bicultural as well as bilingual to avoid misunderstandings caused by nuances of meaning. Lynch (1992) and Paniagua (1998) provided excellent guidelines for working with interpreters, and we suggest that the reader consult their work prior to using an interpreter.

One study of physicians (Robert Wood Johnson Foundation, 2004) found that focus-group participants believed that time and cost were the biggest barriers to improving communication with non- or limited-English-proficient patients. In particular, professional interpretation services were cited as being too costly. Unfortunately, insurance reimbursement is often not available for such services.

3. *Indigenous professionals, paraprofessionals, and consultants should be used as much as possible.* Although professionals can learn about the language and culture of the families they serve, they can never acquire the cultural worldview to the same extent as one raised in the culture. Families also feel more comfortable interacting with their peers. Quesada (1976) thus recommended the use of community representatives as teachers and consultants or the employment of local community representatives at the paraprofessional level.

4. *Professionals must meet the needs of culturally diverse parents for information, belonging, and self-esteem.* These parents are often excluded from advocacy organizations and support groups and feel isolated as a result. They may come from powerless segments of society and have little knowledge of their rights to educational and other services for their children. Professionals must be supportive of these families' cultural values and work toward integrating them into support and service networks located in the cultural mainstream. Harry (1992a) suggested that information could be disseminated through traditional community supports, such as churches, or through community leaders.

5. *Scheduling should be flexible.* Families in the early intervention program formerly directed by one of us (R. B. D.) must often travel to the closest large medical center for consultation and treatment. Some of the clinics there schedule only early-morning appointments. Because they have no other means of transportation, lower-SES families often must rely on a bus to travel to these clinics, and the earliest bus of the day does not arrive until afternoon. As a result, at least one family has had to spend the night at the bus station. Others simply avoid making the trip. Quesada (1976) noted, too, that people working on an hourly basis may not be able to afford to spend entire days at a clinic. He recommended a system of routine call-backs in order to reschedule missed appointments. In addition, as Harry (1992a) suggested, providing access to supports such as transportation or child care may be necessary in assuring the participation of some families in treatment programs.

6. *Attempts must be made to elicit the family's definition of the situation.* Although important for all professional–family interactions, this guideline is especially salient in the case of culturally diverse families. Montalvo (1974) presented a number of cases of Puerto Rican children who had difficulties in school because well-intentioned school personnel failed to take into account the meanings attached by the family to a child's language or style of dress. Similarly, Anderson (1988) noted that an early intervention program could not be established in a Native American community until the support of the elders was obtained. Likewise, Harry, Allen, and McLaughlin (1995) reported that African American parents withdrew their support when their children's preschool program labeled their children in ways they perceived as inappropriately negative. In general, professionals must take what Mercer (1965) called a *social system* (rather than a clinical) perspective when working with culturally diverse populations. To the greatest extent possible, professionals must assume the family's point

of view. Helping cannot occur without understanding. Before professionals can begin to meet the needs of families of children with disabilities, they must determine how those needs are defined by the family itself, within the context of the subcultural world that shapes its daily round of life.

Professionals can take certain steps to better educate themselves about the subcultures of the families they serve (Harry, 1992b). Harry, Otrguson, Katkavich, and Guerrero (1993) described, for example, a teacher training program that requires students to spend time with a culturally different family, including interviewing the parents and participating in a community-based activity.

Lynch (1992) suggested five areas that should be addressed in training early interventionists to work with culturally diverse families. These areas are relevant to other helping professionals as well:

- Self-awareness: The professional should first be able to articulate the relevant norms, values, and beliefs of his or her *own* culture.
- Awareness of other cultures, in general.
- Awareness of other cultures' views of children and childrearing, disability, family roles and structures, healing practices, and intervention by professionals.
- Cross-cultural communication, including verbal and nonverbal messages such as eye contact, proximity and touching, gestures, and listening skills.
- Acknowledgment of cultural differences.

Wayman, Lynch, and Hanson (1991) suggested a series of questions for home visitors in early intervention to ask themselves as an aid in understanding a family's values and lifestyle. The questions address areas such as sleeping patterns, mealtime rituals, and other aspects of life that might be relevant to a family's participation in a program. Eliades and Suitor (1994) also suggested some differences in relation to eating that might have relevance for professional–family interaction.

Jezewski and Sotnik (2005, pp. 52–53) suggested some questions for eliciting a family's view of disability:

- What do you think caused [your child's] condition?
- How does [your child's] disability affect your everyday life?

- How severe do you consider [your child's] disability to be?
- What are the chief problems caused by this disability?
- What do you fear most about [your child's] disability?
- What kind of services do you think you should receive [in relation to your child's disability]?

7. *Professionals must recognize that issues of survival may have to be given precedence over intervention concerns* and be willing to assist families in obtaining material resources, as stated earlier and as Harry (1992a) noted. Families with major needs for food, clothing, shelter, or health care will not have the time or energy for, or interest in, discussing their concerns in relation to their child's disability.

8. *Professionals must adapt their communication style to the expectations of the family*, when possible. Kavanagh and Kennedy (1992) suggested numerous strategies for communicating with culturally diverse families. Some examples follow:

- Do not discredit folk theories or remedies unless you *know* they are harmful.
- Establish a personalized relationship by means of disclosing selected, culturally appropriate personal information.
- If appropriate, acknowledge unfamiliarity with the family's culture.
- Ask direct questions only if appropriate to the family's cultural and linguistic expectations. (Direct questioning should be avoided with some Asian, Latino, or Native American families.)
- Adjust the tone of your voice and your body position to synchronize with those of family members.
- Include extended family members or others in an interview if they are normally part of the family's support system.
- Be willing to tolerate periods of silence.

The authors recommended role playing and other exercises to practice these techniques before they are needed in a professional interaction situation.

For professionals who routinely work with culturally diverse families, this overview of principles and techniques should be supplemented with further reading in some of the sources noted above. In addition, the professional may want to consult one or more of the following:

Brislin, R. W., & Yoshida, T. (1993). *Improving intercultural communications: Modules for cross-cultural training programs.* Thousand Oaks, CA: Sage.

Brislin, R. W., & Yoshida, T. (1994). *Intercultural communication training: An introduction.* Thousand Oaks, CA: Sage.

Canino, I. A., & Spurlock, J. (2000). *Culturally diverse children and adolescents: Assessment, diagnosis, and treatment* (2nd ed.). New York: Guilford Press.

Chang, H. N. L. (Ed.). (1993). *Affirming children's roots: Cultural and linguistic diversity in early care and education.* San Francisco: California Tomorrow (Fort Mason Center, Building B, San Francisco, CA 94123).

Dominguez, S., & Watkins, C. (2003). Creating networks for survival and mobility: Social capital among African-American and Latin-American low-income mothers. *Social Problems, 50*(1), 111–135.

McGoldrick, M. (1993). Ethnicity, cultural diversity, and normality. In F. Walsh (Ed.), *Normal family processes* (2nd ed., pp. 331–360). New York: Guilford Press.

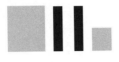

THE FAMILY LIFE CYCLE

4

Becoming the Parent of a Child with a Disability

Reactions to First Information

Various writers have suggested that certain crisis periods are especially traumatic for parents of children with disabilities (see Chapter 2, this volume), including when parents first learn or suspect that their child has a disability, school-entry age, time of leaving school, and when parents become older. Of these, the crisis of first information or suspicion of disability is probably the most difficult, and families' needs for support are greatest at that time. In this chapter we present a sociological view of family reactions to the news of their child's disability and suggest a model of family reactions during the infancy period using an interactionist perspective.

Several psychological theories have attempted to explain family reactions to the birth of a child with a disability (see Chapter 2). Perhaps the most popular is "stage theory" (see Blacher, 1984a, for a review of studies using this model), which suggests that parents progress through a series of "stages" in adapting to a child's diagnosis. As noted in other chapters, some writers have suggested that the sequence is variable, and others have argued that the model does not fit the adaptations of all parents.

Another popular strand in the literature concerns correlates of family adjustment. These studies suggest that certain kinds of families and/or certain kinds of children contribute to a family's ability to accept a child's disability. Some studies, for example, have suggested that a family's size, composition, SES, or ethnicity determines the reaction to the birth of a child with a disability; other studies have suggested a connection between the sex, age, birth-order position, or severity of a child's disability and family acceptance. Some of these studies are presented in Chapter 7.

Because of the great diversity among families, no single reaction or sequence of reactions can be found in all parents of children with disabilities. (The effects of subcultural diversity are explored further in Chapter 3.) In addition to predisposing characteristics that shape parental reactions, situational contingencies, such as coming across a helpful website, play an important role in parental response. These contingencies are discussed later in this chapter.

Symbolic interactionism, the theoretical perspective used here, is a sociological approach to social psychology that derives from the work of George Herbert Mead, Charles Horton Cooley, and others. This approach suggests that beliefs, values, and knowledge are socially determined through interaction and the ability of individuals to "take the role of the other"—that is, understand the meanings attached to situations by other people. The symbolic interactionist view of human behavior focuses on social process rather than on static characteristics of individuals, such as gender, ethnicity, or personality type. When applied to families of children with disabilities, parental reactions would be interpreted within the context of the parents' interactional histories prior to their child's birth and their experiences afterward. Parents attach meanings to their experiences as a result of definitions they have encountered in their interactions with others.

Not all interactions are equally important. Usually the most important are those with *significant others*, typically close family members and friends. When significant others define their situation positively, parents are likely to define it positively as well. The effects of interactions with significant others, along with the broader interactional context, are explored throughout this chapter as we trace the development of parental reactions from the prenatal through the postpartum periods.

THE PRENATAL PERIOD

Prior Knowledge about Disability

Prior to their child's birth, most parents have had only limited experience with individuals with disabilities. In general, they have been exposed primarily to the stereotypes and stigmatizing attitudes toward disability that pervade our culture. During the prenatal period, then, most parents dread the possibility of giving birth to a child with a disability. As one mother of a child with Down syndrome said, "I remember thinking, before I got married, it would be the worst thing that could ever happen to me" (Darling, 1979, p. 124). Parents' concerns are sometimes even greater when they know of other families who have had children with disabilities: "I've always been worried about having a child who was handicapped—one of our friends has a terribly retarded child, terribly retarded. We were concerned. We just wanted a healthy child" (parent of a child without a disability, cited in Darling, 1979, p. 127). In some cases, mothers claim to have had premonitions that something was wrong with their baby:

> I always said if it wasn't a girl, there was something wrong [this mother already had two boys without disabilities]. It just felt different from my other pregnancies, and my sister-in-law had just lost a baby at seven months.
>
> I felt very strongly that she was deformed. . . . She didn't kick as much as I thought she should.
>
> I thought something might be wrong because I was sick all the time and I wasn't sick at all during my first pregnancy. (Darling, 1979, pp. 125–126)

In these cases, concerns seem to be based on experience. These mothers' definitions of "what pregnancy should be like" did not fit their actual experience of pregnancy. Such parents are not typical, however, and most anticipate the birth of a typical baby.

When parents express concerns about the health of their unborn child, these concerns are usually discounted by friends, relatives, and others. Even a mother who had four children with the same genetic disorder managed to rationalize her fears during each successive pregnancy with the help of physicians who assured her that her "bad luck" was not likely to recur. With regard to her third pregnancy, she said: "I was unrealistic. I said, 'He's going to be a Christmas baby. There won't be anything wrong with him' " (Darling, 1979, p. 143). In general, then, parents' fears about the health or disability status of their unborn baby are usually neutralized through interactions with others.

Expectations that a baby will be "normal" are also promoted by childbirth classes. Although these classes typically cover the possibility of unexpected events during labor and delivery, the end product of the birth process that is presented to prospective parents is generally a typical, healthy baby. The possibility of congenital impairment is usually not mentioned at all.

Most parents, then, are poorly prepared for the birth of a child with a disability. In the past, parents generally were not aware of the existence of their child's disability prior to the baby's birth. As one parent said, "I never heard of Down's. . . . Mental retardation wasn't something you talked about in the house. . . . There wasn't much exposure" (Darling, 1979, p. 124). Similarly the parent of a child with dwarfism recalled this initial reaction: "I heard Dr. Z use the word 'dwarf' outside the room when he was talking to the resident. When he came in, I said, 'Dwarf? Are you saying my child's a dwarf?' What dwarf meant to me was a leprechaun. Whatever would that mean? Would you have to send them to a circus?" (Ablon, 1982, p. 36) In other cases, parents can recall having heard of a disability, but only in a limited, and typically negative, way: "I'd heard of it from a book. It was just a terrible picture on a certain page of an abnormal psych book that I can still sort of picture" (Darling, 1979, p. 25).

With the advent of modern technology, some childhood disabilities are diagnosed prenatally. Through techniques such as amniocentesis, ultrasound, the FISH (fluorescence *in situ* hybridization) test, and maternal serum testing, parents are able to learn of atypical conditions prior to their child's birth. In cases of prenatal diagnosis, anticipatory grieving may be tempered by the hope that "maybe they made a mistake," and the baby will be "all right" after all. One mother, who was told after an ultrasound screening late in her pregnancy that her baby had hydrocephalus, said she was "shocked, sad, and depressed" after hearing the news but "hoped they were wrong" at the same time (Darling & Darling, 1982, p. 98). After she saw the baby's enlarged head in the delivery room, she no longer doubted the diagnosis. Similarly, a couple described by Zuckoff (2002) kept hoping that early test results indicating Down syndrome were wrong but finally accepted the diagnosis after receiving the results of an additional test: "As the results sank in, Tierney knew she needed to stop hoping it wouldn't be Down syndrome" (Zuckoff, 2002, p.51).

However, even with prenatal diagnosis, some uncertainty remains. As one father said, "But still there's a fear of the unknown. . . . They can't tell us how mentally retarded she'll be, how severe the effects of Down syndrome will be, and that's hard" (Zuckoff, 2002, p. 120). Of course, even in the case of postnatal diagnosis, predictions about the future typically cannot be made with certainty.

Occasionally, a prenatal prognosis may actually be more dire than the real outcome. In these cases, parents may actually be relieved to receive the diagnosis of a less severe impairment:

> At 37 weeks, I was told that my child had a chromosome problem and that his brain did not develop. They told me he would not live beyond birth. . . . The week between the first diagnosis and when Dylan was actually born were easily the worst times of our lives. It was absolutely devastating to think that you had carried this child, and now all your hopes and dreams for him were gone. We prepared to bury our child. So when Dylan was actually born and we were told he had [spina bifida], we were thrilled! We were going to have a child! We didn't care what the problems were, we were just thrilled to have him! (Hickman, 2000, pp. 14–15)

Early prenatal diagnosis often allows for the option of pregnancy termination but also allows parents who choose to continue the pregnancy to get used to the diagnosis and its implications before having to care for the actual child. Issues relating to informing friends and relatives also can be resolved prior to the birth. In general, families who learn about an impairment through prenatal diagnosis adopt the same rationalizations and adjustment strategies as families who learn later. The advantage is one of timing.

Pregnancy as a Social Role: Expectations and Dreams

LaRossa (1977) argued that a couple's first pregnancy creates a crisis that is a potential strain on the marital relationship. Similarly, Doering, Entwisle, and Quinlan (1980) claimed that a first pregnancy is a progressively developing crisis. The threat is generally not serious enough to destroy an otherwise strong marriage, but we should keep in mind that pregnancy and birth are stress-producing situations, even when a baby has no impairments.

Expectant parents also typically fantasize about their unborn baby. They may imagine the baby's gender, appearance, personality, or other attributes:

> This is the dream child you have been waiting for since you yourself were a little girl playing with dolls. At long last, you will become the perfect mom. . . . Preparations begin . . . Lamaze classes, wallpaper, baby clothes, wooden cradle. . . . You fantasize about who this dream child will be. Tennis star, astronaut, literary genius. You read volumes of books on child care and parenting. . . . A colicky baby is your worst fear. (Spano, 1994, p. 29)

Interactions with friends and relatives help to shape parents' fantasies. Folk wisdom sometimes plays a role, interpreting the pregnant woman's shape or size or the baby's prenatal movements as indicative of the child's gender, size, or temperament. Parents enter the birth situation, then, with a particular base of knowledge, attitudes, expectations, and hopes. They possess varying degrees of knowledge about disabilities; various attitudes toward people with disabilities and toward their own status as expectant parents; differing expectations about the birth situation, parenthood, and the attributes of their unborn child; as well as hopes and wishes relating to those attributes.

THE BIRTH SITUATION

Except in the case of obvious impairments, typically concerns about a baby are not revealed directly to parents in the delivery room. Rather, parents may become suspicious as a result of unintentional clues given by physicians and nurses:

> I remember very vividly. The doctor did not say anything at all when the baby was born. Then he said, "It's a boy," and the way he hesitated, I immediately said, "Is he all right?" And he said, "He has ten fingers and ten toes," so in the back of my mind I knew there was something wrong. (Darling, 1979, p. 129)

D'Arcy (1968) and Walker (1971) noted clues, such as "the look on the nurse's face," consultations between nurses in hushed voices, and nurses who "looked at each other and pointed to something." In rarer cases, the clues are not so subtle:

> When the baby was born, they said, "Oh my God, put her out." That's the first thing they said, "Oh my God, put her out" . . . and the next thing

I remember was waking up in the recovery room. . . . I had my priest on my left hand and my pediatrician on my right hand . . . and they were trying to get me to sign a piece of paper. . . . I just couldn't believe that this was happening to me and I said to my priest, "Father, what's the matter?" and he said, "You have to sign this release. Your daughter is very sick," and I said to the pediatrician, "What's the matter with her?" and he said . . . she had something that was too much to talk about, that I shouldn't worry myself. . . . Nobody was telling me what this was. . . . I was very depressed. (Darling, 1979, p. 130)

Fortunately, such extreme examples of professionals withholding information from parents occur less frequently today.

Parental reactions in the immediate postpartum situation may be characterized by the sociological concept of *anomie*, or normlessness. Because even prepared parents are unable to make sense of atypical events in the delivery room, the birth experience is stressful for almost all parents of children whose impairments can be detected immediately by medical personnel. McHugh (1968) noted that the components of anomie are *meaninglessness* and *powerlessness*, and both are commonly experienced by parents of newborns with disabilities.

As Chapter 11 demonstrates, physicians sometimes deliberately create meaninglessness and powerlessness in the belief that they are protecting parents, who are deemed "not ready to hear the truth" so soon after birth. Yet, as Chapter 11 also reveals, studies show that most parents do want to know their child's diagnosis right from the beginning; uncertainty and suspicion may be more stressful than bad news. As one father wrote, "To me, not knowing was worse than knowing. Until the tests were completed, I didn't know if our child would live a normal life, live his life with a serious disability, or not live at all. All I know was that I was scared" (Freedman, 2001, p. 39).

Parents' immediate reactions to the birth of a child with an impairment, then, may involve suspicions created by interactions with professionals. The birth situation generally occurs in medically controlled settings in our society, placing parents in a state of submission to professional authority. As a result, they are likely to feel powerless and to experience stress when events do not proceed according to their expectations. As the next section shows, the sense of anomie may continue even after a diagnosis has been established.

THE POSTPARTUM PERIOD

Early Reactions

As many studies cited throughout this volume have shown, parents' initial reaction to the news that their child has an impairment is likely to be negative. Rejection of the baby during the early postpartum period is common, as these statements illustrate:

> I was kind of turned off. I didn't want to go near her. It was like she had a disease or something, and I didn't want to catch it. I didn't want to touch her. (Mother of a child with Down syndrome)

> I saw her for the first time when she was 10 days old. . . . She was much more deformed than I had been told. At the time I thought, "Oh my God, what have I done?" (Mother of a child with spina bifida) (Darling, 1979, pp. 135–136)

The fact that parents chose to deny life-saving treatment to such children in the well-publicized "Baby Doe" cases of the early 1980s is not surprising. Attachment to the baby is probably lowest during the first few hours after birth. Parents are also very vulnerable during the immediate postpartum period and likely to be highly susceptible to suggestions by professionals that their children not be treated. Lorber (1971), a British physician who advocated "selective treatment" for children born with spina bifida, has written that he preferred to present his case for nontreatment to parents immediately after birth, before bonding had occurred.

With any baby, disabled or not, attachment grows out of the process of parent–child interaction. When babies respond to parental attempts to feed and cuddle them, parents feel rewarded. Attachment is further enhanced when babies begin smiling and making sounds in response to parental gestures. Infants with disabilities, however, may not be able to respond to their parents' efforts. Bailey and Wolery (1984), Blacher (1984c), Collins-Moore (1984), Robson and Moss (1970), Waechter (1977), and others have suggested that the following characteristics of some childhood impairments may impede the formation of parent–child attachment:

- The child's appearance, especially facial disfigurement
- Negative response to being handled (stiffness, tenseness, limpness, lack of responsiveness)

- Unpleasant crying
- Atypical activity level—either lowered activity or hyperactivity
- High threshold for arousal
- No response to communication
- Delayed smiling
- Feeding difficulties
- Medical fragility
- Presence of medical equipment, such as feeding tubes or oxygen supplies
- Life-threatening conditions
- Prolonged hospitalization and consequent separation
- Impaired ability to vocalize
- Inability to maintain eye contact
- Unpleasant behaviors, such as frequent seizures

Commonly, children with disabilities spend the first weeks or months of their lives in neonatal intensive care units (NICUs). The unnatural surroundings of NICUs, as well as equipment such as monitors and feeding tubes, not only impede parent–child bonding but may cause parents to question their ability to care for the child after release: "A child who requires such handling can become pretty intimidating in the minds of his parents. How could mere mortals like us ever hope to take care of Nicholas?" (Arango, 2001, p. 2).

The tremendous adaptive capacity of families is evidenced by the fact that, given all the obstacles to parent–child attachment present in the case of childhood disability, the vast majority of parents *do* form strong attachments to their infants with impairments. In general, all but the children with the most severe disabilities are able to respond to their parents to some extent—by sound, gesture, or other indication of recognition. In addition, attachment is usually encouraged by supportive interactions with other people. For example, members of parent-to-parent groups in many communities visit parents of newborns with disabilities shortly after birth. The mother of the infant with Down syndrome quoted earlier explained:

> I talked to a nurse and then I felt less resentment. I said I was afraid, and she helped me feed the baby. . . . Then my girlfriend came to see me. She had just lost her husband, and we sort of supported each other. . . . By the time she came home I loved her. When I held her the first time, I felt love and I worried if she'd live. (Darling, 1979, p. 136)

Similarly, the mother of the child with spina bifida reported: "As time goes on, you fall in love. You think, 'This kid's mine, and nobody's gonna take her away from me.' I think by the time she was two weeks old I wasn't appalled by her anymore" (Darling, 1979, p. 136).

Attachment is difficult in the medically controlled setting of the hospital. Even after discharge, medical concerns may consume the first few weeks at home. As one parent of a child with spina bifida said:

> It's difficult when children are first born and they are infants and everything is kind of biological needs and stuff. . . . All the doctors' appointments and therapy and the millions of things we were doing were so overwhelming at the beginning. I was less afraid of them, I guess, when her personality started to emerge. I felt more confident about learning more about her disability than I did right away. (Personal communication, 2003)

Waisbren (1980), Marsh (1992), and others have described the important role of social support in promoting parents' positive feelings about their children. One father of a child with Down syndrome said that, at first, he and his wife had decided not to send birth announcements, but then "everybody was saying he was so lucky to have us as parents." The parents then printed announcements that looked like theater tickets for a hypothetical play entitled "A Very Special Person" (Darling, 1979, p. 136).

Although most parents are not prepared for the birth of a child with a disability and hold negative views toward disability, in general, some parents have different definitions of the situation. In some cases, they have friends or family members with disabilities; in others, they have work or other experience with people with disabilities who are doing well. Some common disabilities such as Down syndrome have received more positive attention in the media, resulting in less dread among new parents. As one mother who learned of her son's diagnosis at 18 weeks' gestation wrote: "The diagnosis of Down syndrome was almost good news, we told ourselves. Given the other possibilities—chromosomal abnormalities incompatible with life—we figured that if we had to have something, at least he, and we, could live with Down syndrome" (Arango, 2001, p. 1).

The Case of Delayed Diagnosis

Not all disabilities are diagnosed in the prenatal or immediate postpartum period. Some developmental disabilities, such as autism, cerebral palsy, or intellectual disability, may not be readily apparent shortly after birth. Other disabilities occur as a result of accidents or illnesses later in infancy or childhood. In still other cases, professionals delay their communicating of a known diagnosis to parents for a variety of reasons (these are discussed in greater detail in Chapter 11). In general, parents have said that they were better able to adjust when they were aware of their child's diagnosis from the beginning. The process of redefining as disabled a child once defined as "normal" appears to be a very difficult one for parents. As a father who learned of his son's disability when the child was 18 months old wrote, "I felt a grief beyond words—as if someone had died—but my child was very much alive" (Naseef, 2001a, p. 206).

Most of the time, however, parents suspect that a problem exists before they receive a diagnosis, and diagnostic delay only protracts the period of suspicion and its attendant stress. The experience of one family is illustrative:

> [After] he was born I realized that something was wrong because I nursed him, and he wasn't catching on. . . . I had problems with him feeding early on, but the doctor said that he appeared normal, that they didn't see anything out of the ordinary. . . . When B got a couple months older, he started doing this jerking like a startle motion . . . and then it . . . . increased and increased. I kept telling the doctor about it and about how he wasn't doing the developmental things like a two month old should do, a four month old should do. You know, there's different stages. And even . . . at six months old he couldn't hold his own head up. I expressed this to the doctor, and the doctor kept saying, '. . . maybe because he was premature, he's going to have a harder time catching up. When he's a year old, you'll never know.' . . . [The jerking movements continued], and I knew that wasn't normal and I told that to the doctor, but he just kept . . . saying everything was OK. . . . You know deep down inside [something is not right], but when a doctor says everything is all right you don't know what to think. (Mother of a child with severe disabilities interviewed by Jon Darling, personal communication, August 25, 2005)

In such cases parents tend to be relieved rather than shocked when they finally receive a diagnosis. This reaction is apparent in these families of children with intellectual disability, quoted by Dickman and Gordon (1985):

> When the doctor told us he couldn't believe how well we accepted the diagnosis. All I can say is that it was such a relief to have someone finally

just come out and say what we had feared so long! We felt now that we could move ahead and do the best we could for Timmy.

When James turned six months old, my husband and I decided to change pediatricians. The second doctor was an angel in disguise. She spotted the problem immediately. . . . The reason I called her an angel was that she finally put an end to the unknown. The not knowing exactly what was wrong was driving me crazy. (pp. 31–32)

Similarly, the parent of a child with autism wrote, "My reaction [to the diagnosis] was relief. Finally, a label for what he had. If you have a label, you have something to research, and some way to help" (Hickman, 2000, p. 37).

Likewise, in a study of 131 families with children who have intellectual disability, Baxter (1986) found that most parents who experienced little or no worry after a diagnostic encounter had gradually become aware of their child's "differentness" or had sought a diagnosis to confirm their own suspicions. With the increasing availability of the Internet, many parents confirm their suspicions before receiving a formal diagnosis:

Actually, Maria had come to the conclusion that James fell along the autistic spectrum several months prior to his formal diagnosis. . . . She had spent countless hours reading current literature and surfing the Internet, gathering as much information as possible. (Beveridge, 2001, p. 83)

I had found the Williams syndrome site on the Internet a week before our actual appointment with [the doctor] and had a strong suspicion that this was the answer we had been looking for. Therefore, I was somewhat prepared when he told us he suspected it, and then it was confirmed with the FISH [test]. (Hickman, 2000, p. 28)

Sometimes, a child's diagnosis is elusive, even when medical professionals are sharing all of their knowledge and suspicions with parents. Medical knowledge simply is not yet at the point where all childhood impairments can be definitively labeled. In such cases, anomie-related stress may be protracted indefinitely. A parent writes about her need for a "label":

Sometimes I wish my son had cerebral palsy or Down syndrome—something definite and preferably a little visible. . . . It is . . . the elusiveness of our son's problems that causes so much pain. So, as awful as it sounds, I have thought of what it might be like to have a child with a defined disability. (Gundry, 1989, pp. 22–24)

In cases of disability resulting from accidents or illnesses occurring later in infancy or childhood, parents typically react in ways similar to those of parents receiving diagnoses earlier in infancy. In some cases, the sense of loss may be even greater, because the child has already been defined and experienced as "normal." However, parents still feel a sense of meaninglessness and powerlessness until they completely understand the nature of their child's disability and have embarked on a course of treatment.

THE POSTDIAGNOSIS EXPERIENCE

Although a diagnosis may relieve the stress associated with meaninglessness and the suspicion that something is wrong, parents generally continue to experience anomie, to some extent, until issues of prognosis have been resolved and the child is enrolled in an intervention program.

The Need for Prognostic Information

A father who had been told that his son would be "a slow learner" expressed the following concerns: "[I was most worried about] how he would develop. It was the uncertainty of not knowing whether he'd be able to go to school and get a job or whether he'd always be dependent upon us. It was just not knowing what was likely to happen and what the future held for him and for us" (Baxter, 1986, p. 85).

Today, many families do not experience a protracted period of concern about prognosis because they are typically enrolled in early intervention programs that provide answers to their questions. However, when parents receive only a diagnostic label or limited information from professionals, they generally continue to wonder, and worry, about what their child will be like in the future. Most parents are especially concerned about whether the child will be able to walk and talk, go to school, and play typical adult occupational and marital roles. In some cases, they are worried about whether the child will even survive infancy. Baxter (1986) noted that the basic underlying factor in all expressions of parental worry is uncertainty. Parents of children with disabilities experience an ongoing need for information about the meaning of their child's condition—a need that professionals must meet. The parents in Baxter's study indicated that the most important type of help they had received from professionals was *information*, and that this help was more important than sympathy and emotional support. Similarly, Gowen, Christy, and Sparling (1993), and Darling and Baxter (1996) report that parents' greatest need, especially during the infant, toddler, and preschool periods, is for information. Even today, with increased access to the Internet, this need continues to be paramount for many parents (see, e.g., Hickman, 2000).

The Quest for Intervention

In addition to providing information, professionals (early interventionists; speech, physical, and occupational therapists; physicians and other medical professionals) are also able to provide therapeutic intervention that will minimize the effects of a child's disability. Once they learn that their child has a disability, virtually all parents are eager to begin a program of treatment. When they receive diagnostic information, parents are relieved of the stress of meaninglessness; until they begin to do something about their child's disability, however, they may continue to experience anomie in the form of powerlessness. As one parent wrote, "By this time, we knew something was wrong and were anxious to do something to help out the situation; to take control, I suppose. It was a relief to finally have a professional agree that something was wrong so we could start to 'fix it' " (Hickman, 2000, p. 33).

Some of the early literature in this field suggested that parents sought treatment because they unrealistically wanted their children to be cured. Numerous studies referred to parents' "shopping around" for a professional or a program that would make their child "normal." When parents are questioned about such "shopping" behavior, however, most do not report curing as their goal. Rather, like parents of children without disabilities in our society, they are simply trying to be "good" parents and do whatever they can to improve their children's quality of life. This mother's explanation of her motivation for seeking treatment is typical:

> Because nothing was happening, and I was just sitting there with this baby, we got involved with the patterning program. . . . We were never told he would be cured. They were the first people who reacted to Billy as a person or called him by name. Up to that time he had done nothing.

My pediatrician said, "You're just looking for hopes." I said, "No, I'm just looking to *do* something for him. I'm sitting at home doing nothing." (Darling, 1979, p. 153)

Similarly, the mother of a child with intellectual disability in an early intervention program directed by one of the authors (R. B. D.) said, after her baby had died, that she was grateful for the program. She felt no guilt at the baby's death because she had done everything she could for him while he was alive.

As early intervention programs have become more widespread and publicity about them has increased, parents' quests for services have become shorter. Yet most continue to search until they are satisfied with their children's medical care and have secured needed services, such as physical therapy or special stimulation programs. The extent of parents' quests for services will be based largely on the resources available to them. Most families have financial and geographic limitations that prevent them from searching endlessly for the "best" program for their child. Competing needs, such as other children at home or ill relatives, may also prevent parents from enrolling their child in a time-consuming program or one far from home.

Sometimes parents are overwhelmed by *too much* information. When daily schedules involve many therapy sessions (sometimes at different locations), in addition to normal routines of work and household responsibilities, parents may again experience anomie in the form of powerlessness. As one mother explained, "Your mind leaps forwards, backwards and sideways trying to sort out the deluge of information—the doctors' reports, nurses' instructions, conflicting or ambiguous diagnoses, appointment, feeding and laundry schedules" (McAnaney, 1990, p. 21).

During the early months, then, parents are typically motivated by a strong need to reduce their anomie, their sense of meaninglessness and powerlessness. As one mother said, "We wanted to get *us* in control instead of everybody else" (Darling, 1979, p. 147). Professionals can be most helpful to parents at this time by providing as much information as possible about diagnosis, prognosis, and the availability of intervention programs and other resources in the community—in as humane a manner as possible. However, professionals should be careful about overloading parents with too much information at any one time. In general, professionals should take their lead from the family by asking about the kind and amount of information desired.

The Need for Emotional Support

One mother said:

> I met other parents of the retarded after we moved here. I felt that made the biggest difference in my life. . . . Down there [where we lived before], with my husband working so much and no other families with retarded children, I felt that I was just singled out for something, that I was weird. I felt a lot of isolation and bitterness. (Darling, 1979, pp. 162–163)

Similarly, another parent wrote:

> My five-year-old son has Down syndrome. . . . Craig is a very hyper child. He goes in his room and dumps toys all over the floor and throws things everywhere. . . . My husband works all day and most evenings until 10 P.M., and I feel like I'm going crazy! . . . I must keep my eyes on him every minute, so I never get my work done. I can't even go to the bathroom by myself! . . . I feel like I'm the only one in the world going through this. No one understands. ("Down Syndrome," 1991, pp. 12–13)

The importance of social support in alleviating stress in families of children with disabilities has been well documented (e.g., Dyson & Fewell, 1986; Trivette & Dunst, 1982). Trivette and Dunst (1982) have shown that parents' personal well-being, perceptions of child functioning, and family integration are positively influenced by a family's informal social support network. They concluded that the negative consequences often associated with the birth and rearing of a child with developmental delays can be lessened or even alleviated to the extent that the members of a family's informal support network are mobilized to strengthen personal and familial well-being and buffer negative effects.

In some cases the birth of a child with a disability creates a rift in a family's relationship with former friends and family members. In other cases, even though friends and family are supportive, parents still need the special kind of support offered by others with children like their own.

SUPPORT WITHIN THE FAMILY
AND OTHER EXISTING NETWORKS

One of the most difficult tasks facing new parents of children with disabilities is telling other family members and friends about their child's impairment for the first time. Many have said that they "just didn't want to explain." In some cases, parents are afraid of upsetting elderly relatives or family members who are expecting the birth of their own child.

Negative reactions from extended family members (see Chapter 10, which discusses grandparents) and friends range from denial of the child's disability to rejection of the child:

> My family had a hard time recognizing the genetic aspects. To this day, my mother wants to believe it came from my dad's family, when I am certain it came from hers. (Hickman, 2000, p. 40)

> We have a rather large family and most members seemed to choose not to believe the diagnosis, saying such things as, "She'll catch up" or "Just wait, she'll get better," etc. This, of course, was frustrating, since we knew her genetic makeup would never change. (Hickman, 2000, p. 43)

> [My in-laws] to this day will not accept her as retarded. They will not say the word. They don't like us to talk about retardation. . . . She's their only grandchild. My mother thought that if she prayed hard enough Susan would be O.K.

> People think that retardation is a contagious disease. . . . I don't understand how it threatens them . . . the fact that a van pulls up in our driveway, picks up our daughter, and takes her to a program.

> When she was little, people were afraid to say anything. They would ask how [her typically developing brother] was doing, but just asking about Julie was like a personal question. (Darling, 1979, pp. 145, 159, 160)

In some cases, family members or friends appear to be unable to understand the nature of a child's disability: "Most were supportive but had no clue what we were trying to explain. The best example of this is my grandfather. We have told him many times what's wrong with Austin and that he's strictly tube-fed and central line, yet he gave him McDonald's gift certificates for Christmas" (Hickman, 2000, p. 53).

On the other hand, many families report that friends and relatives have been very supportive and helpful:

> I called my mother as soon as I knew, and she came over. She was very supportive.

> My father said, "What's the difference? She's yours."

> The thing that surprised me was that everyone accepted it right off. (Darling, 1979, p. 146)

> We are very fortunate to have a supportive and loving extended family living close by. Our parents were, of course, grieved for us, but have been such a source of strength and love! Their love for Christopher has not altered one little bit just because of a label. We are also blessed by a caring church family, who have given their time and many prayers to help us. (Hickman, 2000, p. 48)

Receiving the support of family members may be more important among rural and small-town families, where extended family members tend to live in close proximity and serve as significant others and resources for one another. Heller, Quesada, Harvey, and Wagner (1981) found, for example, that among families living in the Blue Ridge Mountains of Virginia, the identities of nuclear and extended families were fused. Kin were the major source of social support, and involvement with relatives was obligatory. Urban "middle-American" families, on the other hand, were more "primary-kin oriented," and the opinions of extended family members were not as important to them. The relative importance of the extended family in various subcultures is discussed further in Chapter 3.

Another source of support for some families is the church. Both clergy and fellow church members may rally around the family when a child has a disability. One mother explains how she became especially close to those church members who had children with disabilities after her daughter was born with spina bifida:

> Our church family is a very close family . . . I talk to them at least once or twice a week. . . . My friend, Nancy, she actually watches Riley for me one morning a week; she has an adult daughter with MR, mental retardation. . . . Even though Riley and Kim's situations are miles apart, I still have learned a lot from Nancy because I see that my friend has made a huge effort to let her daughter find meaning in things. . . . Like Kim has a lot of responsibilities in church, she does a lot . . . she spends a lot of time with our family, so it's been really valuable for me. (Personal communication, 2003)

However, other families we know have reported negative experiences with churches that were not accepting of their children with disabilities.

SUPPORT GROUPS

Most parents are able to get the support they need from friends and family. However, when friends and family react negatively or are unavailable, parents must look elsewhere for support. Even when members of existing social networks try to be helpful, parents may still feel that they do not *really* understand their situation. Meeting other parents of children with disabilities thus becomes very important to some parents after they learn about their child's disability. As one parent explained:

> Our families were very supportive, yet I think they also had it hard trying to understand. . . . Most of our friends disappeared from our lives. . . . I have an entirely new circle of friends. . . . I think part of the friends-disappearing-act had a lot to do with the fact that no one really knew how to support me. . . . More often than not, I saw pity in their eyes or heard it in their voices. Pity was the last thing I needed because I thought my life wasn't all that bad. I guess to an outsider it was. (Hickman, 2000, pp. 41–42)

Support groups composed of adults with disabilities and/or parents of children with disabilities serve a number of functions, including (1) alleviating loneliness and isolation, (2) providing information, (3) providing role models, and (4) providing a basis for comparison.

As a mother quoted earlier said, before she became involved in a support group, she felt as though she were "singled out for something." Another mother said, "I was in a once-a-week mothers' group, and it was very helpful. You find out you're not the only person with this problem" (Darling, 1979, p. 161). This function appears to be served equally well by groups of parents of children with similar and diverse impairments. The fact of having a child who is "different" provides a common bond among these families. Many parents also report feeling more comfortable in the presence of others who "understand":

> We've spent a lot of time with some families in the spina bifida community. We do a lot with them, and in some ways, it's almost easier to be around people like that when you're out and about because you know that your kid's going to be a little bit slower and they're going to need a little bit more of this or that, and a parent like that is going to have that instinct and already know that. (Personal communication, 2003)

Support groups also serve as sources of practical information. As the parent of a child with dwarfism explained: "The technical aspect is the easiest thing. The doctors can tell you all about that. What makes it so difficult is what you do everyday and how you raise the child. And no one can tell you that except right here at this meeting" (Ablon, 1982, p. 43). Similarly, the mother of a child with cerebral palsy said, "Meeting other parents you get the practical hints—like how someone got their child to chew—that normal parents take for granted" (Darling, 1979, p. 163).

At meetings, too, parents have an opportunity to see others who are coping successfully with their situation. These others provide a model for them to emulate. Sometimes parents who have been too timid to change physicians or seek additional services for their child may have the courage to do so after hearing how other parents have successfully challenged the system. The positive effects of encountering successful models among adults with disabilities is apparent in this statement by a parent of a child with dwarfism:

> At first we could not bring ourselves to go [to the meeting]. Maybe we didn't want to see what she was going to look like. . . . We . . . did go to the next meeting. . . . That was the turning point, because at that meeting we began talking to a number of dwarfs. That's when we found out it was going to be O.K.: that dwarfs live like other people—they married, they drove cars, they took vacations, they held jobs—they could be like other people. (Ablon, 1982, p. 38)

On the other hand, some parents are reluctant to meet adults with disabilities while their own children are still very young. (See Chapter 6 for a further discussion of this issue.)

Finally, when they meet other families, parents discover not only those who are coping successfully but also those whose children's problems are worse than theirs. Most develop a greater appreciation of their own situation as a result:

> You don't feel sorry for yourself when you see some children that are just vegetables.

> We went to a couples' group where we saw that other children were a lot worse than Peter.

> I was active in the parents' association at the beginning. I needed the help more then. . . . Some had much more severe children than I did. I

felt lucky to have Elizabeth. . . . Now I don't feel so sorry for myself. (Darling, 1979, pp. 161–162)

These parents are typically surrounded by friends and relatives whose children do not have disabilities, who may achieve developmental milestones much more quickly than their own children. Many have difficulty watching their children's slow progress in comparison with the accomplishments of their friends' and relatives' children. Comparisons with other children with disabilities, on the other hand, may be much more favorable. The support group thus becomes an important reference group for these families.

Although professionals may not be able to serve as a reference group for parents, they can play an important role by helping parents locate existing support groups—or starting new groups where none exists. A number of parents have reported difficulty in finding other parents like themselves. These stories are illustrative:

> We were walking on the beach and we saw four little people. I decided I'd follow them. I had to talk to them. I followed them a long way then I went up to the woman and said, "Excuse me, but I think my son is a little person"—I don't know what word I used, maybe "dwarf"—"like you are." The woman told us about Little People of America [LPA]. I had read about LPA in *Life* magazine before, but I didn't know how to contact them. When we got back we wrote to B. and she had a mother call us in a few days. (Ablon, 1982, p. 37)

> A friend of mine called and said she thought she saw a girlfriend of ours that we had gone to school with in the doctor's office, and she said that her daughter said there was a little girl that looked like Michelle. I thought about it . . . I hadn't talked to this girl since we graduated from high school. I called her up and said, "You have a daughter, right? . . . I want to ask you a question. I don't want you to feel offended," I said, "If I'm wrong I'm sorry." I said, "[Doesn't] your daughter [have Down syndrome]?" She said, "Yes she [does]. How did you know?" . . . She was our first exposure to other retarded people. . . . She told us about . . . the Association for the Retarded. (Darling, 1979, p. 148)

Professionals who inform parents about the existence of support groups early in a child's life can be very helpful in avoiding the need for protracted and often stressful searches. When no support groups exist in an area, the professional should consider starting one. A further discussion of the professional role in relation to parent support groups and of the functioning of support groups, in general, can be found in Chapter 12.

"Parent-to-parent" groups have also been effective in meeting the information and support needs of parents, and many such groups now exist throughout the country. Thus professional control of support groups does not appear to be necessary. Professional control, at least in the early stages of group development, may be more important in the case of parents who are less well educated or feel powerless for other reasons.

Today, in addition to face-to-face groups, many Internet-based support groups exist. These groups usually function through listservs or chat rooms and may be impairment-specific or for parents of children with disabilities in general. Electronic support is especially valuable in the case of families living in isolated rural areas or those whose children have unusual impairments: "My support group exists on line. I am truly grateful to have the opportunity through technology to be connected with other parents of children with my daughter's rare disorder. It has been a great comfort to know we are not alone" (Sivola, 2001, p. 11). Professionals can make parents aware of opportunities for "long-distance" support through electronic mail networks, the pen pals column in *Exceptional Parent* magazine, and national support groups and organizations of parents of children with rare disorders.

INTERACTIONS WITH STRANGERS

After they have told friends and family members about their child's disability, parents must face having to explain to strangers on the street, in restaurants, and in shopping malls. Most parents have said that taking their child out in public was very difficult for them in the beginning. These reports are illustrative:

> We took her to a store downtown, and she had a hat. . . . I wanted to make sure that hat would stay on so no one would see her ears. . . . We didn't want people to look at her. We didn't want to explain.

> I used to go to the laundromat . . . and so many people would say, "Your little girl is so good to sit there so quietly in the stroller." . . . I would just like, sit there, and my insides were like knots, and I would think, "Oh no, do I have to tell them about the cerebral palsy? Should I or shouldn't I? Should I just let it pass? . . . " All this is going through my mind. . . . I never told anybody. (Darling, 1979, pp. 155, 156)

Because children with disabilities sometimes look younger than their age, parents commonly avoid explanations by lying to strangers:

> He just looked like a little baby, even at two or three. People would ask how old he was—especially waitresses—and then they were embarrassed. So I started lying, and the waitresses would say, "Oh, he's so cute!"

> We bought a car last February. Joey was 15 or 16 months old, and the salesman asked, "Is the baby eight or nine months old?" I said, "Yes." [My daughter] said, "He's one." I said, "Sh." I've been a little too hesitant about telling people. (Darling, 1979, p. 157)

Some come to resent this situation:

> For five years I drew in my breath, narrowed my eyes, and proceeded to explain, in grim detail, Annie's premature birth, from weight and length right down to time spent on a ventilator. The EXPLANATION. Complete with the harrowing account I felt I was required to give to perfect strangers, as though this information was due them. And all because of the simple question, "How old is she?" (Nelson, 1991, p. 23)

Eventually, most parents become more comfortable explaining to strangers about their children's disabilities. Professionals can help them develop explanations they can use in these situations; support groups can also be helpful in sharing explanations that other parents have used. One parent adopted the following solution: "Nowadays, I have small business cards with printed information about my son's diagnoses so if strangers stare, I invite them to ask questions. People are afraid of what they don't know, and it's inherent to human nature to be curious. I would prefer that they ask questions" (Hickman, 2000, p. 40).

LEAVING INFANCY: MOVING TOWARD NORMALIZATION

Parents' reactions to the news that their child has a disability, then, will vary according to their interactions with other people—before, during, and after the time that the news is received. The meanings they attach to their child's disability will continue to change as their child grows and they encounter new interaction situations.

The ability of individuals to cope with any situation depends on how they define or make sense of the situation. Definition of the situation is one of the most difficult tasks facing new parents because of the degree of meaninglessness and powerlessness usually present. Because the birth of a child with a disability is generally an unanticipated event, parents must rely on other people to establish meaning for them. Professionals play an important role by providing parents with diagnostic, prognostic, and treatment information.

By the end of the infancy period, most parents have resolved their anomie. They may still be angry or disappointed by their children's disabilities, but they are beginning to understand them. If their search for an intervention program for the child has been successful, they are also beginning to feel in control of their situation. At this point, the child's disability may decline in importance in their lives; the all-consuming need to make sense of an unexpected and painful event will eventually be replaced by the resumption of concerns with other family members, careers, and leisure activities. The extent to which families will be able to return to a "normalized" lifestyle after the infancy period will vary according to the nature of a child's disability, available social supports, and other factors. These are discussed in the next chapter.

5

Childhood

Continuing Adaptation

NORMALIZATION: GOAL OF THE CHILDHOOD YEARS

By the end of the infancy period, the resolution of anomie is complete for most families. As their children move through the preschool years, parents generally try to resume activities that were disrupted by their child's birth and the period of anomie that followed. The mother who has left a job may wish to return to work; the parents may resume social activities; the family may want to take a vacation or pursue other recreational activities. Other parents, friends, and professionals encourage parents to maintain a "normal-appearing round of life" (Birenbaum, 1970, 1971). Paun (2006) argued that parents have a normality perspective because they are *expected* to be "normal" by other agents in society: parents' associations, magazine articles, clergy, and various helping professionals. These agents help parents rationalize their situation and teach them that they are *supposed* to be "coping splendidly" with their child's disability. Paun stated that families develop an ideology of normalization, which contains the following elements: (1) acceptance of the inevitable ("It could happen to anyone"); (2) partial loss of the taken-for-granted ("taking it day to day"); (3) redefinition of good and evil ("There's always someone worse

off"); (4) discovery of true values ("You appreciate your child's progress more when you don't just take it for granted"); (5) positive value
of suffering ("It brings you closer together"); and (6) positive value of
differentness ("It's for his own good").

The concept of normalization has been used in a variety of ways.
The classical definition in the field of developmental disability is
Wolfensberger's (1972). He argued that individuals with intellectual
disability should have access to the same opportunities for social participation as people without disabilities. Our use of the term here is a
little broader. We view normalization as a social construction, that is,
as a way of defining reality adopted by a social group. Conceptions of
"normal" social life vary from one group to another. For example,
members of an observant Islamic or Jewish group might believe that
normality includes praying several times a day, whereas in some other
groups, prayer may not be an expected component of the daily routine
at all. Thus normalization is consensually defined.

Although the components of normalization vary by social class
and other subcultural factors, in general a normalized lifestyle for
families with school-age children in U.S. society includes the following:

- Employment for either or both parents
- Appropriate educational placement for children
- Access to appropriate medical care
- Adequate housing
- Social relationships with family and friends
- Leisure time
- Freedom of movement in public places
- Sufficient financial resources to maintain basic lifestyle

Gray (1997) has shown that in one sample of Australian families
of children with Asperger syndrome, some components of normalization were more salient than others. For most families in his sample
"social outings and activities" far outranked other criteria as evidence
of "normal family life." He found also that mothers and fathers did
not necessarily agree about whether the family had achieved normalization. The presence of a child with a disability in the home can prevent a family from attaining any or all of the components of normalization, as the family members define it.

The ability of families to achieve a normalized lifestyle is determined by their opportunity structure, that is, their access to resources.
Society provides a variety of resources, ranging from financial aid to

respite care for children with disabilities. These resources are not equally distributed in the population, however, and for many families, life is a constant struggle. We suggest in this chapter that, regardless of the nature of a child's disability or of the personality or coping ability of the parents, the most important determinant of normalization for most families of children with disabilities is the availability of supportive resources in the community.

OBSTACLES TO NORMALIZATION

In a study of 330 parents of children with intellectual disability, Suelzle and Keenan (1981) found that perceptions of unmet needs varied over the life cycle. Perceived needs for family support, respite care, and counseling services were higher among parents of preschoolers and young adults and lowest among parents of school-age children. In a study of families of children with autism, DeMyer and Goldberg (1983) found that the need for respite remained relatively constant during childhood and adolescence. In general, practical problems seem to replace coping difficulties as parents' primary concern as their children get older. These include (Morney, as cited in Mori, 1983) additional financial hardships, stigma, extraordinary demands on time, difficulties in such caregiver tasks as feeding, diminished time for sleeping, social isolation, less time for recreational pursuits, difficulties managing behavior, and difficulties performing routine household chores, among others. These and other problems, which serve as barriers to normalization, are discussed in greater detail below.

Continuing Medical Needs

Children with disabilities generally require more specialized medical care and more frequent hospitalizations than others. In addition, these children may need medically related services, such as physical, occupational, and speech therapy. The availability of these services varies from one geographic location to another. Butler, Rosenbaum, and Palfrey (1987) noted that "where a child lives has become more than ever a predictor of the affordability and accessibility of care" (p. 163). They noted a study showing that 12% of low-income children among the most severely disabled third of special education students in Rochester, New York, did not have a regular physician, and 7% did not have insurance coverage; in Charlotte, North Carolina, 34% of the same group had no regular physician, and 32% had no insurance coverage. The study showed further that use of health care services was related to access: "Even for the most severely impaired group, the likelihood of seeing a physician was 3.5 times higher if the child had insurance coverage" (p. 163).

Obtaining insurance coverage for children with disabilities is often problematic. Some private insurance plans automatically exclude children with disabilities, and not all children are eligible for government-sponsored assistance, such as Medicaid. Some children "fall through the cracks," as illustrated by the following Internet communication (Internet, Children with Special Health Care Needs list, December 14, 1994):

> Linda and her husband have a four-year old daughter with Down syndrome. She has been denied medical insurance coverage under the family's group (employee funded) medical plan (because she has Down syndrome) and has also been denied coverage by New Jersey's ACCESS plan (state funded high-risk pool) because she is her father's dependent and "should be" covered under his plan.

One recent study (Davidoff, 2004) found that children with special health care needs (CSHCN) had higher rates of public insurance and lower rates of private insurance than other children. More than 13% of low-income CSHCN were uninsured, and out-of-pocket spending was significantly higher for families with these children than for other families. Maag (2003) found that unmet needs varied by insurance type, with nearly twice the proportion of disabled children with public health insurance experiencing unmet needs as similar children with private insurance. However, the children with public insurance also used more services.

Even in areas where health care is readily available, parents may have difficulty locating a physician who is interested in treating children with disabilities. Pediatricians especially tend to prefer treating nondisabled children with acute, curable diseases (Darling, 1979; 1994). As a result, parents of children with disabilities may engage in lengthy searches before they find a physician with whom they are satisfied. As one disgruntled father of a youngster with a severe disability commented, "It's like when you take your dog to the vet. . . . Not many doctors pick him up and try to communicate with him as a child" (Darling, 1979, p. 151). For a discussion of other issues relating to health care difficulties for children with disabilities, see Darling and Peter (1994).

Eventually, most parents do obtain satisfactory health care for their child. After their search is ended, parents may be reluctant to move to a new location, where they would have to search once again. Opportunities for career advancement may be limited as a result. Families' freedom of movement may also be limited in other ways by their children's special medical needs:

> There are things we'd like to do with [our two nondisabled children]. We'd like to take some trips before [our daughter] goes to college. . . . But we can't do that now. . . . It's hard to travel with Billy now. . . . Because of his medical problems, I'm fearful to leave. I don't want to end up in a strange hospital somewhere. Everyone knows Billy at University Hospital now, and that's very relieving. (Darling, 1979, p. 182)

Special Educational Needs

The quest for medical services may become less of a priority as children approach school age, but the search for appropriate educational programs often becomes more important at that time.

Preschool Education

For the child with a disability, formal education may begin shortly after birth. With the proliferation of early intervention programs in recent years, many children have begun receiving services soon after, or even before, they are diagnosed. These programs may be either home based or center based, although programs of both kinds typically involve parents as teachers for their own children. Some programs include specialists, such as physical or speech therapists, in addition to specially trained teachers. In some cases, however, parents do not discover early intervention programs until well into their children's preschool years. As one mother said: "[The doctor] said, 'Just take him home and love him.' . . . I wondered, Isn't there anything more? . . . When he was 2, I read in the newspaper about a preschool program for retarded children" (Darling & Darling, 1982, p. 133).

Most families begin early intervention as a home-based service, with developmental specialists and therapists coming to their homes to work with their children and to teach the parents special skills. For many families, home-based services continue in the form of support staff and nurses who assist with child care after their children have entered a center-based program or school. Although parents generally appreciate the help and support they receive from these home visitors, the presence of "strangers" in the home creates its own set of concerns, as the following excerpt from a parent report suggests:

> Hi! Welcome to my home, I think. I mean, maybe you're welcome. I'm not sure yet. When I get to know you, I'll know for sure. My child is disabled, and I need help to do all the things she needs done. So I need you. . . .
>
> Your agency sent you here. I called for help but I don't get a choice of who comes into my home and my life. . . . You call and tell me you're coming Tuesday morning, so I put the stack of unanswered mail and the unpaid bills in the cabinet with the cereal bowls. I race dirty and clean clothes up and down the stairs, shove toys and unmatched shoes in the closet and under the beds, and run the gauntlet with Fantastic to get fingerprints off everything, and then you call and tell me you have to cancel. . . .
>
> My husband resents people coming in and out of our home. He says he feels as though he is living in a goldfish bowl. He says getting help means sacrificing our privacy and spontaneity. (Unpublished document, n.d.)

Professionals need to be aware that the process of receiving services is more complex for service recipients than they might think.

Generally, by the end of the preschool years, parents have found a satisfactory program for their children. However, concerns about the quality of available educational programs are likely to arise again when children reach kindergarten age. Parents of children without disabilities may take for granted the fact that the school system will provide an appropriate education for their children; parents of children with special needs who have similar assumptions often learn that local programs do not meet those needs.

The School Years

Prior to the passage in 1975 of Public Law 94-142, the Education of All Handicapped Children Act (later renamed the Individuals with Disabilities Education Act), guidelines for the education of children with disabilities were vague, and parents' rights were not clearly stated.

Because of difficulties they had in obtaining an appropriate education for their children, many parents of adult children feel bitter and resentful toward the school system and, in some cases, even toward parents of younger children who have benefited from newer legislation and programs.

Special education legislation of the 1970s, 1980s, and 1990s (Public Laws 94-142, 99-457, 102-119) has mandated that children with disabilities receive a free and appropriate public education in the "least restrictive environment." However, for a number of reasons, including ignorance, fear, and the limited resources of school districts, the promise of the legislation has not become a reality for many children. Because of poor knowledge about their legal rights, many parents have not challenged their children's educational placements. Public awareness has been growing, however, and more and more parents are questioning educators about their children's programs. One study (Covert, as cited in Alper, Schloss, & Schloss, 1996) found that more than half of the families interviewed had resorted to either due process hearings or court proceedings to obtain needed services.

Parents may challenge their children's educational plans for a variety of reasons. One common complaint involves placement in an inappropriate setting. Parents may wish to have their child placed in an inclusive setting with typically developing children rather than a special school or classroom; in other cases, they want more special programming for their children. The former case is illustrated by this experience, related by the mother of a child with spina bifida:

> When Ellen entered kindergarten, she was in a special needs class in the morning and mainstreamed in the afternoon. . . . [In the special needs class], she was with children whose needs were much more demanding than Ellen's. . . . Some were retarded. . . . At the end of the year we had a meeting. The first grade was on the second floor [Ellen was in a wheelchair]. . . . They said we should keep her in the special needs class. I was furious. . . . She had done so well in the mainstreaming class. . . . I wanted her in a regular first grade and I suggested moving the class downstairs. . . . They wanted Ellen in the special needs class because it was easier for them, not for any other reason. (Darling & Darling, 1982, p. 140)

Another common parental complaint involves the lack of coordination among the various educational settings through which children move during the school day. In the past, when children in special education were completely segregated from children in regular instruction, coordination was not a problem. With the implementation of newer legislation, however, working relationships have had to be developed between special education administrators, evaluators, and teachers, on the one hand, and regular classroom teachers, principals, and guidance counselors, on the other. As Scanlon, Arick, and Phelps (1981) have shown, regular classroom teachers often do not attend conferences at which children's Individualized Education Plans are developed. Parents commonly complain that regular classroom teachers are not prepared for children with disabilities.

Another type of problem involves disagreements about the kinds of services schools are required to provide to children with disabilities. Parents may believe that related services, such as physical therapy, are needed in order for their children to receive an appropriate education; school systems may disagree. Some children require special health services in order to attend school. Children with spina bifida, for example, may require catheterization one or more times a day. In the past, parents had to come to the school to perform this simple procedure, often at great inconvenience. As a result of one family's persistence, however, the U.S. Supreme Court ruled a while ago that clean intermittent catheterization is indeed a necessary related service that must be provided by the school district ("Related Services and the Supreme Court," 1984).

When they encounter difficulties obtaining appropriate medical, educational, or therapeutic services for their children, many parents learn to become advocates, a role with which they may have no previous experience. One mother wrote:

> [After learning to fight for appropriate medical services] I had to turn over my Ph.D. in *Michael* for a Ph.D. in Education Law. From the beginning, everything about school was a fight. I had to learn the process of writing an IEP, which is an actual legal document. I had to know the law inside and out, so my kid didn't get screwed. . . . Maybe it is because I'm his mom . . . , or maybe it's because he had proven everyone wrong so many times . . . , but I am compelled to find a way for him. (Hickman, 2000, p. 95)

Parent advocacy and activism in educational and other realms are discussed further in Chapter 11.

In some cases, families living in rural areas have had more difficulty than urban families in obtaining appropriate educational services for their children (Capper, 1990). Kelker, Garthwait, and

Seligman's (1992) quote from a mother living in rural Montana is illustrative: " 'We like this small community. Mark and I both grew up in this area and we want our children to experience the same close-knit, family-oriented upbringing that we enjoyed as children. However, with Jeff's special needs we are questioning more and more whether we are doing the right thing by staying here' " (p. 14). Some of the problems faced by rural school districts include difficulty in finding qualified staff, funding inadequacies, and transportation difficulties (Helge, 1984). As a result, rural families of children with disabilities often face special challenges.

Behavior Problems

In a study of families of children with intellectual disability, Baxter (1986) found that the major stressors associated with the care and management of the child were (1) behavior management problems and (2) the child's continued dependence. The first is discussed here and the second, in the next section.

Baxter found that although concern about the child's physical needs tended to decrease with age, worry about the child's behavior in public increased over time. Behavior management problems commonly occur in conjunction with such disabilities as intellectual disability and autism. The following description of a child with both deafness and blindness illustrates some of the forms that these problems may take:

> When he gets off the bus Friday afternoon after a week at the residential school for the blind, he lies on the sidewalk kicking and screaming while his mother runs frantically to and from the house with various foods which might appease his anger. Over the weekend no one in the household is permitted to make program selections on the television because Johnny takes charge of the dial. Most of the night the family lies awake to the sound of ear-piercing screams, and the hours of quiet when they at last lapse into grateful sleep bring the morning rewards of ransacked kitchen shelves and mutilated books. (Klein, 1977, p. 310)

Similarly, a mother describes a need for respite from the demands of caring for a child with difficult behaviors: "How about respite from being repeatedly dive-bombed by an obsessive, perseverative, highly strung, hair-trigger sensitive, empathy-less when stressed, illogical, mind-numbingly boring and repetitive, chaos-making, labour intensive, screechy voiced demanding little person who never sleeps???" (A posting on the *Disability-Research Discussion Listserv*, July 24, 1999). Such nonnormative, disruptive behavior may limit the family's opportunities for social participation. As one mother of a child with intellectual disability and cerebral palsy explained: "He's hard to take with us. I always have to get a babysitter or I'll stay home. . . . It's really like having a little baby, only he doesn't outgrow it. . . . And we don't as a rule have people over—because he doesn't go to sleep" (Darling, 1979, p. 171). Still other parents write:

> The obsessive–compulsive behaviors and emotional outbursts make it difficult for me to take him to the grocery store, to a restaurant, or to friends' houses. We hardly go anywhere. In fact, we went to McDonald's today and he screamed in a high pitch a couple of different times when something wasn't right. . . . He uses inappropriate language, and won't stop if we tell him to not say something. . . . His developmental delays are nothing compared to the daily behavioral outbursts we put up with. (Hickman, 2000, p. 97)

> In social situations, it's hard to explain to people. . . . When you are at a birthday party, or a holiday gathering, and you are in a small area with people you don't know, and you are forced to be there for some time, people stare. . . . I choose to stay home most of the time. It's easier that way. (Hickman, 2000, pp. 183–184)

> As a family, we are all disabled in a way. There are certain things we can't do, places we can't go, and we are not welcome in most of my brothers' and sisters' homes. They say things like, "We'd have you over but we know Cody wouldn't have a good time. We don't have anything here for him to do." (Hickman, 2000, p. 112)

DeMyer and Goldberg (1983) reported that the aspect of family life most affected by a child with autism is family recreation. Baxter (1986) noted that parents are most willing to take such children to gatherings involving family and friends and least willing to take them to places involving other persons. Baxter found that certain social situations produced considerable stress:

- Formal social occasions where the child does not conform to norms.
- Other persons' homes where coping with the child's behavior is difficult.

- Public settings where behavior management is a problem.
- Restrictive settings that do not readily allow parents to withdraw from the situation.
- Social situations where the child engages in deviant forms of interaction with other people.

Parents feel stress when their child's behavior calls attention to the family. Although most try to explain the child's disability to friends or strangers, some simply control their feelings and say nothing or move away from the distressing encounter. Birenbaum (1970) has shown that some parents may try to hide their children's behavior problems by cleaning the house before the guests arrive or controlling the home setting in other ways.

Although the extent of a child's behavior problems may be related to the nature of his or her impairment, even families with children who have severe impairments may be able to achieve some degree of normalization if they have adequate social support. Bristol and Schopler (1984) have shown that family adaptation is more closely related to perceived adequacy of informal support than to the severity of the child's disability in the case of children with autism, and families without support may suffer considerable social isolation as a result of their children's behavior. As Bristol (1987) has shown, single parents may be especially vulnerable to such stress, although we should not assume that social support is lacking in all such cases. Baxter (1986) has shown, too, that small families tend to experience greater stress in care and management than larger families.

Often, family members and other potential caregivers are put off by challenging behaviors. As one parent explained, "I have often received financial and verbal support from family, but hands-on support is rare. None of them can deal with it. I feel angry about that sometimes while at the same time I understand it" (Hickman, 2000, p. 142).

Continuing Dependence

As children without disabilities grow older, they become less dependent on their parents. By the end of the preschool years, they are able to feed and dress themselves and take care of their toileting needs. Later they can go about the neighborhood without supervision, and eventually they can stay home alone, without the need for babysitters. Demands on parents' time thus decrease. Disabilities may limit the ability of children to achieve such increasing independence, however. One study (Barnett, 1995) found, for example, that, in comparison with other parents, those who had children with Down syndrome spent more time on child care and less time in social activities. Mothers allocated less time to paid employment as well.

The following description by the mother of a school-age child illustrates the extra caregiving needs of families of children with significant disabilities and suggests a simulation "exercise" that provides insight into the family experience:

> I tell myself I shouldn't need help, maybe in hopes that it will make me stronger. The fact of the matter is, I feel strong and in control—when I have help. . . . Just because I am a mom and a parent of a child with multiple needs does not mean I am automatically suited for this job. Don't get me wrong. I would not trade my daughter for anything in the world. I am a good mother, but this caregiving role is more than both my husband and I can handle by ourselves. . . . The following is a rough simulation that gives somewhat of a glimpse into the pressures of caregiving.
>
> 1. Pick a work day to try the following. It is important that you select a day that you are absolutely too busy to try this. "Your child" will be two 30 lbs. bags of bird seed, or something similar that is bulky and not easy to move around.
> 2. Get up early. You will need to get yourself ready and "your child" ready. It takes your child at least three times as long to do anything.
> 3. Sit in the bathroom 2 times, each for 20 minutes, doing nothing but holding the bags.
> 4. Get your child dressed. Wait for the count of at least 20 for each limb. No cheating. Your child needs underclothing as well as clothing and outerwear. . . .
> 5. Write a note saying what your child did the previous night and pass on any important information that would be helpful at school, especially since your child has limited means of communicating.
> 6. Pack a special lunch. Gather your child's equipment, at least three large bags of stuff (for my daughter this includes her brace bag, her DynaVox—an augmentative communication board, and her suction machine, as well as her power chair on Mondays and Fridays). Make sure she has these three large bags, her backpack with school journal and homework, and lunch bag.
> 7. It's library day. Find last week's library book and put in her backpack. Wait at the door at least five minutes past 9:00 A.M. for the late bus.
> 8. Finish up last minute details and get yourself to work.
> 9. Leave work one hour early. You're needed to carry out your daughter's care.
> 10. Reverse the morning routines. Put away bags and equipment, go

over school notes, and talk about the day; spend 20 minutes at least three times during the evening sitting in front of the toilet. . . .

11. Eat twice. Once for yourself, once for your child. (The point is not to eat again but to spend the extra time, getting nothing else done.) . . .

12. Dump four dozen small objects on the floor. Then try to get something done. Stop once per minute to pick up one item. (We are constantly wiping her mouth, picking up an item she dropped, repositioning her, or assisting her in some way.)

13. Do an extra load of laundry, even if it means you have to wash sheets and clothing you just washed. . . .

14. Don't neglect the rest of the family. . . . Take the children to their functions and/or run your errands. Use a wagon or something with wheels to transport your weighted bags. Each and every time you get in or out of the car, get the wagon and bags in and out of the car too. . . .

15. Spend a half hour patting someone's rib cage (to avoid pneumonia) and exercising their arms and legs.

16. Get yourself ready for bed. Start all over getting ready for bed (you are doing the care for two people).

17. Now, after everyone is in bed, take the time to get something done from work or home that needs immediate attention. (Adapted from a posting on the *Children with Special Health Care Needs Listserv*, November 20, 1998)

Similarly, the mother of two young adults (ages 21 and 23) wrote:

Both require assistance/support to be available to them 24 hrs/day. . . . Because we are family we are expected by society and governments to keep on keeping on with the intense parental role that would normally be associated with young children. If my son and daughter did not have a disability and were still living at home I would expect to be able to be part of the paid workforce, to accept spontaneous invitations and lead my own life as would they. The last time I had a holiday without my offspring was in 1982 and this was only for a week. (A posting on the *Disability-Research Discussion List*, 1999)

Even families with highly dependent children can achieve normalization if they have access to good support services such as low-cost, specially trained babysitters or respite care. A special camp in Arkansas, for example, cares for school-age children with disabilities 48 weekends a year in order to provide relief for the families:

Julie Mills, a severely mentally handicapped 10-year-old with a speech impairment, attends the camp.

"It allows us to be together the whole weekend, to go shopping at our will or just sit around and watch television," Julie's mother, Sherry Mills, said of time alone with her husband, Carl. "We become a little closer, get to know each other. It's almost like a date."

Susan and Mike Walker send their 7-year-old daughter Rachel to the camp so they can spend time with their 9-year-old daughter Dawn.

Rachel suffers from seizure disorders and mental and physical disabilities, Mrs. Walker said, and caring for her can deprive Dawn of attention. ("Camp Cares," 1986)

On the other hand, when such resources are not available, maintaining a normalized lifestyle can be difficult. Some of the difficulties involved in obtaining assistance with care include:

1. *Lack of sufficient funding.* Although many government programs provide in-home or out-of-home respite care, these programs typically are not entitlements. Consequently, funds are limited, and even qualified families may not receive all the help they need.
2. *Bureaucratic red tape.* Qualifying for assistance typically involves a considerable amount of paperwork and long waiting times. Families with low literacy levels are especially unlikely to be able to understand and complete complex application procedures.
3. *High turnover.* The individuals who provide caregiving assistance tend to be paid little and often leave to take more lucrative positions. Thus, even families who can afford to pay privately for care are often without help.

Because of the lack of needed assistance, most families survive by making accommodations such as working fewer hours, adapting family routines, forgoing social activities, or moving closer to family (see Gallimore, Weisner, Bernheimer, Guthrie, & Nihira, 1993, for a longer list of accommodations made by these families). Some of these accommodations have a direct impact on a family's financial well-being, as the next section will show.

Financial Burden

Childhood disabilities have an economic impact on families in addition to their psychosocial costs. This impact includes both direct costs, such as expenses for child care, medical care, therapy, and special equipment, and indirect costs, such as lost work time, special residential needs, and interference with career advancement. In a study of over 3,000 families of children with disabilities, Rogers and Hogan (2003) found that the existence of an impairment was associated with an increased likelihood that a family would experience job changes, and physical impairments were also associated with financial problems. One study of both direct and indirect costs (Honeycutt et al., 2003) found that the lifetime costs for a person with a developmental disability, in excess of those for a person without a developmental disability, were approximately $870,000 for a person with intellectual disability and $800,000 for a person with cerebral palsy (in 2000 dollars).

Direct Costs

In a British study, Dobson and Middleton (1998) found that the cost to bring up a child with a severe disability was three times as great as the amount required to bring up a child without a disability. Yet these families generally could not increase their income through paid employment because of the need to stay at home to care for their children.

In a nationwide survey of 1,709 families with children with physical disabilities, Harbaugh (1984) found that the largest single out-of-pocket expense was for babysitting. This finding is not surprising, considering the continued dependence of children with disabilities discussed in the last section. Yet because of the costs involved, some parents of children with disabilities may actually use babysitters less than parents of children without disabilities, even though their needs are greater. Harbaugh reported that, after babysitting, physical and occupational therapy costs were the greatest out-of-pocket expenses of the families in his study. These and other medically related services are not always covered by health insurance. Rogers and Hogan (2003) reported that the families they studied spent $1,096 a year for rehabilitation services.

Physician visits and hospitalizations are also expensive for these families, especially when they are not covered by private health insurance or public medical assistance. In one study (Butler et al., 1987) only 22% of privately insured children with disabilities had all their visits to physicians paid by their insurance plans. A survey by the National Center for Health Statistics (NCHS; reported in "NCHS Studies," 1992) indicated that low-income and Latino chronically ill children with special needs were less likely to have insurance coverage than other children. Butler and colleagues (1987) also noted that continuity of insurance coverage is a problem for both publicly and privately insured families. For privately insured families, job changes may mean discontinuity in coverage. (For a further discussion of hospital costs, see Darling, 1987.)

Medical equipment and supplies are also very expensive. The cost of a child-sized power wheelchair, for example, is currently approximately $7,000–8,000. Children with severe physical disabilities may also need special equipment for feeding, toileting, and other activities of daily living. Computerized equipment, which can greatly improve quality of life, is even more expensive. A computerized system that can be controlled by eye gaze (for individuals with little or no motor ability), for example, currently costs about $15,000. Most health insurance plans do not yet cover such items. Many insurance plans have limits as to the dollar amounts they will cover. Health maintenance organizations (HMOs) often have similar limits. As one grandmother related:

> My 7-year-old granddaughter's HMO limits the amount of PT [physical therapy] she can get (she was born with spina bifida). . . . My daughter has been "banking" her PT as she is going to need surgery for scoliosis and will need a great deal of PT then. . . . We find the HMO most restrictive. For instance, they have a $5,000 cap on wheelchairs. She's still using the first chair she received through a different coverage but has had to have new seating on it through her new HMO so is already into her $5,000 max by about $3,000. Consequently when she gets her next chair, within a year or two, she is [going to exceed the cap]. (A posting on the *Children with Special Health Care Needs Listserv*, November 22, 1994)

Medical costs are related to both the nature of an impairment and the age of a child. For example, one study found that the per capita medical cost averaged $20,658 per year for an infant with spina bifida and $16,560 for an infant with Down syndrome, whereas the comparable costs for a school-age child were $8,022 and $1,355, respectively (Waitzman, Scheffler, & Romano, 1996).

Other Direct Costs

A child's disability may also require housing or vehicular modifications, such as ramps, lifts, or widened doorways to accommodate a wheelchair. Klein (1977) noted, too, items such as locks for cabinets and bars for windows in the case of children who are deaf–blind. The father of four teenagers with a cerebral palsy-like syndrome explained:

"[We] can't afford the swimming pool, but water's the best therapy. . . . Where else can they go and swim almost every day in the summer? The city don't have it, so I have it" (Darling, 1979, p. 180).

Indirect Costs

Other, hidden costs may also be associated with childhood disability. Because these children require access to services and greater commitments of their parents' time than other children, the family's overall economic situation may be adversely affected. A mother, quoted in an earlier edition of this book, noted that her family moved to a more expensive community than they could afford because a good preschool program was located there. Similarly, another parent wrote:

> We were forced to leave the Aurora . . . Public School District for the express purpose of obtaining an appropriate public school education for our son. . . . The private sector is willing to educate these children—at huge expense. As one professional said to me: "Our attitude even here is, we'll take your house and your second car. Your husband has to get a second job; then we'll help you with your child." Thus, we left Aurora . . . knowing that we would eventually lose our home if we didn't. ("Readers' Forum," 1985, p. 7)

Some parents may reject opportunities for career advancement because services for their children may not be as good in a new location. The amount of parents' time required by a child's special needs may also interfere with career advancement or a parent's having a job at all. Lipscomb, Kolimaga, Sperduto, Minnich, and Fontenot (1983) found that the average weekly work reduction among parents of children with spina bifida was 5 hours for fathers and 14 hours for mothers. In 1982, the resulting average annual income loss for these families ranged from $8,000 to $17,000. Morris (1987) noted the cases of a mother who forfeited an annual salary of $30,000 to transport her child to speech and physical therapy and a parent who quit work and stayed home for 15 years to care for her disabled child.

More recently, one father wrote:

> I think there is a common perception amongst the public that the costs of raising a child with a disability are only in the costs incurred for medical care, etc. This is hardly true.
>
> We know exactly what the loss to society, and our family was, in dollar terms: $5.2 million. (Our daughter is a quad.) We know because a cer-

tified economist carefully considered all factors involved in the loss as part of legal proceedings. . . .

In terms of the things we definitely notice every day, however: my spouse had to drop to half-time. . . . Because she had to drop to half-time, and because there is a bias against half-time people, and because our frantic schedule means we don't have time for commuting so we need to work close to home, she earns significantly less than half of what she could full-time. Originally, we had both planned on working full-time after the kids were 10 or so, to provide for the kids' college, get ready for retirement, and do some things we had wanted to do while we were still young enough to have the physical vigor to do them.

I have not advanced as far in my work as I had expected to, before the birth of our daughter. I believe my salary is significantly lower than it would be otherwise, because my first priority is care provision and advocacy, not what I do at work. Many of the people I work with know and respect that, however the bottom-line is that you get paid for what you do at work, not for what you do at home. (A posting on the *Children with Special Health Care Needs Listserv*, March 15, 1995)

In another case, a family depended on public assistance because of the parent's inability to work: "I can work, I am educated, yet we live in poverty. He needs full-time availability and I can't do it all. This is a struggle. . . . Being on public assistance has its own stigma; having a child with behavioral difficulties appears to fit all the stereotypes of a welfare mom with a kid running amok on taxpayer money" (Hickman, 2000, p. 105).

Continuing Needs for Support

Needs for social support may be ongoing in families whose opportunities for inclusion in "normal" society remain limited. Such families may be geographically or linguistically isolated or may have children whose disabilities are rare or pose unusual difficulties in obtaining needed services. The following electronic mail requests (all from the *Children with Special Health Care Needs Listserv*) are illustrative:

One of my son's therapists called me yesterday and asked me if I had any ideas about finding some support for one of her families. . . . The family would love to find someone to talk to but have been unable to find any other people locally. . . . Speaking from experience (my son has an even rarer syndrome . . .) it makes *so* much difference in your coping abilities when you have someone to talk to who has *been* there. (January 26, 1995)

One of my son's therapists . . . asked me to put in another request about this, because they are having trouble finding someone to interact with a family of a . . . child. The major problem in this instance is that the family speaks almost no English at all—they are Hispanic. There is another child in this area with the same syndrome, but they don't speak Spanish. (April 27, 1995)

Thanks to all who sent me private e-mails about my [children's disabilities]. It really made me feel less alone, and I got some useful resources to look into (it is hard to find out about resources when you don't live in a big city). (November 10, 1994)

Stigma and Its Consequences

As noted in earlier chapters, individuals with disabilities in our society are likely to encounter stigma in their interactions with others. Moreover, Goffman (1963) has classically shown that parents and others who associate with people with disabilities are likely to bear a "courtesy stigma" of their own. As children get older, their disabilities commonly become more visible and therefore more stigmatizing.

Baxter (1986) found that the attribute most likely to attract attention to a child with a disability was speech, not appearance or behavior. Parental stress was also related to the quality of their child's speech. In order to prevent stigma-producing encounters, then, families may have to structure their lives to avoid social situations that would require their children to speak or perform roles that would otherwise call attention to their disabilities. Such children, then, may not be taken to see Santa Claus at Christmastime or to visit casual acquaintances. Parents' lifestyles may be limited as a result. (See Chapter 12 for a discussion of some interventions to assist families in responding to stigma.)

Physical Barriers

A final, major obstacle to normalization involves physical barriers in the environment. Individuals with disabilities and their families may be prevented from full social participation by stairs, narrow doorways, and hilly terrain. Our society is structured, both socially and physically, to meet the needs of people without disabilities. Although accessibility has increased in recent years, families of children with disabilities are still limited in their housing choices, vacation destinations, and general freedom of movement.

In a small number of families, normalization is delayed when family members themselves do not agree about their needs and their child's needs. For example, parents may disagree about the appropriate school placement for a child. In such cases, professional counseling may be required to resolve the difference. This option is discussed in Chapter 12. In general, though, socially imposed obstacles are the major deterrents to normalization for most families.

CATALYSTS TO NORMALIZATION

The strength of families is demonstrated by the fact that, given the many obstacles that exist, most are still able to achieve a nearly typical lifestyle: Normalization is, in fact, the most common mode of adaptation in our society. Achievement of a normalized lifestyle may be related less to the degree of a child's disability or parents' coping abilities than to the *opportunity structure* within which the family resides.

Opportunity Structures

All families do not have equal access to opportunities for normalization. These opportunities include the following:

- Access to satisfactory medical care and medically related services
- Availability of an appropriate educational program
- Supportive relatives and friends
- Access to respite care and day care, if needed
- Adequate financial resources
- Presence of accepting neighbors
- Adequate quantity and quality of household help
- Access to behavior management programs, if needed
- Availability of appropriate recreational programs
- Access to special equipment, if needed
- Presence of friends and social opportunities for the child
- Adequate and available transportation

Families' opportunity structures can be changed. Such changes may occur when a family moves to a new neighborhood or encounters a helpful professional. Opportunity structures are also changed by new laws and court decisions and through parental activism and disability rights movements. Professionals can play an important role in working with families to change their access to existing opportunities and to help them create opportunities where none exists.

Changes in Support Networks

As we noted in the last chapter, parents commonly become immersed in support groups consisting of others like themselves when their children are young and newly diagnosed. Continued immersion in such homogeneous groups can eventually become an obstacle to normalization, or integration in "normal" society, however. As a result, parents often decrease their involvement in segregated support networks as their children get older. As one mother explained: "We went to the Association pretty regularly for two years. But after awhile we felt that they did not have that much to offer . . . as far as help to us. . . . We just got too busy to go to the meetings. Karen didn't have a lot of problems" (Darling, 1979, pp. 161–162).

Parents may also decrease their involvement with other families of children with disabilities by encouraging their children's friendships with children who do not have disabilities in the neighborhood or at school. As one mother of a child with spina bifida explained, her daughter has some friends at "myelo" clinic, but she does not see them elsewhere. "They live too far away," and the mother will not go out of her way because she wants her daughter to be "as normal as possible" (Darling, 1979, p. 193).

Although parents may choose to become integrated into "normal" society, their success will depend on their opportunity structures—that is, "normal" society must accept them. A summary description of the family of the child with spina bifida, described above, illustrates such a successful adaptation:

> The mother reported that relatives thought the baby was "fantastic" and were very supportive during the first few months. Elizabeth attended a nursery school with children without disabilities and was then in an inclusive public school classroom. She has always been well accepted by the other children. Grandparents and other family members live nearby and continue to be highly supportive. They babysit so that the parents can take short vacations alone. The parents have decreased their involvement in a parents' association and, at the time they were interviewed,

were preoccupied with the "normal" concerns of running a business, wanting to buy a house, and preparing for a new baby. (Based on Darling, 1979, pp. 191–193)

Even low-income families may be able to achieve normalization with enough support, as illustrated by the following description:

> This family (interviewed in 2005 by R. B. D.) consists of a single mother, 19-year-old twins, and 16-year-old Robbie (a pseudonym), who has signifi-cant developmental delays and a seizure disorder. Because of his poorly controlled seizures, Robbie receives home-based instruction. Although the mother does not work, the family is able to make ends meet with the aid of government assistance (SSI for Robbie, Medical Assistance, food stamps, and a program that pays for a nurse to care for Robbie 5 hours a day), child support payments from the children's father (who works sev-eral jobs in order to meet his obligation), and financial and caregiving assistance from the grandparents, who live across the street. The family lives in a house owned by the grandparents. With the aid of these sup-ports, along with government grants and loans, this mother has been able to enroll in a local university, where she is studying to be a teacher. However, if she were to lose any of these supports, her future would likely be very different.

Furthermore, families who do not achieve normalization for other rea-sons may still enjoy the support of friends. As one parent of a child with significant impairments wrote:

> [Our friends] have supported us in many ways, from mowing our lawn to leaving money in our mailbox with no name on it. Some friends held a benefit for T and the money is being held in an account to be used at the time of her transplant. When T is in the hospital, folks from our commu-nity will drive 3 hours just to "pop in" and say "Hi." (Hickman, 2000, p. 145)

In some cases, the support comes from a church:

> Our church is the very best! Every surgery, every illness, every setback, they are there. The ministers call, the members call, they send cards, they offer to help, they bring food. . . . The most important thing, they offer help before I ask. They offer to travel the 3 hours with me to appointments. . . . They don't assume just because my parents are here, I am taken care of. (Hickman, 2000, p. 186)

When families do not receive the support they need in informal ways from family, friends, or fellow church members, professionals may need to assist them in locating other forms of support. Referrals to agencies that provide formal supports, such as respite care, financial aid, assistance with transportation, or supportive counseling, can expand the opportunity structure for these families.

Placement Out of the Home: A Form of Normalization

The placement of children with disabilities in institutional or foster care settings is relatively rare today because of changing norms and the increased availability of support services. However, some families who are unable to achieve normalization in other ways may choose this option. Residential placement may occur more frequently at turning points in the lives of children and their parents—at school-entry age, at the time of leaving school, when parents become older and unable to care for their child at home. If a mother becomes chronically ill, for example, she may not be able to continue caring for a child with a disability. Similarly, if a family's support network changes (e.g., the death of a grandparent who had helped with child care), the parents will be more likely to opt for an alternative such as institutionalization of the child.

Changes in the child can also lead to placement out of the home. As nonambulatory children grow and become heavier, caring for them at home becomes more difficult. Some children with severe intellectual disability also become more difficult to handle as they grow and become more mobile. In some cases, parents may come to believe that a child's special needs can be better met in a residential treatment facility than at home. Meyers and colleagues (as cited in Blacher, 1984a) have noted that the proportion of children with severe and profound intellectual disability who reside in their natural homes drops sharply at school age.

Seltzer and Krauss (1984) noted four categories of characteristics that contribute to residential placement decisions:

1. Child characteristics (level of retardation, behavioral problems, age, degree of care needed)
2. Family characteristics (SES, race, marital satisfaction)
3. Informal supports (friends and family)
4. Formal supports (social and psychological services, respite care, skills training)

MacKeith (1973) suggested three generalizations that can be presented to families to help them make decisions about residential placement:

1. In our culture most people live with their families and do better if they do so.
2. People go away from home if they are thereby able to get treatment and education that are better—and sufficiently better to outweigh the disadvantages of being away from home.
3. People go away from home if other people in the family are suffering from their continued presence.

Through some means, then—social support, access to resources, or removal of the child from the home—most families are able to achieve a normalized lifestyle. *Normalization is the most common mode of adaptation among families with children with disabilities during the childhood years.* In the next section we consider other adaptations and present a typology of family adaptations based on a model of differential opportunity structures.

TYPOLOGY OF ADAPTATIONS

In an earlier work, one of us (Darling, 1979) proposed a typology of adaptations observed in parents of children with disabilities. This typology was included in the two earlier editions of this book. More recently, she and a colleague conducted a study of 72 parents to see whether the ideology of normalization and other forms of adaptation continued to exist. The impetus for the study was a movement away from normalization toward "disability pride" among some segments of the population of adults with disabilities (this movement is discussed further in Chapter 6). The sample consisted mostly (92%) of mothers and was acquired through solicitation at early intervention programs, parent advocacy organizations, and a disability listserv.

The parents anonymously completed the parent version of an instrument, the Questionnaire on Disability Identity and Opportunity (QDIO), which had also been administered to adults with disability. The QDIO consists of a 30-item scale measuring attitudes toward disability and 15 additional questions about demographic characteristics, activism, and social participation. More information about the instrument is provided in Chapter 6.

A form of statistical analysis, called k-means cluster analysis, was used to determine whether the parents in the sample could be grouped in meaningful ways according to their responses to the QDIO. The cluster analysis suggested three groups. The largest group (about 61% of the sample) fit the normalization mode in most ways. These parents were more likely than those in other groups to work full time. They also were the most socially active, with 44% engaging in activities outside the home more than once a week. Moreover, they were the most likely to attend religious services on a regular basis. As might be expected, their children's disabilities tended to be less significant than those of parents in the other clusters (39% reported that their children needed no assistance at all in performing daily activities). They were relatively satisfied with their lives and were relatively unlikely to engage in various forms of activism, such as writing letters or participating in demonstrations to increase the opportunities available to children or adults with disabilities. Findings about the other clusters are included in the discussion below.

The Crusadership Mode

Although normalization is the most common parental adaptation through most of the childhood years, for some parents normalized routines are not readily achieved. As Gray (1997) noted regarding his study of families of children with autism, "normal family life was an elusive goal for many of the parents in this study. It was something that they all aspired to, but often failed to achieve" (p. 1105). In particular, parents whose children have unusual disabilities, continuing medical problems, or unresolved behavioral problems may have difficulty finding the social supports necessary for normalization. Some of these families adopt a *crusadership* mode of adjustment in an attempt to improve their situation.

Unlike parents who have achieved normalization, these parents may become *more* involved in disability associations and segregated support groups as their children get older. In a study of families of children with congenital impairments, Goodman (1980) found that parents who acknowledged serious problems in their lives and the lives of their children were more likely to be involved in parent groups. Parents' associations tend to draw their active membership from parents of younger children (who have not yet achieved normalization) and a smaller number of parents of older children with unresolved problems. When normalization cannot be attained, associations and the activities they provide may fill important needs. As the father of four teenagers with disabilities said: "The [association] is our kids' only social life. . . . I'm on the Board and I'm referee of the soccer team" (Darling, 1979, p. 162). Such parents sometimes come to play leadership roles in state and national disability groups.

Interaction with other parents of children with disabilities also provides ongoing support. As one parent wrote:

> [Other parents] are the tape that binds! Without some of my close friends, I would not know which direction I am supposed to be going! . . . One day my girlfriend called; she was having trouble with her son in school (he also has Down syndrome). . . . I reminded her that all parents get bad reports from their child's teacher and not to let it get in the way of her thinking. . . . On other occasions, she has helped me to think more clearly. (Hickman, 2000, p. 148)

Continued involvement in disability organizations is also an important source of information when parents advocate for their children's rights:

> There was a pupil personnel worker (PPW) who felt that our son belonged in a school for the handicapped instead of a regular public school, because he did not walk well. . . . To this PPW, a 33-inch 25-pound child would have a problem coping in a public school, but thanks to Little People of America, we already knew this wasn't true . . . parents should not stop pursuing important items just because someone says, "No." (Hickman, 2000, p. 159)

The goal of crusadership is normalization, and families who adopt this mode strive to achieve that goal in a variety of ways. Some become involved in campaigns to increase public awareness of their child's disability. Others testify before congressional committees in an attempt to promote legislation favorable to people with disabilities. Still others wage legal battles or challenge the school system to establish new programs. Crusaders, then, are advocates who try to change the opportunity structure for their own and other people's children. Some eventually achieve normalization and withdraw from involvement in advocacy groups and roles; a few, however, may continue to advocate on behalf of others in an altruistic mode (discussed in the next section).

In the cluster analysis described above, 12.5% of the sample seemed to adopt a crusadership orientation. Most of these parents were employed part time, and their household incomes were the lowest of any of the groups. Their children had the most significant disabilities, with *all* needing assistance with daily activities; their children also had *more* impairments than those of parents in the other groups. These parents tended to have less education than those in the other clusters, suggesting that they did not have access to as many resources to help them achieve normalization. Although they were the least knowledgeable about disability rights legislation, they were the most active in terms of engaging in activities to increase opportunities for their children and others. They were likely to feel sorry for people with disabilities and to subscribe to a medical model that espouses a goal of finding a cure.

Altruism

Because the ultimate goal of most parents is normalization, altruism is not common. As noted above, parents generally decrease their involvement in organizations and activities that emphasize their stigmatized status in society as their children get older. The departure of families who have achieved normalization from these organizations is unfortunate for the parents of younger children in need of successful role models. Not all such families abandon organizational activity, however.

A small percentage of families who have achieved normalization remain active in segregated groups for the sake of others, and individuals from such families are often found in leadership roles in national disability associations. Their motivations vary. Some are truly caring, humanistic people; some have a strong sense of justice; some are applying the principles of their religion; and others simply enjoy the social aspects of participation or the prestige resulting from their leadership roles. Altruists, then, are those who *choose*, for whatever reason, to associate with people with disabilities and their families even though they have access to opportunities for integration into "normal" society. In the study described above, none of the clusters approximated the altruism orientation. The small size of the sample may account for this finding, as the number of families in the larger society who adopt this orientation is probably not large. Perhaps families adopting the altruism mode of adaptation will increase in coming years as the disability rights movement becomes more and more successful in removing some of the stigma associated with disability in our society.

Resignation

At the opposite pole from the altruists are the families who, despite their inability to achieve normalization, never become involved in crusadership activity at all. Such parents are doubly isolated: They are stigmatized by "normal" society, and yet they never become integrated into alternative support groups. Some may become fatalistic, whereas others may have mental health problems resulting from stress.

Parents who become resigned to their problematic existence may lack access to supportive resources for a number of reasons. Some may live in isolated rural areas where no parent groups exist. Others may not be able to search for support because of poor health, lack of transportation, or family problems apart from the child with a disability. In the lower socioeconomic classes, especially, the burdens of daily life—of simple survival—may take precedence over concerns relating to a child's disability. Families who are isolated from the mainstream of society, because they do not speak English or because the parents themselves have disabilities, may not have access to the lay or professional referral networks that provide information on available resources. Crusadership and altruism are "luxuries" that presuppose some free time and the absence of competing demands on that time, often making those orientations unattainable for families living in poverty.

The results of the study described above are interesting in this regard. Although the sample selection process tended to exclude families living well below the poverty line, those with the lowest incomes in the sample tended to adopt a crusadership mode, not resignation. The third cluster, which did approximate resignation in many ways, consisted of mostly suburban women who were college graduates but unemployed. These parents reported the lowest level of social participation of any cluster (32% rarely or never participated in activities outside the home). Although some of these parents were activists, many were not. Perhaps the best way to characterize this group would be to say that they tend toward neutrality. They were especially likely to neither agree nor disagree with statements such as, "I am often excluded from activities because of my child's disability" or "My child's disability keeps me from working." Although generalizing from such a small sample (19 families, 26% of the total) is not appropriate, we wonder whether some parents are simply reticent individuals who avoid participation in many areas of life, regardless of their children's disabilities.

A Model of Modes of Adaptation

As the previous section suggested, by the time their children have entered adolescence, most parents have adopted a characteristic mode or style of adaptation to their disabilities. These modes are shown in Table 5.1. The reader should keep in mind that these modes are ideal types that are only approximated by real families. Some families move back and forth between modes as their needs and opportunities change. Ideal types help us to identify different family lifestyles, but they should not be used to stereotype families or to predict their responses in any given situation.

All parents, then, have differential levels of access to two opportunity structures: (1) "normal," or mainstream, society and (2) the smaller disability subculture, consisting of parent support groups, advocacy organizations, special-needs media, and state and national associations. In general, parents who have equal access to both structures will choose a normalization mode rather than the segregated mode of altruism. Parents who do not have equal access to both structures will choose crusadership, if their access to normalized structures is severely restricted, and resignation, if their access to both structures is limited or if they choose to remain uninvolved. Further research is needed to help us understand the interaction between opportunities and choices.

As children with disabilities approach adolescence, the adjustment strategies adopted by their families during the childhood years may become problematic. When children leave school, parents are

TABLE 5.1. Modes of Adaptation among Parents of Children with Disabilities

| | Type of integration[a] | |
Mode of adaptation	"Normal" society	Alternative subculture (disability as a "career")
Altruism	+	+
Normalization	+	−
Crusadership	−	+
Resignation	−	−

[a] +, integration achieved; −, integration not achieved, rejected, or withdrawn

faced with planning for the future and confronting questions about whether their children will be able to play adult roles. These concerns are discussed in Chapter 6.

A SUMMARY OF FAMILY CAREERS IN PROCESS: AN OVERVIEW OF EMERGENT PATTERNS

Several consistent patterns or styles of adaptation emerge from a review of the lifestyle changes over time, or *careers*, of many families of children with disabilities. This usage of the term *career* derives from the sociological literature and does not refer to an occupational sequence. Rather, the concept suggests an increasing commitment to a particular identity and role. The major determinant of the career path that any given family will follow is the social opportunity structure. When supportive resources and services are available to parents, they are most likely to choose a lifestyle based on normalization. When the opportunity structure is limited, on the other hand, they may engage in various forms of seekership (discussed below) or crusadership in an attempt to achieve normalization. The modes of adaptation that families adopt commonly change in a patterned sequence over the course of a child's life cycle.

Immediately after a diagnosis has been issued, parents are generally in a state of anomie; that is, they experience both meaninglessness and powerlessness in relation to their situation. Anomie is also felt by parents who suspect that something is wrong with their child and whose suspicions are not confirmed by a physician or other professional. Most parents experience meaninglessness because they have little knowledge about disabilities, in general, or their child's disability, in particular.

Parents typically feel powerlessness even after they have satisfied their need for meaning. Once they have obtained a diagnosis, most parents ask, "What can I do about it?" Parents have a strong need to do all that they can to help their children. However, most parents of infants with disabilities have little knowledge of intervention programs or educational or supportive services. All too often the professionals who issue the diagnoses are themselves unaware of available programs.

Human beings constantly strive to make sense of their experiences. When events seem random and we feel out of control, most of us try to rationalize our experiences and reestablish order in our lives. Consequently, when parents feel anomie, they are likely to engage in behaviors that will restore their sense of meaning and purpose. During their children's infancy, then, most of these parents become engaged in a process of *seekership*—they read books, they search the Internet, they consult experts, they write letters, and they make telephone calls—in an attempt to find answers to their questions and alleviate the anomie that they feel.

Most parents find the answers they are seeking. As a result, most parental quests end in *normalization*. By the time their children have reached school age, most parents have obtained an accurate diagnosis, found an acceptable pediatrician, and enrolled their child in an appropriate educational program. Many parents have also found support through talking to other parents of children with similar disabilities. Most parents, then, are able to achieve a nearly typical style of life during the childhood years.

Although the majority of parents choose normalization when it is available to them, a few may remain active in parent groups or other advocacy organizations in an attempt to help other people achieve normalization. Such parents forgo the comforts of a normalized routine and adopt an *altruistic* mode of adaptation.

Because of a limited opportunity structure, some families are unable to achieve normalization. Sometimes their children have more severe or unusual disabilities, or they live far away from treatment facilities. When parents do not have access to good medical care, appropriate educational programs, or other services, they may adopt a mode of prolonged seekership, or *crusadership*, and attempt to change the opportunity structure. These parents may join national organizations, go to court to demand that their children's needs be met, or use other means to create necessary services.

Finally, some parents who may not have access to services for their children may also not have access to the means for bringing about change. These parents, who are doubly isolated, adopt a mode of *resignation*. They struggle alone with difficulties created by the child's disability and often with other problems as well. Other parents may choose resignation or passivity simply because they tend not to participate actively in many areas of life, and disability activism is no exception.

When the child with a disability reaches adolescence, normalization is likely to be threatened. During the childhood years, most parents adopt an ideology of "living one day at a time." Once a child approaches adulthood, however, problems raised by the child's continuing dependence must be faced. Regardless of the adaptation they adopted during the childhood years, then, all parents must eventually make decisions about their child's future. At this time, seekership commonly resumes, as parents search for living arrangements, employment opportunities, or other services that their children will need when they are no longer willing or able to care for them. These searches and their outcomes are discussed in the next chapter.

6

Looking to the Future

Adolescence and Adulthood

When Aidan was newly born, "Down syndrome" was all I saw when I looked at him. But now I see that the syndrome is just a small part of who he is and what he will become.

—DWIGHT (2001, pp. 35–36)

In this chapter we consider the next two periods in the life span, adolescence and adulthood. Adolescence is typically a time of transition for families, as childhood ends and adulthood begins. Because children are "future adults," successful adults serve as role models for them and their families. For typical children, role models are not usually hard to find, even in their own families and neighborhoods. However, children with disabilities and their families may not have much interaction with adults with disabilities. Especially in families that have adopted an orientation of normalization, contact with disabled adults may be unlikely. Yet, in looking ahead to their children's futures, parents need to know about the diversity of outcomes that exist in the population of adults with disabilities today. After a discussion of adolescence, the remainder of this chapter considers these outcomes.

APPROACHING ADULTHOOD: A THREAT TO NORMALIZATION

Adolescence is a stressful time for most families, whether their children have disabilities or not. Blumberg, Lewis, and Susman (1984) identified a number of tasks that adolescents must accomplish: (1) establish identity, (2) achieve independence, (3) adjust to sexual maturation, (4) prepare for the future, (5) develop mature relationships with peers, and (6) develop a positive self-image and body image. In addition, Brotherson, Backus, Summers, and Turnbull (1986) noted tasks that are unique to families with young adults who have developmental disabilities:

- Adjusting to the adult implications of disability
- Deciding on an appropriate residence
- Initiating vocational involvement
- Dealing with special issues of sexuality
- Recognizing the need for continuing family responsibility
- Dealing with the continued financial implications of dependency
- Dealing with a lack of socialization opportunities for people with disabilities outside of the family
- Planning for guardianship

One mother wrote: "Outside of the initial diagnosis, families believe the most difficult time in the life of a parent of a child with a developmental disability, is the transition from school to adult life" (Simons, 2004, p. 4). She goes on to suggest a process of "person-centered planning," which focuses on the child's interests and abilities rather than on the parent's desires (and includes in her article a checklist for determining a child's skills). Although most parents want the best for their children, parents and children, including children with developmental disabilities, do not always agree. In a study of 71 teens with varying disabilities, Morningstar (Beach Center on Families and Disability, 1997) found that disagreements between the teens and their families were a common barrier in the transition process.

Continuing Dependence

> The hardest part is at night, when he's lying there peacefully and you're thinking the 100,000 thoughts of what could have been and all the reasons why this happened. You think that from day one, and I think you ask that all your life. And it goes on 24 hours. It does not end. (A 72-year-old mother of a 49-year-old son with mental retardation; Krauss & Seltzer, 1993)

In the typical family, the "launching" stage, when children leave home, creates stresses that have been called the "empty-nest syndrome." As the child becomes an adult, all of the parental energies that have been bound up for so long in childrearing are no longer needed for that purpose. Many parents, and especially those who have not developed occupational or other interests outside the home, experience some anomie during this period in their lives. On the other hand, Clemens and Axelson (1985) noted that in families of children *without disabilities*, the continued presence of adult children in the home can be stressful because it violates social expectations—parents *expect* the empty-nest syndrome to be only a temporary crisis in their lives. Parents of children with disabilities may find themselves in a similar situation as their children approach adulthood. The empty-nest syndrome is an experience they would welcome. As one father said: "We'll never reach the stage that other people reach when their children leave home, and that's depressing. . . . I wonder what will happen to Brian when he no longer looks like a child" (Darling, 1979, p. 184). The reader should be cautioned, however, that, as Turnbull and Turnbull (1996) and others have suggested (see Chapter 3, this volume), expectations about independence are culturally determined and not all families react negatively to an adult child's continuing dependence.

Although some children with disabilities *do* achieve independence during later adolescence and adulthood, many are not able to do so. Those with significant developmental delays or physical impairments that prevent the mastery of self-help skills will continue to be dependent on others, to some extent, for the rest of their lives. Most parents of children with disabilities begin to have concerns about the future from the day they suspect that "something is wrong" with the child. Some have suggested that these concerns occur more commonly among fathers than mothers during the early years (e.g., Meyer, 1995). During the infancy and childhood periods, however, parents develop rationalizations ("It could always be worse"; "Society will be more accepting by then") that enable them to see the future in positive terms, or they push it out of their minds. Until their children reach middle adolescence, most parents of children with disabilities seem to adopt an ideology of, as previously noted, "living one day at a time." This perspective is expressed by the mother of a 9-year-old with spina bifida:

> In high school, Ellen's going to be excluded. I always picture Ellen as being left out. So far, it hasn't happened, but as kids get older, being alike is so much more important. She'll probably have trouble in school—and what happens when she gets out of school? I don't like to think about it. We just take each year as it comes. (Darling & Darling, 1982, p. 155)

As a child moves through adolescence and approaches adulthood, parents are forced to begin thinking more seriously about the future. Some parents who had hoped that their child would someday be independent may reassess their situation at this time and come to realize that independence is an unrealistic goal. The parents of a 15-year-old expressed these concerns:

> We've been a little down . . . in the past year. . . . He's getting to be an adult. . . . He's never going to make it on his own. . . . The present is fine. We can manage it. . . . Our basic concern is the future. . . . We are getting older. We need babysitters constantly. . . . It's a continuation of care. . . . Joe really can't be left alone. . . . What if something happens to us? That's our basic fear. (Darling & Darling, 1982, p. 156)

Some families envision economic and lifestyle consequences as a result of their child's continuing dependence:

> When our daughter is through the school system, it's highly likely my spouse will have to stop working altogether, and I may try to go to a 32-hour week, due to the wretched support for adults with severe disabilities in this state. We might consider moving to another state at that point. Among older people we know with severely handicapped children, except those who are wealthy, the norm seems to be to care for the child at home as long as possible—often well into the 70s or even 80s. (Posting by a father on *Children with Special Health Care Needs Listserv*, March 15, 1995)

Parents such as these typically embark on a search for solutions that is similar in some ways to the searches undertaken by younger parents whose children have just been diagnosed. They search for such things as appropriate living and employment arrangements; financial and legal advice; and social, recreational, and, when deemed appropriate, sexual opportunities for their children. Suelzle and Keenan (1981) found that perceptions of unmet service needs were more widespread among parents of young adults than among parents at any other time in the life cycle. They found that needs for family support and services, such as counseling and respite care, exhibited a U-shaped function: They were high among parents of preschoolers and young adults and lower among parents of school-age children. As adulthood approaches, then, the normalization adaptation, so common among families during the childhood years, is likely to be threatened by a new awareness of unmet needs.

LIVING ARRANGEMENTS

Although they may have physical disabilities, many adults without significant intellectual limitations are able to live independently with supports such as personal assistants or modified housing, equipment, or vehicles. These individuals need to be included in planning for their own futures, and some may become involved, like their parents, in advocacy and activism to make normalized ways of life more accessible to them.

Currently, many adults with disabilities are involved in a movement to create more opportunities for personal assistant services. Many otherwise capable individuals are institutionalized simply because of a lack of availability of funding for personal assistants to help with routine tasks such as dressing or cooking. Personal assistants are paid employees who work for the disabled individual, allowing the individual to achieve a normalized lifestyle. The late poet Mark O'Brien is a good example of someone with severe impairments (including the use of an iron lung), who was able to live independently with the aid of a personal assistant.

For adults who cannot achieve true independence, a number of alternatives may be available, depending on where they live and their financial resources. At one extreme is institutionalization; at the other are various forms of community living arrangements. Although residential alternatives have continued to increase during the last two decades, many adults with major disabilities still reside in relatively large settings. Waiting lists for group homes and other smaller, community-based programs and for personal assistant services are often long. In some areas, such facilities may not even exist. Parents also have expressed concerns about the high rate of personnel turn-over in some group homes and the qualifications of staff there (Darling & Darling, 1982). In addition, Simons (2004) noted that in vendor-owned homes or apartments, the provider determines who will be hired, and families and residents have only limited input or control. She suggested alternatives such as personally owned housing, shared living, and foster homes; however, individuals with limited financial resources may not be able to take advantage of these options.

In cases such as the one noted above, parents decide to keep their adult children with them for as long as they live. Some expect siblings to accept or share this responsibility, and others rely on various members of the extended family. Most parents realize that none of these arrangements is necessarily permanent, yet many delay in exploring residential alternatives, continuing the wait-and-see ideology so common among parents of younger children. Many of these parents are ambivalent—knowing that eventually their child will have to enter another living situation but also dreading that time. These remarks by the parents of an adolescent with moderate intellectual disability are illustrative:

> He's never going to be self-sufficient, which means as long as we are alive, he'll be with us. I'll never permit institutionalization. Perhaps eventually he'll be in a group home situation . . . maybe an adult day program. . . . His brother and sister are being trained to want to take care of him. I don't want them to have him live with them but I want them to keep close ties. . . . We haven't really explored things for the future. . . . We live for today. (Darling & Darling, 1982, p. 158)

EMPLOYMENT OPPORTUNITIES

Normalization for adults in most segments of society includes independent employment. Yet individuals with disabilities may be limited, either by their disabilities or by employer attitudes, in their quest for jobs. Parents' concerns about their children's ability to achieve independence generally include the world of work, as evidenced in these comments by the mother of a young adult with spina bifida:

> Right now we're not sure what he'll be able to do and what's available for him to do. . . . I've thought for years, "What will Paul do?" His father and I won't always be around to take care of him. Paul's got to have a reason to get up in the morning. . . .

Eighteen seemed like a long time away when he was four years old. . . . Now he doesn't have any inkling as to the value of a dollar. . . . I'm concerned about what he will do. . . . Sometimes, I get so angry at Paul. . . . He's waiting for me to come up with an answer. (Darling & Darling, 1982, p. 162)

In some cases parents must readjust their goals for their children in accordance with their children's disabilities. The mother of a child with Down syndrome said: "There was a Down's woman who was a dishwasher at work. My first reaction was, 'My daughter will not wash dishes for somebody else.' Later, I thought, 'Well, maybe she'd like washing dishes.' I just want her to do whatever she wants to do" (Darling, 1979, p. 184).

Other parents may become involved in efforts to enforce the implementation of the Americans with Disabilities Act (ADA) in order to increase their children's opportunities for employment. Although the ADA requires employers to make reasonable accommodations for employees with disabilities, in practice many employers fear increased costs or other difficulties that keep them from hiring individuals with disabilities. Loprest and Maag (2003) reported that about a third of a large nonworking sample of adults with disabilities indicated a need for accommodations, including accessible parking, transportation, elevators, and modified work stations. They found that reporting a need for accommodation was negatively correlated with the probability of working. Thus, advocacy and activism are needed to increase opportunities for employment in this population.

Some individuals with disabilities may not be able to achieve competitive employment at all but may be able to work in sheltered or supported employment situations. Still others may not be capable of any kind of work. Being able to work for a living is a basic expectation deeply rooted in the American way of life. The capitalist ethic suggests that those who do not work are in some way morally inferior to those who are employed. Consequently, the realization that a child might not ever be able to do any work that is deemed socially productive is a difficult one for some parents.

SOCIAL OPPORTUNITIES

Parents' concerns about social acceptance for their children cover a variety of interactional areas: friendship, dating, marriage, recreational opportunities, and opportunities for sexual activity. As one mother noted, "Most families find the loss of the activities of school life difficult to replicate" (Simons, 2004, p. 11). Moreover, getting information may be difficult. As one mother said:

> I made a feeble attempt to discuss Bruce's sexual development with the pediatrician, but he seemed more embarrassed than I and suggested that I not borrow trouble. . . . Few medical and other professional people seemed interested in the impact which sexuality has on the entire family of a retarded person. (Meyer, 1978, p. 108)

Media images that reflect societal appearance norms make adolescence an especially difficult time for those with disabilities. As one adult wrote:

> The people on television, in movies, and in the music industry . . . seemed to be so beautiful, so perfect, so flawless. It seemed as if society and the media were saying that you had to look perfect in order to succeed in life. It didn't help that people with disabilities were rarely shown or mentioned, and, if they were, they were portrayed as helpless and asexual. (Abbott, 2004, p. 141)

Adolescents' attempts to achieve normalization have included rejection of the "disabled" peer group:

> When I graduated from special school, I said, "Thank God, no more handicapped people." And I slipped into college. The first year I didn't have any friends. My parents said, "Why don't you invite the old high school friends?" I said, "No, I'm not going to be associated with handicapped people anymore. I'm finished with that." (Richardson, 1972, p. 530)

In other cases, the peer group of others with disabilities becomes the locus of the adolescent's social life:

> His best friend has spina bifida too. He lives [nearby], and they talk all the time. He doesn't really have any other friends that he sees. . . . He goes to a spina bifida meeting once a month at City Children's Hospital. . . . He has a girlfriend in the spina bifida group. They write and talk on the phone between meetings. (Darling & Darling, 1982, p. 166)

More recently, some parents of young adults who were in inclusive settings in school have attempted to create opportunities for social inclusion for their children after they have finished school. University of Kansas researcher Ann Turnbull, for example, has spoken at conferences about her family's attempts to create an inclusive peer group for her adult son by involving college students in the community. Others have tried to combine living arrangements with opportunities for social inclusion by finding roommates without disabilities for their adult children with developmental disabilities.

LEGAL/FINANCIAL NEEDS

When parents realize that their children with disabilities may outlive them, they usually become concerned about providing for their children's future legal and financial security. Finding an estate-planning specialist who can help them plan for the future is not always easy. As one such specialist noted, "Planning for these families is planning for two generations" (Whitaker, 1996, p. 1). The writer noted further the importance of a long-term savings plan.

Beyer (1986) noted that if parents leave their assets directly to their child, the child may not be eligible for government benefits, such as SSI or Medicaid. He recommended instead that parents establish a trust for the child, naming a sibling or other person as the trustee. A special-needs trust specifies permissible expenses such as recreation and clothing that are not covered through government programs. Other options include master cooperative trusts, which pool the resources of a number of families. These trusts are set up by organizations such as the Arc. In all cases, parents should seek out a good lawyer, preferably one experienced in planning for situations involving disability.

An alternative to family or public guardianship of the individual with a disability is corporate guardianship (Appolloni, 1987). These programs have been developing in various areas throughout the United States and have a number of advantages, including standards relating to quality of life and the possibility of a lifetime commitment.

THE DIGNITY OF RISK

Perske (1972) argued that normalization includes the opportunity to make and learn from mistakes. Often, parents of adults with developmental disabilities try to protect their offspring from some situations they believe to pose risks to individuals with impaired judgment and reasoning ability. Perske argued that failure, however, is a normal part of adult life and that individuals with disabilities should have the right to experience failure along with success.

In a study of parents and their young adult children with developmental disabilities, McConkey and Smyth (2003) found that the parents' perceptions of risk were different from, and greater than, those of their children. The parents were especially concerned about hazards such as getting hurt crossing the street or sexual predation; however, actual reports suggested that these fears were exaggerated, given the experiences of most young adults with developmental disabilities. One mother of a teenage son described her fears:

> For most of his life, I have served my son, Nat, a buttered bagel for breakfast. . . . I never thought much of it. But now that he is 14, the breakfast has become a moment to worry.
>
> I find myself thinking about how I have to start helping him to perfect his use of a knife or he will never be able to live by himself. He is autistic. . . .
>
> I lay my hand over his to give him the orientation of knife to bagel. . . . But always I realize that if one thing goes wrong, he will end up with a terrible cut. How will he know if he needs a Band-Aid or if it's bad enough to warrant stitches?
>
> O.K., I say to myself, taking a deep breath and folding away the rising despair like the breakfast napkins. . . . We can always get him a bagel slicer. But my mind races. Toaster burns, electric shocks, power failures. And what about lunch? (Senator, 2004, p. 34)

Another mother described how risk is an important part of successful independent living for her young adult son with Down syndrome: "A cell phone provides all of us with some increased measure of comfort. It helped when he was lost at the Fleet Center and when he lost power in his house. But, everyday, since he lives two hours from us, Jon is allowed to take the risks that come with increased dignity and for that he is very proud" (Simons, 2004, p. 11).

DISABILITY IDENTITIES AND ORIENTATIONS

In order to assist their children in achieving success as adults, parents need to be aware of the ways of life and disability orientations of disabled adults. One recent qualitative study (Gilson & DePoy, 2004) suggested that adults with disabilities had diverse orientations. In a recent article (Darling, 2003), one of us proposed a typology of orientations toward disability. In order to determine whether this theoretical, literature-based typology could be tested empirically, I (R. B. D.) and a colleague conducted a pilot study involving a sample of people with disabilities (Darling & Heckert, 2004). The results of this study supported the typology and suggested directions for future research. These results are summarized below. (The descriptive information about the various types draws heavily on Darling, 2003.)

Background

As noted in Chapter 1, in the past, most orientations toward disability were based on a medical model, and people with disabilities and their families were commonly categorized on the basis of whether or not they had "accepted" and adapted to their limitations. More recently, a social or sociological model, which shifts the focus from the individual to the larger society, has become popular. However, not all people with disabilities share a common perspective. Because research and practice need to address diverse segments of this population, models that reflect the entire range of disability orientations are important.

Chapter 5 presented a typology of "adaptations" among parents of children with disabilities, based on opportunity structure theory in sociology. This theory is derived, in turn, from anomie theory, which assumes that most people in society desire the same goals. In the case of people with disabilities (or their parents), those goals seemed to center on "normalization"—that is, a lifestyle that was similar to that of people who did not have disabilities.

Is Anomie Theory Still Relevant Today?

During the past 20 years, largely through the efforts of the disability rights movement (e.g., Charlton, 1998; Shapiro, 1994; Stroman, 2003), the identities of at least some individuals with disabilities has changed, and a stigma-based identity model has been replaced by "disability pride" (e.g., Linton, 1998). Proponents of the newer model reject the norms of the larger society that label disabilities as failings and persons with disabilities as morally inferior to "normals." Swain and French (2000) described an "affirmation model," which views disability as part of a positive social identity and rejects older models that view disabilities as personal tragedies. They argue that disability is increasingly being recognized as a normal form of human diversity rather than as a condition that needs to be changed or eliminated. People with disabilities who adopt this view have been characterized as "proud, angry, and strong."

The affirmation model clearly rejects the notion, based in anomie theory, that everyone in society accepts the dominant cultural norms with regard to abilities and appearances. Although many disability activists clearly adhere to the newer model, large numbers of individuals with disabilities who are not part of recent social movements may continue to accept the older views and regard themselves as victims of personal misfortune.

A typology of current disability orientations would need to include both the normalization and affirmation models, along with any other orientations that were found to exist. In order to develop such a typology, one of us (R. B. D.) reviewed a considerable amount of recent literature about and by adults with disabilities. This literature included numerous autobiographical accounts (e.g., Kisor, 1990; Kuusisto, 1998; Mairs, 1996), media accounts for both lay and professional audiences, writings by movement activists, and published studies of various disabled populations by social scientists and other academic researchers. This literature review suggested that orientations to disability do indeed reflect differential access to opportunities to achieve either (or both) normalization or the alternative, affirmative definitions promoted through disability culture and the disability rights movement.

Table 6.1 is based on the finding that two primary orientations to disability appear to exist. The first, or "cultural majority," orientation includes acceptance of, and/or access to, generally accepted norms about appearance and ability, based on cultural values of attractiveness and achievement. The minority, or subcultural, orientation involves acceptance of, and/or access to, alternative norms about appearance and ability, based on a value of diversity. Access and acceptance are not necessarily coexistent in the same individual. In some cases individuals may have access to opportunities for success in the societal mainstream but may choose to reject mainstream norms in favor of identification with the minority. Conversely, individuals who do not have opportunities for inclusion in mainstream society may identify with the majority nonetheless. On the other hand, individuals may have access to the minority subculture but

TABLE 6.1. A Typology of Disability Orientations

	Norms/goals of cultural majority		Norms/goals of disability subculture	
	Access	Acceptance	Access	Acceptance
Normalization	+	+	+/−	−
Crusadership	−	−	+	−
Affirmation	+/−	−	+	+
Situational identification	+	+	+	+
Resignation	−	+	−	−
Apathy	+/−	−	+/−	−
Isolated affirmation	−	−	−	+

Note. +, has access or accepts; −, does not have access or does not accept; +/−, may or may not have access.

may not choose to identify with it or may accept its norms even though they are isolated from it. Each of these types is described in greater detail below, along with illustrative examples from the literature review.

Normalization

Individuals who adopt this orientation accept the norms of the larger society with regard to appearance and/or ability and achieve lifestyles that are similar to those of individuals of their social status who do not have disabilities. Those who have disabilities that are not highly visible may even choose to "pass" as "normal." Typically, these individuals have supportive families and employers and have sufficient financial resources to purchase other supports that may be needed, such as accessible housing. They are likely to welcome rehabilitation efforts by professionals, as well as technological advances (e.g., cochlear implants) that allow them to function more "normally." Conversely, they may reject "stigma symbols," such as white canes or orthopedic appliances. Most of their social interactions are likely to center around individuals without disabilities. A good example of this orientation is that of Henry Kisor (Kisor, 1990), a deaf journalist working for a major newspaper who functions well orally, who is married to a hearing person, and whose social life is almost exclusively within the hearing world.

Crusadership

As described in Chapter 5, "crusaders" accept the norms of the cultural majority but do not have access to a normalized lifestyle. Consequently, they become involved in the disability subculture in an attempt to achieve normalization. Their activities may include self-advocacy as well as involvement in larger social movements in order to create normalization-promoting social change. For example, during the 1970s, parents of children with spina bifida engaged in court battles to force school personnel to perform clean intermittent catheterization to enable their children to receive regular public education. Typically, when their crusades were successful, these individuals would adopt a normalization orientation.

A recent example of a crusadership orientation would be that of the deceased actor Christopher Reeve. After his paralysis in an equestrian accident, Reeve was prominent in the media as a campaigner for research into a cure for spinal injuries. Although his celebrity afforded him access to a wealth of resources, the visibility and extent of his disability prevented him from achieving the normalization he desired. Consequently, he espoused a medical model rather than simply affirming his new identity as a person with a disability.

Affirmation

Like crusaders, "affirmers" identify with the disability subculture in order to achieve their goals. However, unlike crusaders, their identification is not temporary. The goal for these individuals is not normalization. Although they may seek access to the right to participate fully in society, they continue to view their disability in positive terms as their primary identity. For example, a study of high-functioning adults with autism (Hurlbutt & Chalmers, 2002) found that they were proud to have autism and did not desire to be "neurotypical." Some writers have referred to this orientation in terms of "coming out" as a person with a disability (e.g., C. J. Gill, 1997).

Disability pride seems to include two aspects: self-esteem and separation. Russell (1994) likened disability pride to the "black pride" that arose from the civil rights movement, noting, "like Malcolm [X], disabled people must learn to celebrate our own bodies and respect who we are" (p. 13). The second aspect involves the rejection of assimilation or the notion of a "melting pot." Gill (1994) argued that ability and disability do not exist on a continuum and that people who are labeled by society occupy a separate and distinct social status. People who do not share this experience of oppression cannot identify as disabled. She wrote: "Politically and psychologically our power will come from celebrating who we are as a distinct people" (p. 49). Many of the leaders of the disability rights movement seem to share this view, and disability movements and the rise of a "disability culture" clearly have contributed to a positive view of disability. However, the view is not new; Anspach (1979) used the concept of "identity politics" to describe the connection between political activism and the repudiation of societal conceptions of disability.

Situational Identification

People are chameleons, able to maintain multiple identities or to adopt whatever identity seems appropriate or expedient at any given time. In some cases, these identity shifts simply reflect ambivalence or the inability or unwillingness to choose between competing norms. Thus some disabled individuals who have access to full inclusion in society may choose normalization when interacting with individuals without disabilities but may reject norms of "fitting in" to society when interacting with their disabled peers.

Resignation

Some individuals who desire, but are unable to achieve, normalization do not have access to the disability subculture either. They may be illiterate or living in poverty or in isolated rural areas without access to a computer. Such individuals are more likely to be exposed to the norms of the majority culture than to those of the disability subculture, because of the dominance of the majority view in the media and in society in general. Thus they do not have the resources to achieve normalization and also lack opportunities for learning about affirmation. This population is perhaps the least studied group of people with disabilities and the least likely to be empowered to speak for itself.

In one of only a few studies of African Americans with disabilities, Devlieger and Albrecht (2000) suggested that the inner-city individuals they interviewed were more focused on issues of poverty and racism than they were on their disabilities. They wrote: "In a way, one could say that in the inner-city cultural context, there is no time to deal with a disability" (p. 58). In some ways, their respondents had more of a normalization than a resignation orientation, because they did not define themselves primarily in terms of their disabilities.

Apathy

To include all logical possibilities in the typology, one would need to acknowledge that some individuals might simply be apathetic or completely uninformed. This category might include people with significant intellectual or emotional disability. Such individuals might be truly unaware of the norms of either the majority culture or the disability subculture. This lack of awareness would be unrelated to their access to opportunities for normalization.

Isolated Affirmation

Finally, some individuals who do not have access to the disability subculture may, on their own, arrive at an affirmation orientation. Sociological knowledge about the processes of socialization would suggest that such an outcome is highly unlikely. However, the possibility of innovation based on ideas derived from other social movements or related social situations cannot be excluded. The founders of the disability rights movement would exemplify this type. Early leaders of the movement in the United States, such as Ed Roberts, advocated affirmation long before it was a common disability identity. Today, isolated affirmers would be likely to join the disability subculture upon learning of its existence.

Empirical Evidence

Although no study has determined the percentages of the disabled population that would fit into each of the types described above, some evidence suggests that the affirmation categories may represent a larger share of the population today than they did in the past. A recent national survey (*National Organization on Disability/Harris Survey of Americans with Disabilities*, 2000) found that among the disabled population as a whole, 85% shared at least some sense of common identity with other people with disabilities. This percentage is considerably higher than in past years. However, people who identify with other people with disabilities do not necessarily accept the norms and goals of the disability subculture. In fact, the same survey showed that only 63% of disabled respondents had heard of the Americans with Disabilities Act. Many of those who share a sense of common identity may simply see themselves as part of a group of fellow sufferers who are not able to achieve normalization. Further research is needed to clarify the orientations of individuals with various identities.

The affirmation literature is probably the most rapidly growing body of writing in the field of disability studies today. The proponents of the affirmation orientation have tended to be well educated and very adept at communicating their message. Much of this literature presents a dualistic view, namely, one of a world in which a social (or affirmation) model is replacing the older medical (or normalization) model. Such a view, suggesting an "in-group" and an "out-group," is not uncharacteristic of social movements, in general, and serves a valuable purpose in promoting the rights of people with disabilities. However, sociologists need to understand all segments of the disabled population. Whether the identities of *most* people with disabilities have changed since the advent of the disability rights movement is an empirical question.

The typology presented above was intended as a framework for guiding future research in the disability field. Large-scale surveys are needed to determine whether, and in what proportion, the orientations described above are present in the current population of people with disabilities. The correlates of identification with each type also are an important research topic. For example, the nature and visibility of an impairment as well as the time of its acquisition (present at birth or acquired later in life) might be important variables in disability orientation. Some evidence suggests that those with more severe impairments (*National Organization on Disability/Harris Survey of Americans with Disabilities*, 2000) and those with congenital impairments are more likely to identify with the disability community. As one individual wrote in a listserv posting, "What have I lost? I was born with . . . my impairment. . . . I . . . am very happy with who I am" (Higgins, 2002). This writer went on to suggest that those who acquire their impairments later in life might be more likely to experience a sense of loss and to identify with the medical model.

The field of disability studies today includes a mix of empirical research and ideological writings. Few studies have attempted to link these strands of work. As a result, although the ideological literature continues to expand, we know very little about the actual identities and roles of different segments of the population or about how those identities and roles develop. In addition, further research is needed to determine whether parents' orientations toward disability, as described in the last chapter, are associated with the orientations their children later develop as adults. Although no large-scale studies of this nature have been undertaken to date, the following section describes a small, pilot study (Darling & Heckert, 2004) that did confirm the existence of a diversity of disability orientations.

The Darling and Heckert (2004) Pilot Study

Methods and Findings

QUALITATIVE COMPONENT

The first phase of the research consisted of a qualitative study involving depth interviews with a convenience sample of 10 individuals. All of these individuals lived in small cities or rural areas. An analysis of the data from this phase of the research supported the literature-based hypothesis that a variety of orientations toward disability exist. In particular, the researchers were able to identify the orientations of normalization, affirmation, crusadership, and resignation. The following quotes are illustrative:

Normalization

[Do you think of yourself as a person with a disability?] Not at all. [Why not?] I function real well. . . . I have a lot of family and my children, and there's nothing wrong with any of them. They don't consider me with a disability either.

Affirmation

(If I didn't have a disability) I think I would be a totally different person. . . . I am a better person. . . . I could never be that way if I were able-bodied.

Resignation

Well, I just love to be out and among people, and it breaks my heart when I can't. I just . . . I know my limits but I wish I didn't have them, but, praise the Lord, he knows best.

Crusadership

We're going to get all these doctors, hopefully, and we're going to give them an office booklet that explains the disease . . . , and, hopefully, it's going to make it a lot easier for people that have the disease, because the problem is the people who are supposed to know something about this stuff, they don't know anything about it. They don't know how to handle these people. . . . Five years, we're gonna have a treatment.

QUANTITATIVE COMPONENT

Based on the literature review described above and the interview results, the researchers developed a survey, the Questionnaire on Disability Identity and Opportunity (QDIO). The questionnaire was divided into two parts. The first consisted of a 30-item Likert scale with five response choices to measure the various dimensions of orientation to disability. The second consisted of 14 questions that identified demographic and behavioral characteristics of the respondents. The instrument was designed to measure the following dimensions of disability orientation:

- Access (to "normal" society, social participation, and the disability subculture)
- Orientation
  - Identity (pride vs. stigma)
  - Model (social vs. personal)
  - Role (activism vs. passivity)

Normalization was expected to be reflected in agreement with items indicating access to "normal" society, rejection of disability pride and the social model, and a lack of activism. Affirmation was expected to be reflected in agreement with items indicating access to the disability subculture and acceptance of disability pride (rejection of stigma), the social model, and activism. Crusadership was expected to be reflected in agreement with items indicating lack of access to "normal" society and acceptance of stigma, the personal model, and activism. Finally, resignation was expected to be reflected in agreement with items indicating lack of access to both "normal" society and the disability subculture, acceptance of stigma and the personal model, and a rejection of activism. Isolated affirmation and apathy were not expected to be found in a sample drawn from participants in disability-related organizations, and situational identification could not be measured by a survey conducted at a single point in time.

The QDIO was distributed anonymously with the assistance of three Centers for Independent Living, a social club and two assistance programs for people with disabilities, and an Internet listserv for people with disabilities. A total of 108 forms was returned.

Respondents ranged in age from young adults to those over 65 and included people from large urban areas as well as from small towns and rural areas. A little more than half (56.7%) of the respondents were women, and the large majority (76.6%) had mobility-related impairments. Like many samples of people with disabilities, these respondents generally had low incomes (65.7% had household incomes of under $25,000 a year). The large majority of the sample (87.6%) was white; 6.7% identified themselves as African American; and the rest identified with other racial backgrounds. About a third were college graduates, and the rest had less education.

Analysis of the data suggests that respondents had widely diverging orientations toward disability. The data were analyzed using k-means cluster analysis, based on the 30-item scale in the QDIO, to determine whether respondents could be grouped in meaningful ways. In addition, clusters were cross-tabulated with responses to the behavioral and demographic items on the questionnaire to determine whether the types that emerged correlated with other characteristics in expected ways.

A four-cluster solution emerged from the exploratory analysis. These clusters largely reflected four of the types in the theoretical typology described above: normalization (13% of the sample), crusadership (26% of the sample), affirmation (28% of the sample), and resignation (33% of the sample), although not in all proposed dimensions. The researchers renamed the types in accordance with the empirical findings; each is described below.

PASSIVE ACCEPTANCE (FORMERLY NORMALIZATION)

Because of the emphasis on this outcome in mainstream society, the researchers were surprised to learn that this cluster was the smallest in their sample. However, the use of disability organizations as a sample source may have biased these results, and we would anticipate that a larger proportion of respondents would fall into this category in a random sample of the general population. The respondents in this cluster were the least likely of any in the sample to have mobility-related impairments, and most reported that they did not require any assistance in performing daily activities. Most had had their disabilities since birth, and only one was over the age of 65. Most of these individuals participated in social activities on a regular basis and generally did not participate in, or support, activism on behalf of people with disabilities, nor did they read disability-related literature.

ACTIVISM WITHOUT AFFIRMATION (FORMERLY CRUSADERSHIP)

This cluster had the least education and the lowest average income in the sample. Moreover, they were the most likely to be unemployed or retired. They generally subscribed to a medical model and strongly desired a cure for their impairments. They were fairly likely to be active in disability organizations and to have participated in demonstrations or other activities to promote the quality of life for people with disabilities. Because the pilot sample was drawn from disability organizations, the researchers believe that this type may have been overrepresented in comparison with the proportion that would occur in a random sample of the population.

AFFIRMATIVE ACTIVISM (FORMERLY AFFIRMATION)

This cluster had the greatest degree of disability pride and the highest levels of activism in the sample. Most were younger, well-educated, and employed, and they had had their disabilities since birth. This cluster was the most likely to participate in social activities on a regular basis and the most likely to engage in various forms of disability rights activism, including use of the Internet to access disability-related websites. Again, because of the sources of the sample, the researchers believe that this orientation may have been overrepresented in the pilot study.

PASSIVITY WITHOUT AFFIRMATION (FORMERLY RESIGNATION)

This, the largest cluster in the sample, needed the most assistance in performing activities of daily living. They also were more likely to have acquired their disabilities during adulthood. Of all the clusters, they were the only ones to indicate dissatisfaction with the quality of their lives and were the least likely to have disability pride. Although they were dissatisfied, they were the least activist of all the clusters. However, their lack of activism did not seem to reflect a lack of awareness (a characteristic assumed in the original typology); they generally were familiar with the Americans with Disabilities Act and the disability rights movement and tended to live in urban areas that typically provide opportunities for involvement in activism. However, about half did not use e-mail or the Internet. Perhaps the individuals in this group were too immersed in coping with the day-to-day difficulties posed by their disabilities to be engaged in activism.

Conclusions and Implications

These findings provide a limited test of the social model of disability and suggest that both the personal (medical) and the social model exist in various segments of the population of people with disabilities in the United States today. In addition, some segments of this population do not appear to fully espouse either model. The study also raises some interesting questions about the interaction among opportunities, orientations, and identities. However, parents of children with disabilities might take comfort in the finding that adults with lifelong disabilities reported higher levels of life satisfaction than those who had acquired their disabilities later in life.

As this volume was going to press, we completed the analysis of data from a larger sample of 390 respondents. This analysis produced findings similar to those reported here. However, one new and interesting finding was the emergence of two normalization orientations, one of which included some disability pride. The primary determinant of a positive identity appeared to be lifelong disability, regardless of other aspects of disability orientation. Respondents who had acquired their disabilities later in life clearly had less pride than those who had their disabilities since birth. Although further research is still needed, these findings suggest that children with disabilities are likely to have positive identities as adults.

A Comparison of the Orientations of Adults with Disabilities and Parents of Children with Disabilities

The results reported above indicate some clear parallels between these adults and the parents of children with disabilities described in Chapter 5. The adult orientations of passive acceptance and activism without affirmation clearly mirror the parent orientations of normalization and crusadership, respectively. Further, the adult orientation of passivity without affirmation shares some, but not all, of its characteristics with the parent orientation of resignation.

The orientation that is conspicuously missing from the parent sample is affirmative activism, suggesting that the social model and disability pride are not common. If this finding were supported by large-scale research with random samples of parents, it would suggest that affirmative activism is learned in adulthood, probably through inter-action among individuals with disabilities in advocacy organizations, on the Internet, or elsewhere. As one man who developed affirmative activism in adulthood wrote: "You cannot have a pride or rights-asserting identity if you do not know that such identities even exist in the world" (*Disability-Research Discussion Listserv*, December 24, 2002).

The lack of a social model perspective among parents is not a sur-prising finding, given that most parents of children with disabilities are not disabled themselves. As Chapter 4 suggested, although most parents are able to adapt to their children's disabilities and achieve normalization, given a choice, they might still prefer a more typical life. One adult with a disability wrote: "Parents need to appreciate that their view of disability may differ radically from their offspring's view. For parents, disability may be an unplanned surprise . . . , a tragedy, touching and poignant. For the child, it may just be a given, something that is natural" (Blumberg, 2004, p. 24).

The research reported above seems to suggest that affirmative activism is the orientation associated with the greatest degree of life satisfaction among adults with disabilities. Consequently, parents may need to learn to foster this orientation in their children, perhaps by focusing less on medical intervention and rehabilitation and more on the value of diversity and the need to promote social change to broaden opportunities for inclusion in employment, recreation, and other areas of life. As one successful adult wrote: "Each week, as we drove long distances to the city for my therapy and medical appoint-ments, [my parents] never focused on the idea of a 'cure.' Their atti-tude helped me feel that while I should work to achieve the best func-tioning possible, I was perfectly OK just the way I was" (Spruill, 2004, p. 93). Another wrote, "Thank you, Dad, for giving me the gift of pride in being equal as well as different" (Kemp, 2004, p. 195).

Providing opportunities for interaction with adult role models might be valuable as well. However, some adults have argued that, as children, they felt uncomfortable in contrived situations that paired them with "role models." As one man wrote: "I felt the idea that they are disabled ergo I should warm to them strange at the time (I was 2 to 16), even a little insulting and still do" (*Disability-Research Discussion Listserv*, December 23, 2002). In contrast, another individual wrote: "Looking back on this period in my life, I really missed having a men-tor with some personal knowledge of disability" (Flood, 2004, p. 4).

One disabled adult suggested that a balance between passive acceptance and affirmative activism might be best:

I think it is an interesting question how best to raise a disabled child to be confident and secure and positive in their identity—whether to minimise [sic] impairment [the same individual writes, "Many of us with visible, congenital impairments are so used to the impairment that we are not constantly aware of it. We have minimised it totally!], or to celebrate a political disabled identity. I think people should have disabled and non-disabled role models. (*Disability-Research Discussion Listserv*, January 2, 2003, January 6, 2003)

Yet another individual asked, "How much [does] the minimisation [sic] of impairment [have] to do with having access to resources rather than having an impairment?" (*Disability-Research Discussion Listserv*, January 7, 2003).

Even those who have grown up with an orientation of passive acceptance may question this orientation as adults at times when they encounter barriers to normalization. As symbolic interaction theory suggests, identity is situational. Thus, exposure to, and consequent awareness of, affirmative activism may be a valuable component of the socialization of all children with disabilities in order to prepare them for situations of exclusion.

The development of disability pride is likely to be especially difficult for adults who were socialized by parents who promoted the acceptance of societal stigma, either actively or tacitly. As one adult explained:

Unfortunately, I . . . learned from my family that my disability, while not a problem at home, was not acceptable in public—as if my [juvenile rheumatoid arthritis; JRA] were a shameful secret. My parents never actually said that to me, but I believed JRA was not acceptable because it was never mentioned at home. . . . By acknowledging my disability at home, my parents could have helped me learn to assert my right to exist. I could have learned to identify my needs and ask for help—valuable skills for an adult with a disability. (Danielson, 2004, p. 9)

QUALITY OF LIFE

As noted in the last section, many adults with disabilities appear to experience high levels of life satisfaction and social participation. For example, a study comparing the life satisfaction of individuals with tetraplegia with the perceptions of professionals (Bach & Tilton, 1994) found that the majority of their respondents were satisfied with their lives and that their satisfaction was significantly underestimated by professionals. These findings support that of Albrecht and Devlieger (1999) regarding the "disability paradox." These researchers found that high reported quality of life is common among individuals with disabilities, including those with moderate to severe impairments. This finding appears paradoxical, because people with disabilities do not enjoy the same access to opportunities as others in society. A recent survey (*National Organization on Disability/Harris Survey of Americans with Disabilities*, 2000) found, for example, that in the population as a whole, only 35% of people with disabilities were employed and a much higher percentage than their nondisabled counterparts lacked adequate transportation and health care. The survey also found that people with disabilities are less likely to socialize, eat out, or attend religious services than people without disabilities, and that only 74% are very satisfied or somewhat satisfied with their lives, compared with 93% of those without disabilities. Although this last finding suggests a fair amount of *relative* dissatisfaction, still almost three-quarters of this population are not dissatisfied with their lives.

Albrecht and Devlieger (1999) reported that in their study, high quality of life appeared to be associated with a sense of control. Conversely, low quality of life was associated with "difficult-to-manage impairments, lack of knowledge and resources, and disabling environments" (p. 986). Here we can see that anomie (see Chapter 4) impairs the quality of life of adults just as it does that of parents of infants and toddlers with disabilities. For both groups powerlessness is reduced when resources become available to facilitate social participation.

PARENTS AND ADULTS: SEPARATE QUESTS FOR RIGHTS

Although disabled adults and parents of children with disabilities have much in common, including societal stigma and barriers to social participation, the disability rights movement has been led mostly by adults, and parent movements have generally excluded disabled adults. In some cases, adult children exclude their parents because they resent their parents' lack of an affirmation orientation. Parents, on the other hand, sometimes have difficulty envisioning their children as adults. Altman (1997) noted that new legal rights provided by the Americans with Disabilities Act and new attitudes toward independent living may provide a basis for shared action.

Turnbull and Turnbull (1993) suggested some bases for *rapprochement* between adults and parents: (1) connecting children and their families with adult role models; (2) fostering decision making and self-determination skills in children, starting from the earliest years; (3) approaching transition as a generic issue by focusing on similarities among transitions at various life stages; (4) focusing on family services and support through the life span, not just during early childhood. In addition, professionals who work with parents might encourage them to get involved in the disability rights movement by pointing out the common issues faced by individuals with disabilities of all ages and by encouraging them to view their children from a life-span perspective.

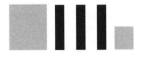

THE FAMILY SYSTEM

7

Effects on the Family
as a System

As in the previous edition of *Ordinary Families, Special Children*, we believe that it is misleading to draw firm conclusions about the extent and depth of the challenges experienced by families of children with disabilities. It is also difficult to ascertain whether these families are better or worse off than comparable families in which no child or adolescent with special needs resides. We believe that these assertions hold true in this edition as well.

Methodological problems (Crnic, Friedrich, & Greenberg, 1983; Berger & Foster, 1986; Trute, 1995; Blacher, 2003; Hatton, Blacher, & Llewellyn, 2003) have resulted in inconclusive results. Some earlier contributors to the professional literature reported that the trauma and unrelenting stress of coping with a child or adolescent with a disability can be difficult at best, if not immobilizing.

Even though there are inconsistent and contradictory findings, in general, the available literature suggests that families of children with mental retardation and other childhood disabilities are at risk for numerous difficulties in comparison to families with children without retardation (Crnic, Friedrich, et al., 1983; Marshak & Prezant, 2007). Patterson (1991) cited studies reporting that parents of children with disabilities have more health and psychological problems and experience a diminished sense of mastery. Furthermore, mothers seem to be vulnerable when they absorb family stress and attempt to protect the rest of the family from it. And although divorce rates of these families are comparable to those of other families, there tends to be more reported marital distress among families of children with disabilities (Marshak & Prezant, 2007). Maternal stress and marital problems are further discussed in subsequent sections of this chapter.

What is known about family adjustment is derived from empirical data and anecdotal accounts authored by family members, especially those from mothers. Poignant accounts written by family members describe their experiences of parenting a child with a disability (see the magazine *The Exceptional Parent*; Turnbull & Turnbull's *Parents Speak Out* [1985]; Helen Featherstone's *A Difference in the Family* [1980]; D. J. Meyer's *Uncommon Fathers* [1995]; Moorman's *My Sister's Keeper* [1992b]; Klein & Schive's *You Will Dream New Dreams* (2001); Klein & Kemp's *Reflections from a Different Journey* (2004); and Ariel and Naseef's *Voices from the Spectrum* [2006], among others). Personal accounts provide rich insights into the questions of impact and coping, yet from a research perspective there are questions about how representative these views are of the broader population of families. For example, many of these personal stories are written by educated, articulate individuals, prompting questions about parents who are in the throes of poverty, otherwise troubled families, and those who are poorly educated. This is not meant to diminish the value of personal testaments. Our intent is to promote the complementary value of both personal observations and research, where each adds to the other.

Much of the research has been from the mother's perspective, and it is not unusual for mothers to be asked about the adjustment of other family members (Hornby, 1994a). A mother's view of another family member's functioning has value, but this type of information should not take the place of, nor should it be interpreted as necessarily accurate information about, other family members. Because of the emphasis on mothers in the literature, many of the studies described in this chapter are based on their perspectives; this emphasis is also why there is no separate chapter on mothers here. The remaining three chapters in this section focus specifically on fathers, siblings, and grandparents.

Much of the early research was conducted on families of children with mental retardation, especially with children with severe retardation (Farber, 1959, 1960b; Ross, 1964), leaving a gap in our understanding of families of children with other disabilities or those with chronic illnesses. There continues to be a disproportionate number of studies published about these families, but the situation is changing as research and commentary in other areas are being published with greater frequency. Publications examining other impairments are appearing in the professional literature; for example, hearing impairment (Israelite, 1985; Sloman, Springer, & Vachon, 1993; Moores, 2006), epilepsy (Lechtenberg, 1984), chronic illness (Thompson & Gustafson, 1996; Pollin, 1995; Rolland, 2003; Travis, 1976; Turk & Kerns, 1985), spina bifida (Fagan & Schor, 1993; Tew, Lawrence, Payne, & Rawnsley, 1977), autism (Harris, 1994; Harris & Glasberg, 2003; Schopler & Mesibov, 1984), hemophilia (Varekamp et al., 1990), and mental illness (MacGregor, 1994; Marsh, 1998; Ufner, 2004). These developments are important, yet their segregated nature implies that families of children with different impairments are more dissimilar than alike. We examine this assumption more closely later in this chapter.

Separate lines of inquiry are developing, which can imply that some impairments exert a more stressful influence on the family than others. In reality we know little about the differential impact of children and youth with dissimilar conditions, but the research, with its segregated literature, may contribute to misleading conclusions. We also have not sufficiently explored the effects of mild–moderate versus severe impairment on the family.

As noted above, mothers' experiences have been explored with far greater frequency than those of other family members, and many of the studies cited in this chapter used mothers as subjects. That focus is beginning to change also, as more attention is directed toward siblings (Grossman, 1972; Seligman, 1991a; Stoneman & Berman, 1993; Wasserman, 1983; McHugh, 1999; Simon, 1997; Safer, 2002; Harris & Glasberg, 2003), fathers (Lamb & Meyer, 1991; Meyer, 1995; Naseef, 2001; Quinn, 1999; Ricci & Hodapp, 2003), and even grandparents and other extended family members (Seligman, 1991a, 1991b; Sonnek, 1986; Green, 2001; Frisco, 2002; Kornhaber, 2002).

The changing nature of the family has made it even more difficult to study the effects of childhood disability on family life. The heterosexual, married, two-child family continues to exist alongside other family configurations (Goldenberg & Goldenberg, 2003; Chapter 3, this volume). Another area that needs more research attention is the question of family adaptation over time. Longitudinal research requires long-term commitment, financial resources, and institutional support to carry out; thus this important long-term perspective tends not to be implemented. Given the stages and transitions families experience, this type of developmental perspective should receive more research attention. Innovative research models also need to be considered more seriously, such as Goode's (1984) in-depth examination of the public presentation of a family with a deaf–blind child. He used a naturalistic/observational research design to study this phenomenon. Only a handful of studies have used observational models. Other research-related problems include an overreliance on self-reports in studies of parental adjustment; as noted, the study of mothers predominates at the expense of information about other family members; and comparison groups are often lacking or poorly selected (Thompson & Gustafson, 1996). Finally, research on families from non-American countries, other cultures, and different ethnic groups is in short supply (Harry, 1992a; Mary, 1990; Turnbull & Turnbull, 2001), but studies are beginning to appear (Hatton et al., 2003; Blacher, 2003; Olsson & Hwang, 2003; Turnbull, Turnbull, Erwin, & Soodak, 2006).

The preceding section represents the backdrop against which the following discussion proceeds. We acknowledge that there are few definitive answers to the vexing questions regarding the impact of childhood disability on family life. However, we discuss notable trends, associations, assertions, and tentative conclusions.

STAGES OF MOURNING

This section addresses the effects of first knowledge of disability on the family. Generally speaking, when a chronic illness or developmental disability is first disclosed, there is a period of disequilibrium and a series of adjustments that need to be made by family members as they negotiate a complicated, sometimes bumpy road to normalization. Here we briefly review the stages parents are thought to experience after learning of their child's disability. This chapter also explores additional concepts related to early knowledge. Unlike the discussion of the reactions to first information in Chapter 4, this discussion is derived from the psychological literature on adjustment and coping.

Stage theory, as it has been applied to parents of children with disabilities, has been subject to some controversy including a lack of empirical support (Blacher, 1984b; Mary, 1990; Olshansky, 1962; Searle, 1978). Malow-Iroff and Johnson (2005) questioned whether parents go through a grieving process as suggested by some. Their belief is that families do not negotiate stages in any particular order. They contended that the parents' response to childhood disability is as varied as the personalities in the family as well as the nature of the disability, the cultural context, and their economic well-being. Stages can be conceptually confusing. For example, "acceptance" may be an end point for one theory and a temporary stop for another. Another problem is that most of the limited studies in this area have been done with European American middle- to upper-middle-class subjects (Cook, Klein, & Tessier, 2004). An exception to this approach is Mary (1990), who found in her small-scale study that only 25% of the African American mothers of children with disabilities felt that they had experienced a progression of emotions (stages) over time, compared to 68% for whites and 75% for the Latino mothers. Mothers with some education and experience in utilizing human services seemed better at articulating a stage theory model—or perhaps in articulating a stage theory model that had been proposed to them. Another investigation, aimed at examining the grief process, studied 130 families (Anderegg, Vergason, & Smith, 1992). The authors produced a three-stage theory that both resembles other theories and differs from them. The stages are (1) confrontation (denial, blame/guilt, shock), (2) adjustment (depression, anger, bargaining), and (3) adaptation (life-cycle changes, realistic planning, adjustment of expectations).

Duncan (1977) adapted Kübler-Ross's (1969) stages, which characterize reactions to impending death, to the event of the diagnosis of childhood disability. As Marshak and Prezant (2007) have pointed out, "Many parents grieve with the same emotion and intensity often experienced when a loved one dies. This intensity of grief is normal, because parents often are mourning the death of the child they had envisioned having and the dreams attached to that child." Due to the complexity and uniqueness of families and the unpredictable impact an event may have, these stages should be applied in a flexible manner. Knowledge of these stages can help professionals understand family response to a crisis in context and not regard their behavior as inappropriate, chaotic, or pathological. Also, being aware of these stages enables professionals to intervene in a timely and appropriate fashion.

Some parents may not be able to accept their child's condition. Cook et al. (2004) asserted that it is the responsibility of service providers to help families cope with the demands of their reality. Grieving for the child they had hoped for is not something that all parents do easily: "Some people brace themselves against mourning even when they feel grief welling up because they equate it with weakness, succumbing, and loss of emotional control" (Marshak & Prezant, 2007). According to Marshak and Prezant, the expression of grief is so individualistic that one should not equate mourning with a barometer of love. That is, one partner may be overwhelmed with grief while the other one is more stoic. It is a mistake to believe that one is grieving while the other one is not, and thus, is less troubled by the loss. Kübler-Ross's (1969) stages are as follows:

1. Denial
2. Bargaining
3. Anger
4. Depression
5. Acceptance

A parent's initial responses tend to be *shock* and *Denial*, just like one's reaction to any traumatic news about a family member. Denial operates on an unconscious level to ward off excessive anxiety. It serves a useful, buffering purpose early on but can cause difficulties if it persists. If in the face of clear evidence and over an extended period, parents continue to deny the existence of their child's disability, the child may be pushed beyond his or her capabilities; parents may fail to enroll their child in beneficial early intervention programs or may make endless and pointless visits to professionals to secure an acceptable diagnosis. Some parents who fail to come to grips with the situation ignore or neglect other family members while attempting to prove that their child's diagnosis was wrong. Sometimes these attempts take the form of intensive self-instruction (Cook et al., 2004). Denial can undermine realistic solutions. How dysfunctional and resistant the denial become depend on the parents' psychological makeup, the nature and severity of the disability, and the types of support and assistance that are available (Hardman, Drew, & Egan, 2002). Marshak and Prezant (2007) found that gender plays a major role in parental response to their child's diagnosis. To quote one of the parents they intervened, "Moms often blame themselves for the child's disability, while the dads are more removed." They cited cross-gender communication experts, Deborah Tannen and John Gray, who assert that men are likely to attack or withdraw from a problem, rather than use emotional expression as their coping style in the face of a crisis.

During this stage, parents report feeling confusion, numbness, emotional disorganization (Blacher, 1984b), and helplessness. Attempts are made to find out what is wrong with their baby—often in the hopes of finding someone who will say that the baby will be fine.

Some parents are unable to hear much of what they are told when the child is diagnosed:

> One mother told me that when the pediatrician told her that her 18-month-old son had cerebral palsy, she "burst into tears" and didn't hear anything else. Another mother recalled how she had listened very calmly as the neurologist explained the extent of the brain damage her 14-year-old daughter had sustained as the result of a car accident. Then she got in her car and began to drive home, but after a few hundred yards, as she was crossing a bridge, she felt sick and her legs felt like they'd turned to jelly, so she got out of the car and leaned over the side of the bridge to get some air. (Hornby, 1994a, p. 16)

It is important for professionals to realize that, after they have communicated a diagnosis, parents may not be in an emotional state that allows them to hear the details or the implications and prognosis (Hardman et al., 2002). The professional can add to parents' discomfort during a diagnostic meeting because, as one therapist said (as quoted in Nissenbaum, Tollefson, & Reese, 2002, p. 36), they can, "sense the tension in our voices and I think they react to it. They know something is wrong with their child just by our behavior. Our anxiety brings out their own anxiety." During this period professionals may avoid making the child's diagnosis explicit and instead mistakenly offer services before parents are ready (Turnbull et al., 2006). Withholding or creating ambiguity about the diagnosis enhances the parents' anxiety. By not communicating the diagnosis, the professional is protecting him- or herself from distressing emotion rather than protecting the parents.

Furthermore, explanations about etiology, course, and prognosis may fall on deaf ears. Professionals need to deliver the diagnosis honestly and with compassion and respond to any questions the parents may have. The questions parents ask at this juncture probably reflect the answers they are prepared to hear. Most importantly, the professional involved during this initial diagnosis stage (usually a physician) should consider scheduling another meeting in which he or she can review the details of the disability and respond to any questions the parents may have.

The *bargaining* phase is characterized by a type of magical or fantasy thinking. The underlying theme is that, if the parent works extra hard, the child will improve. For example, a child's improved condition is compensation for hard work. It is a negotiation with God. Parents may join local groups in activities that benefit a particular cause during this phase. Another manifestation of the bargaining phase is turning to religion or looking for a miracle—which sometimes can result in shopping for an acceptable, or at least more benign, diagnosis. Poston and Turnbull (2004) contended that research has consistently shown that children with disabilities are a catalyst for families to increase their spirituality.

As parents realize that their child will not improve significantly, *anger* develops. There may be anger at God ("Why me?") or at oneself or one's spouse for having produced the child or for not helping. Professionals make convenient targets for not healing the child (doctors) or for not helping their child make significant learning gains (teachers). Anger can also come from the perception of an unsympathetic community, insensitive professionals, inadequate services, fatigue due to long hospital stays, and the like. Excessive guilt can sometimes turn anger inward, so that a parent blames him- or herself for the disability. Anger turned inward often results in depression. Professionals should allow and encourage parents to express their normal and understandable anger, depression, and anxiety. This means that professionals need to be comfortable with these emotions, which is not easy for those who have learned from their families of origin that emotions are not positive and should remain private.

When parents realize that their anger doesn't change their child's condition and they accept the chronic nature of the disability and its implications for the family, *depression* may set in. Depression for most parents is temporary or episodic, possibly coinciding with a particular stage of the family life cycle. Developmental transitions imply change and invite comparisons with other children and families. These periods are time bound, and the seriousness of the depression depends on how family members interpret an event and on their coping abilities. It is important for the professional to be able to distinguish clinical depression from milder forms of dysphoria. Deep sadness, an inability to find joy in life, problems with eating or sleeping, concentration difficulties, and sometimes suicidal thinking characterize clinical depression. When depression is intractable and significantly interferes with life, professional counseling, with or without medication, may be necessary. When appropriate, professionals need to find tactful ways to suggest to parents that counseling can help ease their worries and anxieties (Cook et al., 2004).

For some parents, *detachment* follows anger and they report feeling empty, as if nothing seems to matter (Hornby, 1994a). Life has lost its meaning. This reaction is thought to indicate a turning point in the adaptation process as the parent reluctantly begins to accept the realty of the disability. In the same vein, Hardman et al. (2002) referred to a process of *defensive retreat* that occurs when parents have an urge to avoid the anxiety-provoking realities of their child's disability. Some parents accomplish a retreat by seeking placement for their child or by disappearing temporarily to a safer (i.e., free of the stress of disability) environment.

Acceptance is achieved when parents demonstrate some of the following characteristics:

1. They are able to discuss their child's disabilities with relative ease.
2. They evidence a balance between encouraging independence and showing love.
3. They are able to collaborate with professionals to make realistic short- and long-term plans.
4. They pursue personal interests unrelated to their child.
5. They can discipline appropriately without undue guilt.
6. They can abandon overprotective or unduly harsh behavioral patterns toward their child.

Acceptance is not a surrender to the idea that the disability is unchangeable. "Rather, parents accept the need to learn skillful ways to alter the negative effects of the condition. True acceptance includes the conviction that much needs to be done and that what is done will make a difference" (Cook et al., 2004, p. 44). The acceptance phase can result in a perception or realization that one is blessed in being chosen to be the parent of a child with a disability. Others, however, "experience something vastly different and can't fathom how this could feel like a blessing" (Marshak & Prezant, 2007).

In applying these stages, professionals need to be mindful that families are not homogeneous and that these stages may not be a good fit for some families. For some, these stages are cyclical and recur as new developmental milestones are achieved or when a crisis occurs (e.g., a child's condition worsens). According to Hornby (1994a), "Some parents appear to work the process in a few days, whereas others seem to take years to reach a reasonable level of adaptation. Just as for any major loss it is considered that most people will take around two years to come to terms with the disability. However, some parents seem to take longer and a few possibly never fully adjust to the situation" (p. 20).

Olshansky (1962), a pioneer researcher in the area of families and children with mental retardation, suggested that chronic sorrow is a *normal* reaction to parenting a child with a disability, and it is a more meaningful concept than the overly simplistic notion of acceptance/ rejection. In this view, a parent who continues to experience sadness about a child's disability can still be a competent and caring parent. He asserts, that professionals have been quick to label parents as unaccepting or poorly adjusted when they are, in fact, reacting normally to a challenging situation.

A final variation on the stage model of adjustment suggests that, although one reaction may be the most dominant one, certain amounts of the other reactions will also be present (Hornby, 1994a, 1994b). For example, when parents' predominant emotion is one of anger, they may experience some denial and sadness at the same time.

THE CHALLENGE OF THE ENDLESS CARE

A major feature that distinguishes families of children with disabilities from those confronting other crises is that of the chronicity of care such families face. For some families the care is 24 hours a day, 7 days a week, for many years. The stress can be relentless and drain the family physically and psychologically. In addition, financial worries may exist, and the family becomes at risk of coping difficulties: "Economic difficulties can have a negative effect on family members' social or recreational activities. Likewise, stress related to financial worries can have a negative impact on affection and self-esteem" (Turnbull et al., 2006, p. 50). The degree to which the family is functioning poorly may depend on how it conceptualizes or reframes its life circumstance, how supportive family members are of each other, and how much social support is available outside of the family. The variability of parental response to childhood disability is aptly reflected in the following passage by Trute (1995):

> Having a disabled child in the family will constitute a prolonged and serious stressor for some parents. It will require extraordinary psychological adjustment for these parents and, in some instances, require a major

reorganization of the family system. For other parents, it will not be perceived as a particularly threatening or challenging circumstance, but as a natural occurrence in the life of the family which is met by smooth accommodation and seen as requiring modest adjustment within the family setting. For yet another cluster of parents, taking care of a disabled child will be viewed in positive terms, as an event that provokes personal growth in family members. (pp. 1225–1226)

For some families, the burden of care is chronic. Instead of independence, growth, self-fulfillment, and differentiation, a family may see only despair, dependence, and social isolation. Family members who are distressed and depressed may need family counseling (Elman, 1991). The mental health concerns of parents can be cumulative. That is, living with a child with a disability over many years can take its toll psychologically, physically and financially and can contribute to feelings of exhaustion, despair, and resignation.

In facing the future, family members must decide how they plan to negotiate their special life circumstance. As we noted earlier, flexibility, adaptability, and open communication between family members are important to successful family living. Family members may need to assume roles that were not anticipated. For example, siblings may need to help with caretaking more than they otherwise would, and fathers may need to assist instrumentally more often and also be psychologically supportive of their partners. Mothers, so that they do not become enmeshed, have to learn to facilitate, without undue guilt, as much growth and independence as their child is capable of achieving. All in all, over the family's life span, members need to adapt, negotiate, and communicate. This is sound advice for all families, but it has special relevance for families in which there is a childhood disability or chronic illness.

In addition to seeking help within the family, the family system needs to be permeable enough to allow for outside help, such as respite care, when such help is needed and available. Respite care services are important; Upshur (1991) advocated a spectrum of respite care to meet different family needs. However, not all families are receptive to respite people from services. Some cultures are more comfortable asking for help within the family than outside of it. Furthermore, professionals can help families *create* such resources where they do not exist (Darling & Baxter, 1996; Darling & Darling, 1982; Laborde & Seligman, 1991).

STIGMA

The sociological concept of stigma has important implications for understanding the effects of disability. According to Dovido, Major, and Crocker (2000):

> Stigma is a powerful phenomenon, inextricably linked to the value placed on varying social identities. It is a social construction that involves at least two fundamental components: (1) the recognition of difference based on some distinguishing characteristic, or "mark," and (2) a consequent devaluing of the person. . . . Stigmatized individuals are regarded as flawed, compromised, and somehow less than fully human. (p. 3)

These authors noted that because stigma is defined socially, the variations across cultures vary in terms of what is stigmatizing. Thus attitudes toward homosexuality, disability, obesity, etc., vary according to a culture's definition of valued characteristics. People who are stigmatized are almost always the target of prejudice, avoidance, and rejection.

Stigma is comprised of characteristics such as the visibility of a disability, its perceived controllability, and its perceived danger (Deaux, Reid, Mizrahi, & Ethier, 1995; Crocker, Major, & Steele, 1998). The *visibileness* of a disability is apparent in the differences between someone with autism and a person in a wheelchair. *Controllability* refers to the observer's perception of a person's control over a condition or circumstance. For example, mental illness and alcoholism are often perceived as under one's control, whereas mental retardation or cystic fibrosis is not. Also, in terms of perceived *dangerousness*, mental illness may appear to some to be dangerous, whereas spina bifida would not.

Mark Twain wrote that "there is something that he [man] loves more than he loves peace—the approval of his neighbors and the public. And perhaps there is something which he dreads more than he dreads pain—the disapproval of his neighbors and the public" (Clemens, 1963, p. 344). In U.S. society today, persons with physical and mental disabilities are often judged on the same basis as nondisabled persons, resulting in their degradation or *stigmatization*. To the extent that individuals deviate from the societal norm of physical and mental perfection, they are likely to be shunned, ridiculed, avoided, ostracized, and discriminated against.

Goffman (1963) noted that some disabilities are "discredited," whereas others are "discreditable." A "discreditable" condition is one that is not readily apparent to a lay person. A child with a disfigurement hidden by clothing or a disease such as cystic fibrosis might be able to "pass" as nondisabled or not chronically ill in many situations and thus avoid stigma. On the other hand, a child with a more visible disability, such as Down syndrome or spina bifida, would be "discredited" immediately.

Individuals with discreditable disabilities and their families sometimes engage in what Goffman (1963) called "impression management" to appear normal. Voysey (1972) mentioned the mother of an autistic child who was able to conceal the severity of her child's condition from even the closest family members by cleaning him and the house before visits. Parents may dress a child in contemporary clothes that reflect the mores of the day, or they may groom him or her in a modern hairstyle. These are efforts to offset any noticeable characteristics of the disability. Of course, some parents dress and groom their children well because this is how their other children are clothed and groomed and not because they are particularly concerned about the opinion of others.

For those with hidden disabilities or illnesses, the fear of exposure can be enormous. Nicole Johnson, the winner of the Miss Virginia beauty contest, then Miss America in 1999, hid her diabetes and her dependence on insulin from the public (Szish, 2004). Following a terrifying 40 minutes of unresponsiveness after a diabetic episode during the 1997 Miss Virginia beauty pageant, Johnson awoke and uttered her first words, "Does anybody know?" Johnson's concern about being "found out" was paramount and contributed to the stress of keeping her illness hidden from others who might have judged her harshly. Since that fateful day, she converted her anxieties about being discovered to become a graduate student and an international spokesperson on diabetes education.

In the case of discredited conditions, which are immediately obvious to strangers, the problems of "impression management" are different. "Passing" as "normal" is not possible in these cases. Davis (1961) suggested that when those with visible disabilities come into contact with people who are not disabled, a kind of mutual pretense takes place: Both the stigmatized and the nondisabled person act as though the disability does not exist. Davis calls this mode of interaction *fictional acceptance*, because the nondisabled person does not *really* accept the person with a disability as a moral equal.

The interaction between stigmatized and nonstigmatized persons may never move beyond a superficial level. People may be hesitant to become close to the family of a stigmatized person because they, in turn, might be stigmatized. As noted, Goffman (1963) suggested that close associates of stigmatized persons come to bear a "courtesy stigma" and may suffer similar reactions of avoidance, rejection, or ridicule. For this reason, stigmatized individuals and their families may choose their friends from among what Goffman (1963) called "their own"—others who already share a similar stigma. Family response to stigma is discussed further in Chapter 5.

Miller and Major (2002) marshaled considerable evidence that stigma causes anxiety and stress in those who are stigmatized. According to these authors, anxiety is experienced by stigmatized people when others make derisive comments, or because they are excluded, discriminated against, or are the victims of violence. Self-esteem is assaulted when they believe that others do not like, value, or respect them. There is also an ambiguous anxiety that arises when individuals are unsure whether they are being treated in a prejudicial manner due to stigma. Nonstigmatized persons often disguise their attitudes toward stigmatized people. "This attributional ambiguity and uncertainty that this creates for stigmatized persons is likely to be a source of stress" (Miller & Major, p. 244). Furthermore, because stigmatized persons suffer from discrimination, there are limits on housing, education, health care, and employment. All of these chronic stressors contribute to anxiety, frustration, anger, social isolation, and a loss of social support.

Stigma does not apply exclusively to persons with disabilities but also to other minority group members (Heatherton, Kleck, Hebl, & Hull, 2000). However, persons with a disability differ from other minority groups in that their disability is not likely to be shared by other family members or perhaps even by others in the immediate environment. In contrast, members of minority groups are often surrounded by other persons with whom they share common attributes, such as skin color.

The concept of "spread" applies to children with disabilities and, by association, their families. Dembo, Leviton, and Wright (1956) introduced the term *spread*, which refers to the power of single characteristics to evoke broader inferences about a person. If a person has an undesirable characteristic and is viewed as less adequate only in that regard, the judgment would be a realistic one. But the realistic appraisal of others is more the exception than the rule. Consider physique (being obese or fit and trim), which evokes a wide variety of impressions and feelings about people. Specific characteristics may be inferred from physique (e.g., an obese person may have physical restrictions), but also the person *as a whole* is sometimes evaluated (e.g., the obese person is viewed as depressed, socially isolated, low in self-esteem, and lacking in sexual relationships). Global devaluations are problems of some magnitude, in that persons with atypical characteristics are considered to be less worthy, less valuable, and less desirable (Marshak & Seligman, 1993). Because of spread, the degree of disability is often perceived as more severe than it actually is. An illustration of spread is a sighted person speaking unusually loudly to a person who is blind, as if blindness implies a hearing impairment as well.

The phenomenon of spread is implicated in the way parents of children with disabilities are sometimes viewed. As noted earlier, Goffman (1963) called this phenomenon "courtesy stigma." As a consequence of disability in the family, some parents are as subject to spread as are their sons and daughters with disabilities. Parents of these children may be viewed as deeply troubled and burdened—or as extraordinarily brave and courageous. The numerous factors that contribute to family adjustment, as well as the complex nature of their interactions, are typically disregarded. By association, then, certain characteristics may be attributed to family members of children who have disabilities. The premature and misguided judgment, on the basis of disability in the family, that a person's life is a tragedy from which there is no reprieve may be a fairly common occurrence.

Studies have consistently shown that persons with disabilities are viewed negatively by the general public (Marshak & Seligman, 1993; Resnick, 1984; Heatherton et al., 2000). Furthermore, research has demonstrated that certain disabling conditions are more acceptable than others and that professionals hold attitudes that are negative (Darling, 1979; Resnick, 1984).

In short, the predominant social attitude toward those who are different has been one of stigma, and stigmatized persons are regarded as morally inferior to those who are "normal" (Goffman, 1963). As Chapter 3 suggests and as Newman (1991) pointed out, "In early societies, illness and disability were seen as the work of evil demons and supernatural forces—disease and disability [were seen] as the scourge of God, as punishment for sin" (p. 9). In today's society, stigma may be decreasing as a result of personal experience and greater public awareness. Most of us can think of family members, friends, or acquaintances who have an illness (cancer, arthritis), or a disability (mental retardation, spina bifida). Thus, personal experience with someone who has a disability tends to soften stigma.

Attitudes toward persons with disabilities must be integrated into conceptions of family life when there is a child with a disability. Professionals must examine their own attitudes toward disability and toward families of children with special needs, lest these attitudes interfere with the provision of services in subtle ways. An appropriate arena for beginning to explore attitudes would be in professional training programs.

To conclude this discussion on stigma, it is noteworthy that many adults with disabilities today reject society's stigma and even acquire a sense of pride in their disabled identities. See Chapter 6 for a discussion of variability in the internalization of stigma.

MARITAL ADJUSTMENT, DIVORCE, AND SINGLE PARENTHOOD

Divorce adds to the stress of disability and chronic illness; unfortunately, many such children live in households with only one parent (Hobbs et al., 1986; Chapter 3, this volume). A growing U.S. population of single parents, in general, and single parents of children with disabilities, in particular, would appear to experience greater stresses in the family system than two-parent families (Simpson, 1990; Vadasy, 1986; Teyber, 1992). Because of the high rate of separation and divorce and the growing number of out-of-wedlock births to both older women and teenagers, one-parent families constitute the fastest growing family type in the United States (Cox, 1996). Between 50 and 60% of children born in the 1990s lived in single-family homes at some point (Hetherington, Bridges, & Insabella, 1998). Empirical data on single parenthood and childhood disability are scarce. However, as the September 2004 issue of the *Monitor on Psychology* (a publication of the American Psychological Association) reported, major national efforts are being made to help families cope better with a host of internal and external stressors; this issue on the *Monitor* focused on poverty and single parenthood.

One form of respite care is the availability of a spouse, even one who is not involved in caretaking. "A supportive husband—even one who does not participate in child care—seems to be an important predictor of a mother's sense of well-being" (Turnbull et al., 2006, p. 7). There is a growing need to provide respite services for families; such services provide needed relief from caretaking and promote adult-to-adult communication, socialization, and intimacy (Upshur, 1991). A number of authors claim that divorce and single parenthood lead to financial, psychological, and instrumental problems (Hodapp & Krasner, 1994–1995). However, divorce does not have the same impact on all family members, and the effects of divorce may depend on when it occurs in the family life cycle and the degree of dysfunction in the family prior to the marital breakup (Schulz, 1987; Simpson, 1990). Furthermore, far fewer children with disabilities reside with both biological parents than do nondisabled children (Turnbull et al., 2006). Together both parents can share responsibilities and support each other during difficult times (Scorgie, Wilgosh, & McDonald, 1998).

One outcome of divorce occurs in families in which one or both parents in the original family remarry (Visher & Visher, 1996). Blended families may face an array of familial variations and resulting emotional confusion (Turnbull & Turnbull, 1990; Goldenberg & Goldenberg, 2003). In these families, new rules and roles need to be adopted, loyalty issues to the biological and nonbiological parents need to be negotiated, new lines of authority need to be established, and financial responsibilities need to be reconsidered. When a child with a disability resides in a blended family, other issues, such as caretaking and primary responsibility for the child, need to be negotiated (Turnbull et al., 2006). Furthermore, children from the former relationships need time to bond and negotiate sibling rivalry issues (Friend & Cook, 2002).

In two-parent families, the functions assumed by family members are usually shared, thereby decreasing the burden on any one family member. Children living with two parents are more likely to report that their parents are involved in their school and other activities, and these parents are less likely to worry about their children than their single counterparts (Turnbull, Turnbull, Shank, & Leal, 1999). Perhaps the most support a single parent can expect from family is from his or her own parents. However, help and support can come from a nonresidential parent, grandparents, kin, colleagues, and professionals. Generally speaking, issues for single parents of children with disabilities include economic, physical, and emotional needs.

About one-third of children with disabilities live in a single-parent residence, and the poverty rate for those families is almost 40% (Fujiura & Yamaki, 2000). Furthermore, some single parents do not have the time or emotional energy to be involved in their child's education, an important parental role for all children but especially for children with disabilities (Cigno & Burke, 1997).

The information regarding marital problems and divorce in families of children with disabilities is sparse and contradictory (Patterson,

1991; Marshak & Prezant, 2007). In 1983 Gabel, McDowell, and Cerreto reported that the onset of marital difficulties is one of the more frequently reported adjustment problems. Their research review showed that marital problems included more frequent conflict, feelings of marital dissatisfaction, sexual difficulties, temporary separations, and divorce. In their large-scale study, Hodapp and Krasner (1994–1995) reported that parents of eighth-grade students with disabilities showed higher rates of divorce and separation than the comparison group of parents of nondisabled children. In their study, almost 28% of parents of children with disabilities reported that they had no spouse or partner. This is a significant figure and suggests that more than a quarter of these parents had to seek help and support from someone other than a partner—which, in turn, means that help/support was not necessarily immediately available from a deeply involved and trusted family member.

In his pioneering study, Farber (1959) found marital conflict to be common in families of children with disabilities, especially in families containing a retarded boy age 9 or above. Conversely, some families reported no more frequent problems than comparison families (Bernard, 1974; Dorner, 1975; Martin, 1975; Patterson, 1991; Weisbren, 1980), and some marriages have even been reported to improve after the diagnosis of a child's disability (Schwab, 1989; Klein & Schive, 2001). In regard to the latter point, Marsh (1992) observed that "there is increasing recognition among professionals that catastrophic events are inherently challenges that can serve as catalysts for the emergence of regenerated and enriched lives. Although a diagnosis of mental retardation may involve the disintegration of existing modes of functioning, it also provides opportunities for personal and familial reintegration" (p. 89). We embrace Marsh's sentiment, believing that childhood disability exhorts some families to find meaning and growth—and purpose. Marvelous examples of this perspective can be found in such books as Klein and Shive's (2001) *You Will Dream New Dreams*, a book containing essays from family members of children with impairments; Klein and Kemp's (2004) more recent publication, *Reflections from a Different Journey*; and Meyer's (1995) book of observations from fathers on their lives with their children who have disabilities.

Although the data regarding marital satisfaction and divorce in families of children with disabilities are contradictory, we do know that some marriages are under stress but remain intact, others simply fail, whereas still others survive and are even enhanced. Generally speaking, it is as reasonable to assume that families of children without disabilities also have varied outcomes, as suggested by the high rate of divorce.

In regard to divorce rates, Marshak and Prezant (2007) state,

> Definitive statistics on the divorce rate of couples with children with disabilities are not available, but there is general consensus that it is somewhat higher than in families with typical children. However, we do know that the divorce rate is terribly high for marriages in general; it is reported as approximately 50% for first marriages and close to 75% for second marriages. (p. ?)

We believe that there should be an increasing examination of those family dynamics that can lead to family conflict, increased stress, and marital disintegration. For example, in attending to the needs of an infant or child with impairments, the mother may unwittingly move away from her husband as she attends to her child. Feeling abandoned, a husband may turn to others for solace or at least he may distance himself from the family as a means of self-protection (Houser & Seligman, 1991). A common sibling response to a parent's excessive attention to a brother or sister with a disability is to feel angry and resentful (McHugh, 2003); perhaps the same general dynamic operates with marital partners.

Families can focus on the child with a disability as a source of family problems. This tends to be a red herring that leads the parents away from more fundamental issues about their relationship. It is important to discriminate between family problems brought about by childhood disability and those that would have arisen under any circumstances. Problematic marital relationships can be made considerably worse by the birth of a child with a disability (Marshak & Prezant, 2007). For example, in those families with serious personal and/or financial problems *prior* to the birth of their child with a disability, the child can become "the straw that broke the camel's back." Typically, such a child—or any child, for that matter—does not bring a troubled marriage together although there are reports of families who are strengthened in these circumstances (Ariel & Naseef, 2006). Families often harbor the fantasy that a baby will absorb their attention and divert them from their problems, allowing them to rally around the newborn. There is a sense that their conflicts will magically disappear.

After a thorough review of the literature on families of children with severe and multiple disabilities, Lyon and Lyon (1991) concluded that these families must cope with a number of stressors. They contended that, in general, the research reveals mixed conclusions regarding the impact a child has on the family. In the absence of clear evidence, that (1) these families are coping badly; and (2) professionals should focus on such practical matters as early intervention, concrete information, respite services, financial help, and other supportive services that address logistical problems: "Rather than to continue to view these families as functioning pathologically we might better and more productively focus upon those practical matters that are of great concern to the families themselves" (Lyon & Lyon, 1991, p. 254). We would add, however, that for some families, emotional support and family and individual counseling can also be helpful.

What can we conclude about marital harmony/dysfunction among families of children with disabilities? One conclusion may be that marital dysfunction might have occurred even without the presence of disability. Another is that in some families a child with disabilities may aggravate latent problems. Still another conclusion is that many families can cope successfully with the help of kin and community supports. Finally, marital discord may result in divorce and single parenthood—areas that deserve much more attention than they have thus far received. Certainly it goes without saying that poverty, racism, discrimination, alcoholism, unemployment, or mental illness would further compromise a family's ability to cope with childhood disabilities.

FAMILIES OF CHILDREN WITH DIFFERENT IMPAIRMENTS

The research on the impact of different childhood disabilities continues to be contradictory, which makes it difficult to draw definitive conclusions. Recent investigations conducted on children with a variety of impairments/illnesses have attempted to explore factors across conditions that may influence parental stress and coping. Some studies report on families of children with more than one impairment, and others employ terminology that changes from study to study (e.g., *handicapped, disability, impairment, special needs, developmentally disabled*). Nevertheless, most of these studies explore parental response to a child with a specific impairment or with more than one impairment.

One national study explored the separation/divorce rates among parents of eighth-grade students who had one of four disabilities: visual impairment, hearing impairment, deafness, and orthopedic impairments (Hodapp & Krasner, 1994–1995). These families were also compared to families with nonimpaired children. The researchers found that families of eighth-grade students with impairments had higher rates of divorce/separation than their counterparts with typical children. Further, divorce or separation was most evident in the visual impairment group, followed by the orthopedically impaired, deaf, and hearing impaired. In addition, the families with a child who had an impairment were less well off financially than those in the comparison group. The poorest parents were those of children with visual and hearing impairments, which in part may account for the higher divorce/separation rate among the parents of visually impaired children. Poverty certainly contributes to family stress. Also, there were more single-wage earners in the group of families of children who had an impairment than in the comparison group. Further, there was a disproportionate number of African American and Latino families in the visually impaired group, although their separation/divorce rates were lower than those of the European American families, which the authors attributed to a chance occurrence. The authors felt that because of the divorce/separation rates across families of children with different disabling conditions, research should focus on how such differences contribute to various levels of stress in families.

Developmental Disabilities

In another study, researchers interviewed 24 families of children with a number of developmental disabilities (Kornblatt & Heinrich, 1985). They found that 83% of the families reported high-level needs for care, and 67% said that they were coping at a low level. Families living in the inner city and younger families most often expressed high-intensity needs as well as decreased coping ability. The researchers found that families repeatedly revealed a lack of knowledge about, and utilization of, existing community services. This study demonstrates the importance of communicating the availability of existing services to poor populations, and it highlights the added problems of poverty and the other concomitants of inner-city life. Future research needs to examine the impact of poverty and cultural diversity on the family, major factors that complicate coping (Hatton et al., 2003; Evans, 2004).

Forty-five parents of children with a developmental impairment were compared to 44 control parents of children with no impairments on six instruments designed to examine the impact of children with impairments on the parents (DoAmaral, 2003). The instruments examined parental adjustment, self-esteem, symptoms of stress, and family support. The author reported that the parents of children with impairments had lower levels of parenting satisfaction and higher levels of stress than the comparison group. Fathers and mothers did not differ on the tests, except that the mothers were more at risk for depression in comparison with the control group of mothers and fathers. The researcher recommended a holistic counseling approach to respond to parents' needs, according to their own definition of need.

Trute (1995) evaluated a sample of 73 Canadian families of children with developmental disabilities by using several scales that measured depression, self-esteem, marital adjustment, and perceived support, among others. The interviews with parents were lengthy. The goal of the research was to compare psychological distress in mothers and fathers. A major finding of this study was that mothers reported significantly higher levels of depression, similar to those in DoAmaral's study, noted above, than did fathers, and that mothers had significantly lower self-esteem than fathers. Trute speculated that mothers have a more demanding role than fathers in child care, placing mothers at higher risk. Lower levels of self-esteem may contribute to depression, but we suspect that the question of whether the depression preceded or was subsequent to the child's birth is an open issue. Higher levels of depression in fathers were related to less disabled male children, an association that has been noted previously (Frey, Greenberg, & Fewell, 1989; Tallman, 1965). Trute speculated that fathers may more easily accept a son who is more seriously incapacitated; a son may be more difficult to accept when the impairment is marginal and the future economic and social implications are ambiguous. It seems that fathers take pride in the accomplishments of their children, especially those of their sons. This is not to imply that only fathers revel in their children's accomplishments. Mothers do too, but fathers may struggle more with a son who has a less well-defined disability due to the fathers' expectations of their male offspring. How fathers experience their child's disability is addressed further in Chapter 8.

One study reported on an 11-year follow-up of adoptive and birth families rearing children with intellectual disabilities (Glidden & Schoolcraft, 2003). The focus of the study focused on depression and how, or whether, the symptoms of depression changed over time in a sample of 187 mothers. The results indicated that both adoptive and birth mothers reported low depression, with scores not significantly different from each other at the 11-year follow-up. This study suggests a long-term positive prognosis of adjustment to childhood disability, as the mothers displayed less depression over time. Parents become accustomed to their child over the years after coming to grips with the initial shock, learning to deal with hardships, stigma, and barriers, and perhaps learning about opportunities for support. This study supports the view that the initial stages of adjustment to disability seem to be the most distressing.

Depression can be a serious problem in families of children with disabilities, and it is often undiagnosed in patients seeking medical care. This oversight has led to initiatives to help physicians become more aware of depression and its symptoms in the patients they treat. Depression can contribute to, or even be the main cause of, a medical complaint. However, depressive symptoms can range from mild to severe (called "clinical depression" at the extreme). We do not feel that milder forms of depression, which are often transitory reactions to an external event, necessarily cause problems for spouses or the family. These are reactions that most people experience and are a normal and expected part of life.

Pelchat, Bisson, Ricard, Perreault, and Bouchard (1999) explored the longitudinal (birth through 18 months) effects of an early intervention program in Montreal for mothers and fathers of children who had Down syndrome and cleft lip/palate. The focus of the intervention was to help fathers and mothers when their need for assistance was most pronounced—namely, in the first months after the birth, when they need to adapt to their parental situation, grieve their dreams of a healthy child, and learn to take care of, and become attached to, their baby. The program used six to eight weekly meetings with a trained nurse and provided an emphasis on the strength and adaptive capacities of the family, optimal usage of both internal and external resources, and empowerment of the family in regard to competencies useful in its adaptation and care of the child.

This study had two unique features: It utilized a control group of parents of children with the above-mentioned conditions who did not participate in the intervention, and it was longitudinal in nature, over an 18-month period. A total of 198 mothers and fathers were assessed with several instruments at three periods: when their children were 6, 12, and 18 months. The researchers reported that there was a significant positive effect of the early intervention on parental adaptation. Compared to parents who did not receive the intervention, the group felt less threatened by their parental situation and more willing to accept help from others; reported less distress, anxiety, and depression; and perceived more emotional support from their spouses. The authors argued that the positive effects evident during the three evaluation periods bode well for the future adaptation of these parents, although no further data were collected. Whether or not these positive findings continue with the same level of significance, this approach appears to be useful in helping parents cope with the initial stages of adaptation. Indeed, such interventions for parents, combined with early intervention programs for children, should be a potent package to help parents negotiate the challenges ahead.

Attention-Deficit/Hyperactivity Disorder

In a brief summary of selected research on attention-deficit/hyperactivity disorder (ADHD), Barkley (2004) noted that more severe behavioral symptoms of children can result in mothers who are critical, commanding, and less responsive to their children. After children were given medication, the mothers' behavior toward their offspring improved as the children's behavior improved. We bring Barkley's observations to the reader's attention to highlight the effect children's behavior can have on parents. The author adds another issue to the discussion to help muddy the waters, namely, that ADHD is a highly inheritable disorder and that the parents may have passed it on to their children. The genetic component raises a chicken–egg dilemma that advises against engaging in parent blaming.

Autism

The unpredictability of the behavior of children with autism and the social–interpersonal ramifications experienced by families cause considerable stress (Bristol, 1984; Harris & Glasberg, 2003; Schopler & Mesibov, 1984). McHugh (1999) adds that autism is one of the most challenging disabilities because of the child's behavioral problems. She quotes one of the parents she interviewed for her book: "It's like a three-ring circus day-to-day. There is no way you can ignore somebody who has motor oil for blood, doesn't sleep so nobody sleeps. There's constant turmoil in the house. You either accept it or you flail against it your whole life" (p. 73). For families of children with autism, the following constitute risk factors: ambiguity of diagnosis, severity, behavioral problems, and duration of condition, and lack of community norms (Bristol, 1984; Harris & Glasberg, 2003). Cantwell and Baker (1984) cited research indicating that mothers appear the most severely affected; spousal affectional bonds tend to be weakened; siblings are affected; and family difficulties do not diminish as the child grows older. It is important to acknowledge that autism is a spectrum disorder (Ariel & Naseef, 2006) and that children are differentially affected, with parents reporting mild to severe impairment in social, intellectual, and behavioral spheres.

Deafness

The effects of a child who is deaf on the family are mixed (Luterman, 1991). Deaf children are often impaired in their communication which can be a source of considerable frustration for family members (Sloman et al., 1993; Lane, Hoffmeister, & Bahan, 1996). Most deaf children have hearing parents, which can cause more communication problems than when a child who is deaf is born to deaf parents (Moores, 2006).

Parents typically endure an extended diagnostic journey, which contributes to ambiguity, stress, anxiety—and family conflict. "The final identification of deafness generally represents the culmination of a long, emotional, draining process. Typically the mother has known for some time that something is wrong with the child but she is not exactly sure what it is. Frequently, a pediatrician has offered assurances that the mother is overly concerned and that the child is merely a 'late bloomer' " (Moores, 2006, p. 147). This conflict may be fueled by the denial that often attends ambiguity and by the professional community that often aids parental denial by asserting that their child is not impaired, even in the face of parent reports to the contrary. In addition to the above concerns, conflicts within the deaf community regarding the "best" communication practices for their child leads to increased choices available to the family, but it can also contribute to family conflict in that there may be differing opinions about which method will give their child the best opportunity for self-reliance, employment, and social interaction.

More research is needed into the impact of deafness on nuclear family members, including siblings and grandparents. In the deaf community, especially in families where a child who is deaf is born to parents who are deaf, there is a growing acceptance of deafness as a cultural phenomenon as opposed to a disability or deficit (Lane et al., 1996). The deaf community is viewed by some, especially by those who are deaf, as a cultural group, much like other minority groups, with its own identity, rituals, and communication patterns.

Blindness

In the area of childhood blindness, Fewell (1991) reported that the *degree* of visual loss in children who are usually impaired has important implications both for the child and the family's reaction to the child. Just as children with low vision may try to "pass" as normally sighted, parents too are caught in the dilemma of not wanting to identify their child's differences. Because blind children have normal cognitive abilities, unless there are certain additional impairments, they can communicate and carry on with the chores of daily living, making blindness less devastating to the blind child and the family than other disabilities (Fewell, 1991).

Physical Impairments

Mobility is affected for many children with physical impairments, which, in turn, may affect their ability to perform self-care functions. Physical impairments can take a variety of forms, such as a loss of limbs or a paralysis due to a genetic condition, accident, or disease. The nature, characteristics, and severity of the physical impairment may determine the type of adjustment the child and the family must make (Marshak & Seligman, 1993). For example, a quadriplegic condition holds numerous implications for family members assisting with caretaking duties. Muscular dystrophy, a degenerative disease, creates a need for the child and family to adjust to an increasing level of dependency as the disease progresses. Numerous other physical impairments—many that are rare and leave the family with few others to identify with—create challenges for the family.

Chronic Illness

Approximately 10–25% of children become chronically ill, with asthma as the most common illness (Northy, Griffin, & Krainz, 1998). There are a number of chronic illnesses with varying degrees of impairment, such as cystic fibrosis, cancer, arthritis, and diabetes, among others.

Any chronic illness brings with it considerable financial, logistical, and emotional costs for parents. Stigma can be an issue for siblings whose brother or sister suffers from such illnesses as cancer or AIDS (McHugh, 1999). Sensing the stigma, siblings are reluctant to share this with their friends (Lobato, 1990). In the developmental disability literature the coping issues within the family focus on the child's impact.

Although chronic childhood illness is considered a major stressor, and it is generally assumed that it has a negative impact on the parents' relationship, the research does not support this view (Gordon, Walker, Johnson, Manion, & Cloutier, as cited in Gaither, Bingen, & Hopkins, 2000). The literature cited in Gaither et al. (2000) indicates that couples can have negative, positive, or no effects from caring for children who have a chronic illness. In terms of negative effects, the following seem to be supported by the research (as cited in Gaither et al., 2000):

- Communication problems
- Higher divorce rates
- Increased conflict between spouses
- Decreased relationship satisfaction

The apparently contradictory literature in terms of family coping with childhood chronic illness can be attributed to a number of factors. For one, the illnesses are varied yet share common characteristics that can affect the couple's relationship, such as family stress and burden of care. But illnesses vary in severity, course, and prognosis, which constitutes different challenges for the couple and family (Gaither et al., 2000; Rolland, 2003). For some illnesses, such as certain cancers and cystic fibrosis, the outcome can be death—an atypical outcome in the case of most developmental disabilities.

Cancer

The incidence of childhood cancer is rising, as one in 330 children develops cancer before age 19 (Ross, Severson, Pollock, & Robinson, 1996; Miller, Young, & Nivakovic, 1996, as cited in Vannatta & Gerhardt, 2003). Treatment regimens can be rough, often including surgery, radiation, and chemotherapy, but advances in treatment have improved the survival rate (National Cancer Institute, as cited in Vannatta & Gerhardt, 2003). Children undergoing cancer treatment may be at risk in their relations with peers and in the emotional realm (as cited in Vannatta & Gerhardt, 2003), although the problems in these domains are not pervasive or long-lasting.

Cystic Fibrosis

Cystic fibrosis, one of the most common chronic diseases of childhood, requires the family to comply with a prescribed home regimen. Pulmonary dysfunction characterizes the disease, but it also involves the pancreatic and gastrointestinal systems and presents serious challenges for the coping skills and adjustment of the family as a whole (Brinthaupt, 1991; McHugh, 1999). The home care of the child is difficult and chronic (Dushenko, 1981). In regard to compliance with home treatment for children with cystic fibrosis, Patterson (1985) reported that age is a factor in that children are more reluctant to adhere to prescriptions as they grow older. Communication in these families may decline in a situation that is challenging and requires the continued expression of hope and mutual support (Patterson, 1985). Families with children who have cystic fibrosis have multiple problems, and an adolescent's problems are exacerbated by short stature and appearance of lower maturational level (McCracken, 1984; Offer Ostrov, & Howard, 1984).

Death from Chronic Illness

The death of a child is one of the most profound experiences parents face. Vannetta and Gerhardt (2003) discussed the literature in this area and reported that parents described greater internalizing difficulties (e.g., self-blame, guilt), ongoing family disruption, and a number of emotional problems (e.g., depression, anxiety, anger, and posttraumatic stress disorder). In addition, bereaved families reported increased parental and marital strain, less marital satisfaction, less intimacy, and higher rates of divorce. These parents may be preoccupied with their grief and inadvertently ignore the needs of their other children or become closer and overprotective. Siblings also reported some of the same difficulties as their parents after the death of a brother or sister.

The possibility of death for a minority of children with a chronic disease and the "roller coaster" nature of particular illnesses differentiate these children and their families from the more predictable course in developmental disabilities. This observation is not to diminish the challenges and concomitant medical complications present for some children with developmental disabilities. It is meant to highlight shared challenges as well as the differences families confront in their daily lives.

Conclusions about the Nature of an Impairment

It is impossible to conclude with any certainty how the particular type of a child's impairment will affect a family. Factors other than severity of disability may play an important role in determining family adaptation (Crnic, Friedrich, et al., 1983). We know from Rolland's (2003) model (Chapter 2, this volume) that onset, course, and prognosis, as well as other illness/disability-related variables, may influence family response. Researchers report that the quantity and quality of community resources and family support have an impact on the family's ability to cope with childhood disability (Darling, 1991; Korn et al., 1978; Wortis & Margolies, 1955). Researchers have sought to determine more specifically how, and which aspects of, social support are most helpful to families (Kazak & Marvin, 1984; Kazak & Wilcox, 1984; Krahn, 1993).

According to one researcher, mothers of children with disabilities experienced significantly more stress if their offspring had a greater number of, or unusual, caregiving demands, were less socially responsive, had more difficult temperaments, and displayed more repetitive behavioral patterns (Beckman, 1983). McHugh (1999) asserts that "when a child needs constant physical care, the mother in the family will get less sleep at night, [and] the parents' marriage will be under a lot more stress because of the unrelenting needs of the child with a disability" (p. 67).

In the face of inconclusive research data, we feel that it is incumbent that professionals be aware of the numerous variables that affect family adjustment and to persuade them to keep these variables in mind when evaluating a family's level of functioning. However, as further research avenues are explored, it seems to us that Beckman's (1983) observations, though a quarter of a century old, deserve attention. The effects that specific attributes of children (or the demand characteristics of the impairment) may have on the family is a more productive line of inquiry than to lump all children with a particular label into one diagnostic category and assume that they are all alike.

However, it appears from the review thus far that caregiving demands and aberrant behavior of the child lead to more stress than any other aspects of an impairment.

THE SEVERITY OF DISABILITY

Severity of disability has implications for caregivers in terms of dependency, the need for increased attention for the child with a disability (perhaps at the expense of other family members), frequent contact with medical personnel and other service providers, the prospect of lifelong care, and, in some cases, coping with difficult behavior.

Placing children with mild, moderate, and severe disabilities into categories is somewhat arbitrary. Diagnostic ambiguity is particularly evident between the mild and moderate categories. Nevertheless, Fewell (1991) differentiated these categories:

1. *Mild:* Includes children whose disabilities require special services but who have substantial areas of normal functioning.
2. *Moderate:* Includes children who are markedly different in at least one area while functioning normally in others.
3. *Severe:* Includes children with disabilities that pervade most, if not all, areas of functioning.

Children in the less severe categories are more difficult to assess educationally and in terms of emotional adjustment, and thus treatment alternatives are less obvious, according to Fewell (1991). Furthermore, the ambiguity of the diagnosis may cause families to go to many sources in search of a favorable diagnosis ("shopping"), thus delaying a treatment plan. The more "normal" a child appears, the more likely that parents may be "stuck" in the denial stage and engage in further shopping (Hornby, 1994a; Seligman, 1979). Parents who deny their child's disability seem to experience more tension with professionals (especially school personnel).

For children with mild to moderate disabilities, treatment may need to be modified as they develop and other problems appear, decrease, or increase. Moderate disabilities may worsen or improve over time. Children with mild or moderate disabilities (especially those who fall into the mild category) are often considered "marginal" in that they do not clearly fit into either the disabled or the "normal" category (Marshak & Seligman, 1993). Fewell (1991) argued that people with intermediate disabilities will have more adjustment problems than individuals with more severe disabilities. However, others believe that children with severe disabilities take a greater toll on family resources (McHugh, 1999).

Marginality implies ambiguity not only in terms of diagnosis but also in terms of the parents' concerns about the future, social acceptance, and level of functioning. But it seems that social adjustment may have the most severe impact on the child and family. In this regard, Turnbull et al. (2006) asserted, "Socialization is vital to the overall quality of life for most individuals. Persons of all ages with exceptionalities need opportunities to experience both the joys and disappointments of friendships" (p. 61). In one study, 40% of mothers expressed worries about the rejection their children may face from peers and the impact of this on their children's self-esteem (Guralnick, Connor, & Hammond, 1995). Fewell (1991) made the cogent point that a family's difficulty with the social destiny of its stigmatized child is inevitable and normal, and is not a sign of pathological functioning.

Children with severe disabilities constitute an extremely low incidence population (approximately 1% of the general population) and are really a heterogeneous population comprised of different characteristics, needs, and abilities (Lyon et al., 2005). Although children with severe disabilities are heterogeneous, there are a number of problems and difficulties that characterize them and their families' responses to them. These children may be substantially delayed cognitively and may not acquire even the most rudimentary conceptual abilities. They may also be extremely limited in the acquisition and use of language.

Another problem common among children with severe disabilities is the presence of physical impairments such as walking, use of the hands, speaking, and eating, along with mental retardation. A third characteristic is sensory impairment such as visual and/or auditory disabilities. It is not uncommon for children with sensory impairments also to have varying degrees of retardation and physical impairments as well.

Children with severe disabilities manifest difficulty in developing appropriate social skills. These children may demonstrate bizarre behavior through unintelligible or repetitive speech, self-stimulation, and even self-destructive behavior. These behaviors are difficult to treat and often necessitate extensive effort and commitment for the family to remedy or even tolerate (Harris, 1994; Lyon & Lyon, 1991). We already know from the research of Beckman (1983) and Tartar (1987) that a child's behavior can be a major stressor in the family. Behavioral problems in the school setting can be problematic for both the child with a disability and the other children in the classroom (Turnbull et al., 2006).

It would seem from this review of children with severe disabilities that the consequences for the family would be insurmountable. Indeed, this circumstance requires extensive day-to-day support in order to meet basic needs, as parents attend to their child's medical, educational, and therapy needs. These activities can be isolating and exhausting. For some families this may be so, but the evidence regarding negative impact is unclear because research in this area is not abundant. Lyon and his colleagues (2005) concluded: "Positive outcomes have been reported for people with severe disabilities who live and work in more typical settings and circumstances. There is ample research to indicate that people living in the community with supports can experience an improved quality of life" (p. 833). Nevertheless, the literature does provide some preliminary evidence as to how children with severe disabilities affect the family.

Farber's (1959, 1960b) pioneering studies showed that overall integration of families who kept their children with severe retardation at home was affected negatively. Another early study found that families of children with severe disabilities evidenced more negative emotions (Gath, 1974). Other early researchers have reported role tension, increased divisiveness within the family, negative emotionality, and increased financial burden, as well as restrictions in family activities, more physical health problems, and more marital distress (Caldwell & Guze, 1960; Farber, 1960b; Patterson, 1991). After interviewing marital partners for their book *Married with Special Needs Children*, Marshak and Prezant (2007) contended that:

- Childhood disability does have a major impact on marriage. The impact can be detrimental, beneficial, or mixed.
- A child with a disability "amplifies" what occurs in typical marriages: "Closeness may be stronger, anger intensified, sadness deeper, parenting decisions weightier, and happy times . . . More exhilarating."
- Childhood disability makes marriage more complicated.
- Being a parent of a child with a disability means that one needs to develop even better parenting skills than those who are not.

In a study designed to compare families of children with severe mental retardation, educable mental retardation, and trainable mental retardation, Blacher, Nihira, and Meyers (1987) found that parents of children with severe retardation reported the greatest amount of negative impact on family adjustment. The excessive caretaking responsibilities of family members of children with severe retardation apparently influenced family adjustment. However, on the measures of marital adjustment ("extent to which the retarded child has influenced the parents' marriage" [p. 315]), no differences were found among the three groups. Blacher and colleagues' results reinforce those found by others, who explain that the demanding care of a child with severe disabilities was more likely to disrupt family routines and social lives than contribute to significant marital problems. A further finding was that there were no differences among the three groups on the coping scores, reflecting an equal ability to deal with day-to-day events.

A number of professionals argued that the negative effects have been overstated and the positive effects have been ignored (Jacobson & Humphrey, 1979; Lyon & Lyon, 1991; Schwab, 1989; McHugh, 1999; Turnbull et al., 2006). Lyon et al. (2005) noted that problems frequently reported by families of children with severe disabilities include financial difficulties and the burden on the practical day-to-day operations and logistics of the family. They concurred with others that these families have been pathologized too often in the past and that, with adequate services (and these families need many), families with youth who have severe disabilities do manage to cope. When families experience severe stress, they argued, it is usually due to the failure of the service delivery system and not necessarily a consequence of the child's disability.

In contrast to the aforementioned authors, Blacher (1984b) concluded from her comprehensive literature review that "the impact of a severely impaired child on the family appears to be profound, pervasive, and persistent. It is reasonable to assume that parents feel the effects of such a child throughout infancy, early childhood, during the school years, and beyond into adult life" (p. 41). And Crnic, Friedrich, et al. (1983) commented that the "research in this area suggests that parents of retarded children are at the least a group at high risk for emotional and personality difficulties" (p. 128). Although Blacher (1984b) and Crnic, Friedrich, et al. (1983) tended to view the effect of a child with severe disabilities more negatively than others, they noted that extrafamilial and intrafamilial support can buffer the hardships. The availability and quality of social support are generally viewed as a critical factor in a family's ability to cope—a fact that should be noted by those in a position to affect public policy.

To suggest that the *type of impairment* or *severity of disability* is more debilitating to the family is less useful as determinants of impact. We believe that a more useful construct may come from Hill's (1949) model of stress. Recall from Chapter 2 that a key to a family's experience of stress is the *C* factor, which refers to how the family interprets a particular event. This view of human behavior would suggest that a key intervention with distressed families would be to help them to reorganize their thinking, which in turn would affect their outlook and thus their behavior. Several publications offer a cognitive approach to helping families cope (Singer & Powers, 1993; Turnbull et al., 1993). Of course, when social supports are lacking, changing family members' thinking will not, in itself, diminish their problems. A combination of constructive thinking about their situation and adequate family and community support would constitute a meaningful strategy for professionals to consider in helping these families. However, due to mounting tensions in the family and relentless burdens, a few families may need extensive psychotherapeutic help as well (Marsh, 1992; Marshak & Prezant, 2007).

One conclusion from this review is that it is too simplistic to base one's evaluation of family functioning on whether a child has a particular type of impairment or whether the disability is moderate or severe. Phenomenological thinkers have argued that the most meaningful reality is that which the person, or in this case, the family, perceives. It is only by "walking in the shoes" of another that we can truly understand his or her reality.

OTHER FACTORS THAT AFFECT THE FAMILY

Stress, along with its causes and consequences, has probably been studied more than any other construct with regard to coping in general and in regard to families of children with disabilities (Beckman, 1983; Friedrich, 1979; Friedrich & Friedrich, 1981; Houser & Seligman, 1991; Patterson, 1991; Wikler, 1981; Lustig & Akey, 1999b; Singer et al., 1999).

Some research indicates that stress is a major factor in the lives of family members who deal with disability and that emotional or social supports reduce stress and improve emotional well-being (Boyd, 2002; Evans, 2004). Other studies reported the reverse to be true. Houser

(1987), for example, reported that fathers of adolescent children with mental retardation were no more stressed than a control group of fathers of adolescents without retardation. This positive outcome conflicts with other studies on fathers (Andrew, 1968; Cummings, 1976; Holt, 1958). Dyson and Fewell (1986) found that parents of young children with severe impairments were significantly more stressed than a control group. Beckman (1983) reported that single mothers reported more stress than mothers in two-parent homes but found also that two child characteristics, age and sex, were not related to the amount of stress experienced by mothers—a finding that contradicts that of other studies (Bristol, 1984; Farber, 1959). These studies once again reflect the mixed and contradictory results found in the literature.

It is important to acknowledge that stress is a common human condition and that it is caused by both familial and extrafamilial factors. Furthermore, based on the available evidence we cannot say that these families experience more or less stress than the general population, although certain factors (e.g., lack of support, child characteristics) do add to the stress families experience. However, it is misleading to assume that stress is necessarily dysfunctional. Low levels of stress over relatively short periods of time may be perfectly adaptive. High levels of stress over long periods of time, however, are another matter: We believe that high stress levels, if chronically sustained, contribute significantly to a lowering of energy levels, performance failures, conflict in interpersonal relationships, depression, and other negative outcomes. However, we agree with Turnbull et al. (2006) that the following sources of support contribute to reduced stress and improved coping:

- Within-family support
- Family-to-family support
- Parent-to-parent program support
- Information provided by:
  - Parent training and information centers
  - Community resource centers
  - Clearinghouses
  - Family organizations
  - Books, magazines, and the Internet

Perhaps the research question that needs to be asked is whether stress levels of family members are high or low and whether they are sustained over long periods of time, rather than simply assessing whether stress exists or not. Clearly, the exploration of this phenomenon has captured the interest of researchers, but different questions regarding stress and families need to be formulated before meaningful conclusions can be reached.

The interest in stress research has sparked a corresponding interest in coping behaviors (Folkman, Lazarus, Dunkel-Schelter, De-Longis, & Gruen, 1986; Houser & Seligman, 1991; Turnbull et al., 1993). Coping, which can take several forms, has social support as a major component. Indeed, social support, both within and outside of the family, is generally viewed as buffering the effects of stress. In evaluating families, then, a useful approach would be to evaluate the demand characteristics of the child's disability, determine the coping resources within the family, and ascertain the social supports available to help reduce negative effects. In this regard, Matheny, Aycock, Pugh, Curlette, and Canella (1986) provided an in-depth discussion of coping resources (e.g., social support, beliefs/values, self-esteem) and coping behaviors (e.g., assertive responses, tension reduction strategies, cognitive restructuring). Turnbull et al. (2006) noted life-management skills such as reframing, passive appraisal, professional support, and spiritual support contribute to family coping.

There is some evidence that children with disabilities are at risk for abuse or neglect (Morgan, 1987; White, Benedict, Wulff, & Kelley, 1987). More than 12% of all children were victims of maltreatment in 2002 (NCCAN, 2004). Maltreatment refers to abuse, injury, or neglect that includes physical, emotional, and sexual abuse and neglect. Children with disabilities, however, are two to three times more likely to be victims of maltreatment than children without disabilities (Sullivan & Knudson, 2000). Furthermore, these children are least likely to have their stories of abuse believed.

Child maltreatment accounts for about 15% of new cases of developmental disabilities each year (Malow-Iroff & Johnson, 2005). For those children who are already disabled, the stress of caring for them can lead to abuse. Thus, these authors concluded, that "child maltreatment contributes to developmental disabilities and that children with disabilities are at high risk for child maltreatment" (p. 890).

The most consistently reported demographic factor associated with reported child abuse or neglect is low SES (White et al., 1987). However, child abuse among high-SES families tends to be underreported. Stress is a consequence of poor economic conditions, too much change too quickly, poor general coping, inadequate parenting skills, and social isolation. A major child characteristic in child abuse is low birth weight or prematurity. Premature infants are ill more often, cry more, and are more irritable; they may thus overwhelm their parents (Morgan, 1987). It is also important to keep in mind that some infants and children become disabled after an abusive attack, yet "states do not typically document the number of children whose disabilities were found to be caused by abuse" (Turnbull et al., 2006, p. 226). Childhood abuse continues to be an issue deserving of attention and redress.

Although some of the literature in this field has stressed the negative impact of childhood disability on the family, other studies have noted benefits created by the presence of such a child in the home (Singer & Powers, 1993; Turnbull et al., 1993). Some of the positive aspects include (1) increased family cohesion, (2) increased "involvement," and (3) personal growth (Darling & Baxter, 1986). The literature on the negative impact of children with disabilities must be balanced by a greater recognition of family strengths. More research is needed on the positive effects that arise from childhood disability. We are pleased to report that since the publication of the first edition of *Ordinary Families, Special Children* in 1989, we have detected a move in the direction of discerning family resilience, strengths, and coping abilities.

We conclude this chapter by quoting Marshak and Prezant (2007) about the impact of childhood disability on the spousal subsystem:

> If we use the metaphor of a marriage being like the two of you going down the river on a boat, this phase of life represents the rapids in terms of the speed and intensity of forces that may crash into you. Many of those who experience a rough ride make it through as a strengthed couple. Some are relatively unaffected as a couple, but often sustain damage that threatens to swamp or destroy the marital "boat." The main danger involves breaking apart from each other as a couple. This is often due to a failure to understood or accept differences in emotional coping styles. The lack of comprehension or tolerance in such a stressful emotional time often results in alienation and a widening gap between spouses.

■8

Effects on Fathers

Mothers have been the most studied family members in the area of childhood disability. As noted, mothers are often asked in research studies to evaluate other family members' reactions to their child's disability. Mothers are studied more because they are more accessible. More importantly, attention to mothers reflects the fact that they give birth and are considered natural caregivers and nurturers. Also, mothers stay at home to raise the children more often than their partners, who work outside the home. Within the context of a family systems perspective, which stresses that all family members are affected by a crisis, fathers, siblings, and grandparents are now being considered important influences. Most of the literature reviewed in previous chapters was derived from studies of mothers. This chapter examines one of the lesser studied groups of family members: fathers.

One author observed that fathering is the "single most creative, complicated, fulfilling, frustrating, engrossing, enriching, depleting endeavor of a man's life" (Pruett, 1987, p. 282). After a series of studies on infant attachment and the research on "maternal deprivation" there emerged a realization that in emphasizing mothers, researchers neglected the broader context in which children are raised (Lamb & Meyer, 1991). The role of fathers in child development and family functioning had been undervalued. A significant range of social problems, such as childhood poverty, teenage pregnancy, and poor school performance, can be traced to the absence of fathers in the lives of their children (Silverstein & Auerbach, 1999; Evans, 2004). The term "paternal deprivation" has been applied to this phenomenon (Biller & Klimpton, 1997). The meager interest in the father's influence can be attributed, in part, to Freud's (1926/1936) theories, which promoted the mother as the primary influence in the development of children. One author suggested that the father's role in child development was secondary to that of the mother (Bowlby, 1951). Thus, until the 1970s, the mother's role in the family overshadowed that of the father.

Traditionally, men assumed an instrumental role whereas women were socialized into an expressive one. The instrumental role is task oriented and involves problem solving, independence, rational thought, and an unemotional stance (Darling & Baxter, 1996; Parsons, 1951). Conversely, the expressive role involves attention to communication, feelings, emotional needs, and cooperation. Evidence for the elevation of the importance of fathers has been the escalation of publications on fathers in the last several years (Darling & Baxter, 1996; Hornby, 1995a; Houser & Seligman, 1991; May, 1991; Meyer, 1995; Mahalik, Good, & Englar-Carlson, 2003).

Interest in fathers has come about for several reasons (Hornby, 1988; Pruett, 1987). Accompanying the increase in the number of mothers who work has come a corresponding focus on alternative caregivers for children, and a likely resource for alternative care would be fathers. The shortened work week means that fathers have more time to spend with their families. Changes in child custody laws have contributed to an increase in the number of single fathers who have joint or sole custody of their children. In addition, compelling research on masculine roles and scripts and their relationship to major health problems in men have promoted investigation of this link. Gender roles are more flexible, so that the identification of women with motherhood and caretaking and men with breadwinning is less rigid. The dearth of information on fathers and fathering has encouraged researchers to investigate this family role from a number of perspectives.

THE FATHER'S ROLE

In the past, children were viewed as malleable organisms waiting to be shaped by outside socialization processes. A more contemporary view suggests that each child has individual characteristics that not only affect the way the child is influenced by external forces but that also cause the child to shape the socializers themselves (Lamb, 1983). Therefore, socialization is viewed as a bidirectional process. According to reviews by Lamb (1983), Meyer, Vadasy, Fewell, and Schell (1985), and Lamb and Meyer (1991), nurturing emotions are not unique to mothers; fathers also know instinctively how to interact with their infants and how to care for them. Furthermore, fathers are interested in their infants and want to be actively involved with them. In fact, during infancy the father's sensitivity to his infant's distress is just as acute as the mother's. One study of fathers of children in Kindergarten through third grade showed that fathers spend a comparable amount of time caring for their children and in school-related activities (Turbiville, 1994).

There are differences between mothers' and fathers' behaviors with their infants that begin to emerge shortly after birth. Mothers tend to engage more in caretaking whereas fathers tend to play more with their infants. Fathers are more vigorous with their infants, and they are more likely to pick up and toss their infants and generally be rougher than mothers, who are more likely to play such games as peek-a-boo or hide-and-seek. However, fathers, like mothers, adapt their play to their child's developmental level, suggesting that both fathers and mothers are equally sensitive to their child's developmental changes. These general observations would suggest that fathers are competent nurturers and caretakers.

An important area of research that appears to play a role in the emotions and behaviors of men has emerged. This line of inquiry has to do with the rigid masculine roles and scripts to which men subscribe and that bear a relationship to their families, their work, and social situations. In addition to the effects on interactions with family members and others, the research evidence is compelling that "macho" roles contribute to major health problems in men. In this regard Mahalik et al. (2003) discussed "scripts" that men follow that can lead to unwanted outcomes. We briefly consider the scripts and how they pertain to children with disabilities:

Strong and Silent Script

Masculine role expectations demand that men maintain control of their emotions. Levant and Pollack (1995) coined the term "alexithymia" to denote not having words for emotions. Such restricted emotionality has been linked to fear of intimacy, higher levels of depression, anxiety, and anger. The inability to express one's emotions can cause problems within the family, probably more so if there is a child with a disability. It can be devastating for fathers of children with a disability who would be well served or would benefit from expressing their emotions of anger, sadness, grief, and disappointment.

Tough-Guy Script

Related to the script above is the tough guy who projects fearlessness, aggression, and invulnerability in the face of difficulties. Tough guys take risks and are involved in fatal auto accidents three times more often than women. There are major health consequences related to both the strong and silent and tough-guy scripts. These factors contribute to the challenge some men face in coping with their powerful emotions in the wake of childhood disability (Mahalik et al., 2003).

Give-'Em-Hell Script

Aggression or violence can be sparked by feelings of vulnerability or to cover up uncomfortable feeling (e.g., fear, anxiety, shame). Men see violence or aggression as a way to gain control in interpersonal situations (e.g., conflict with spouse, loss of job; Mahalik et al., 2003). In some instances, when frustration and anger are caused by inadequate services and uninterested professionals, a father's *assertive* though not aggressive, response can be helpful. Families of children with disabilities must cope with a service delivery system that is not always up to the challenges these families face. Thus assertive actions can facilitate better care.

Playboy Script

This script relates, in part, to behaviors related to sexuality. The relevant part of this script to our discussion involves fears of relating to, and connecting with, others. A sense of vulnerability and fear of intimacy can permeate a man's partnership with his spouse. In families of children with disabilities conflicts around issues of intimacy may make it difficult for the partners to provide a relatively conflict-free environment for their children. Intimacy issues can precede or follow a child's birth.

In sum, rigid masculine scripts can compromise men's (fathers') health and can interfere with positive relations within the family. Fears of vulnerability, intimacy, and the difficulty communicating emotions can result in problems such as alcohol abuse, distancing, and problems with intimacy and aggression. Mahalik et al. (2003) cited research that points to the following problems men experience: greater medical concerns, greater distress, problems with violence, greater depression, and difficulties with intimacy.

In regard to fathers of children with disabilities, some of these male attributes may interfere with the mourning process. Many fathers believe they must be strong and in control of their emotions, and to be competitive and fulfill the roles of family protector, provider, and problem solver.

> Just as these role attributes interfere with the mourning process in the case of biological death, they also interfere with the process of adaptation that accompanies the ... [disability] of a child. Their inability to serve as protectors undermines their self esteem; their suppression of affect may prevent them from resolving their emotional burden; and their involvement increases their care giving burden. In addition, the metamorphosis of male roles in recent years has undoubtedly added to the confusion that fathers experience when they are confronted with the disability of a child. (Marsh, 1998, pp. 155–156)

FATHERS AND THE CHILD WITH A DISABILITY

Compared to the research and commentary devoted to maternal adaptation, and even to that of siblings, there is still not enough studies of fathers whose children have disabilities. Therefore, conclusions about fathers' adjustment must be made cautiously. Some of the studies are compromised in a variety of ways (Lamb & Meyer, 1991; Hornby, 1995a). First, there are few observational studies of fathers whose children have disabilities. Findings are sometimes based on maternal reports of paternal reactions. Maternal reports were sought because this perspective was considered sufficient to get an accurate picture of the family (Crowley & Taylor, 1994). However, mothers constitute a secondary source. Second, many studies are methodologically flawed, and often researchers provide few details concerning the procedures used and the range of disabilities represented. Third, studies have focused on the fathers' reaction to the diagnosis and on initial adaptation rather than on the impact on fathers of adolescent or adult children. Finally, there is a disproportionate interest in fathers with children who have intellectual disability, to the exclusion of children with other developmental disabilities or chronic illness.

Fathers and mothers initially respond differently to the news that they have produced a child with a disability (Lamb & Meyer, 1991). Fathers tend to respond less emotionally and focus on possible long-term concerns, whereas mothers respond more emotionally and are concerned about their ability to cope with the burdens of child care. Thus, fathers tend to perceive the diagnosis of the disability as an instrumental crisis, whereas mothers see it as an expressive crisis. Fathers may be more instrumental and mothers more expressive, however, some fathers are concerned about the day-to-day demands of the disability, and some mothers worry about the costs of raising a child with a disability.

Fathers tend to be more concerned than mothers about the adoption of socially acceptable behavior by their children—especially their sons—and they are more anxious about the social status and occupational success of their offspring. As a result, fathers are more concerned about the long-term outcomes of their children with disabilities than mothers are, and they are probably more affected by the visibleness of the disability (Lamb & Meyer, 1991; Tallman, 1965). One study found that fathers of children with severe disabilities were involved in playing, nurturing, discipline, and helping to decide on services (Simmerman, Blacher, & Baker, 2001). In a study of 575 men work and other demands were the most important barriers to fathers' involvement in a child's education (Summers, Boller, & Raikes, 2004).

Differences between mothers and fathers are not necessarily good or bad; they do suggest approaches that may serve to complement each other—or, if there are deep impasses, they can contribute to tension and added stress. In such instances, couple counseling can prove beneficial. Counseling allows parents to view each other's perspectives and expectations in a protected environment. A neutral professional can help sort out and resolve areas of conflict between parents.

In one study mothers considered the child's characteristics as adding to their stress, whereas marital factors were the main source of stress for fathers (Sloper, Knussen, Turner, & Cunningham, 1991). In another study, mothers and fathers demonstrated similar perceptions of sibling relationships and cohesion, but mothers were more likely to perceive external sources of support as helpful and important whereas fathers considered spousal support as more important (Crowley & Taylor, 1994). Other studies have likewise found similarities and differences between spouses, but because different instruments and procedures were used, there is no consensus as to how fathers and mothers perceive the challenges brought about by childhood disability.

However, from their literature review and their own study, Crowley and Taylor (1994) advised the following:

> For practitioners, it is critical to remember that the concerns of mothers and fathers about their child with a disability may be fundamentally different. Effective intervention will require talking to *each* parent regarding his or her or her concerns, and devising specific treatment plans to address these concerns. In terms of support, mothers are more likely to be helped through external sources of support and appropriate referral would be beneficial. Conversely, fathers will feel more supported through strengthening the marital dyad and working to keep the lines of communication between the parents open. (p. 223)

Because of the high expectations fathers have of their sons, they may be especially disappointed when they have a boy with a disability (Farber, 1959; Grossman, 1972). The behavioral consequences of this disappointment are manifested in extremes of intense involvement with, and total withdrawal from, their sons, whereas some early studies showed that fathers seem to have limited, routine involvement with their daughters who are disabled (Chigier, 1972; Grossman, 1972; Tallman, 1965). Recent studies, however, do not support the contention that fathers are more distressed by a boy with a disability than a girl, suggesting that more research is needed in this area (Hornby, 1995a, 1995b; Houser & Seligman, 1991).

Fathers' reactions to their children with special needs have implications for other family members. For example, one early study found a strong relationship between the degree of paternal acceptance toward the child and the amount of acceptance and rejection generally observed in the home (Peck & Stephens, 1960). This suggests that the father's reaction might set the tone for the entire family. Lamb (1983) and Lamb and Meyer (1991) speculated that paternal acceptance reflects the fact that fathers obtain less satisfaction from children with disabilities than from nondisabled children, although this assertion is not necessarily borne out by other research (Ricci & Hodapp, 2003; Lillie, 1993; Klein & Kemp, 2004). Fathers' involvement is discretionary; that is, fathers can increase or decrease their involvement, whereas mothers are expected to show the same commitment to all children (Lamb, 1983). When fathers withdraw, the development of the child is affected and the entire family suffers. Indeed, Houser and Seligman (1991) found that the fathers who experienced higher levels of stress tended to cope by employing escape–avoidance strategies, as in the following illustration: "Rick's father, Ed, coped with his discomfort with his son in a different way. He avoided him. Already busy, Ed became a workaholic. He left the house at six or six-thirty in the morning to prepare for his clients, and returned at seven-thirty at night with his briefcase full" (Greenspan & Wieder, 2003, p. 368).

When fathers pull away, other family members will be affected and will respond in reaction to the father's withdrawal. When fathers withdraw, the burden of care falls to other family members, particularly the mother. The father's distancing behavior, as family members struggle with the added pressures of coping with a child with special needs, will set into motion negative and dysfunctional dynamics. Mothers are forced to cope alone with the emotionally and physically demanding tasks of attending to the child's needs and the needs of other family members when fathers withdraw. Fathers may thus bear a greater responsibility for allowing a child's special needs to have adverse effects on the marriage. If fathers choose to be more involved, their own satisfaction and the integration of the family tends to increase (Lamb & Meyer, 1991; Lillie, 1993; Willoughby & Glidden, 1995; Greenspan & Wieder, 2003).

A father's stoic behavior can be viewed by professionals as a more manageable reaction. The male physicians quoted below seem to feel more comfortable communicating distressing information to fathers than to mothers:

> Usually I prefer to tell the father. The mother is in an emotional state after having just given birth.

> If I had a choice, I'd probably prefer talking with the father first and let him help me make the decision about talking to the mother.

> I call the father and ask him what he wants me to do. I wait until I can reach the father before I talk to the mother.

> I try to talk to the obstetrician to find out if it's the mother's first baby or if she's anxious or apprehensive. I always tell the father right away. (Darling, 1979, p. 206)

However, professionals should be careful about assuming that mothers and fathers will react in stereotypic ways. Sometimes, in fact, the *mother* may play the role of comforter, as this father's account suggests:

[After learning that the baby had Down syndrome,] I must have looked as if I were horribly lost, because through her tears Janet was actually trying to comfort me: "We can handle this," I remember her saying. "We can handle this together. This is not a stopper. We can handle this." (Berube, 1996, p. 6)

Many of the assertions about fathers require considerably more study than what is presently available (Hornby, 1995a, 1995b). In his British study, Hornby evaluated adaptation, marital functioning, social support, stress, and personality of 87 fathers of children with Down syndrome. The mean age of the fathers was 41 years (range = 27–62 years); 64% of the children were boys, with a mean age of 9.2 years and a mean IQ of 40 (range = 7–63). Hornby's research showed the following:

1. Fathers adapted equally well to their sons and daughters.
2. Fathers' adaptation was not related to the severity of their child's disability.
3. The stress experienced by fathers was not related to the ages of their children.
4. Fathers' adaptation was not related to the level of social support they received but to their satisfaction with the support.
5. Fathers' adaptation was significantly related to their levels of neuroticism.
6. The stress experienced by fathers was inversely related to the educational level and perceived financial adequacy, but not to their social class.
7. The majority of fathers did not experience depression or major personality problems.
8. Fathers did not experience higher levels of marital distress, nor were they more prone to divorce than the national average.

In his conclusion, Hornby (1995b) noted:

Clearly these findings regarding fathers of children with Down syndrome provide quite a different view of the effects on fathers of children of disabilities than has appeared in the literature. Therefore, it is possible that the assertions about these fathers, on which there was a consensus in previous reviews of the literature, provide a mostly erroneous view of their experiences. (p. 252)

Hornby's (1995a, 1995b) research supports the contention that the fathers in his studies adjusted quite well to their child with Down syndrome.

In his discussion/support groups, Smith (1981) found that fathers distrusted male displays of emotion and that they had learned as children that "men" are always in control of their emotions and that "big boys" don't cry. Along with others (e.g., Mihalik et al., 2003; Lamb & Meyer, 1991), Smith contended that these masculine behaviors place considerable stress on fathers and make it harder for them to express and be attuned to their own feelings. In an article authored by psychologist, author, and parent Robert Naseef (1999), titled, "Big Boys Don't Cry," he observed that fathers and children have a bidirectional influence on each other; an assertion also made by Lamb and Meyer (1991):

> I thought I would change him and make him the boy I wanted him to be. But he has changed me, and helped me to become the man I needed to be. He taught me the meaning of unconditional love—to honor his sacred right to be loved for who he is, not what he has achieved lately, how he looks, or how much money he will earn. What a priceless lesson that he has taught me in his silence, without words—like a Buddha. (p. 3)

In Smith's discussion groups, those facets of the stereotypic masculine role were restrictive and presented obstacles to the men's coming to terms with their children's disabilities and with their own feelings as parents of children with disabilities. In particular, these men displayed stereotypical instrumental traits, as noted by Mahalik et al. (2003), such as a reluctance to show one's emotions, a need for independence and self-reliance, and a need to "fix" problematic situations.

As fathers of children with disabilities, men experienced a variety of intense emotions that they could not easily express or confront. Some felt anger at physicians who initially informed them of their child's disability, believing that they were unnecessarily abrupt and unsympathetic, a complaint noted by both parents. Furthermore, the fathers found themselves dependent on the expertise of professionals. This dependence made them feel less in control and less competent as parents. Males are socialized to be "fixers" who actively confront problems. Passivity in the face of a crisis is threatening to men who have learned that they must be "strong," not show weakness (mainly by suppressing emotions), and be able to resolve difficult situations competently. The most poignant frustration is that fathers simply cannot "fix" their child's disability, and, despite their anguish about this situation, they may not be able to express how they feel.

Azar (1994) reported that the suppression of emotions contributes to a heightened intrusion of disturbing thoughts: "Keeping thoughts secret creates a suppression cycle: The thought immediately comes to mind, the person tries to suppress it again and the cycle continues. Wegner hypothesizes that disclosing suppressed thoughts may stop this cycle and prevent intrusive thoughts" (p. 25). As we noted earlier, suppressed emotions have medical as well as psychological implications, as noted by Mihalik et al. (2003). Headaches, back pain, and a more vulnerable immune system have been linked to suppressed emotions.

Smith, as well as Seligman and Marshak (2003), believes that support/discussion groups for fathers are an important resource and indirectly will have a positive effect on the entire family. The support that fathers can provide to their wives and other family members is another reason it is important that they learn to cope with their child's disability.

In terms of the vulnerability fathers experience in the face of childhood disability, Marsh (1992) wrote:

> Their [fathers'] inability to serve as protectors undermines their self-esteem; their suppression of affect may prevent them from resolving their emotional burden; and their involvement increases their caregiving burden. In addition, the metamorphosis of male roles in recent years has undoubtedly added to the confusion that fathers experience when they are confronted with the disability of a child. (p. 155)

As noted, we believe that contemporary views of fathers reflect a more flexible and nurturing role as opposed to the rigid, instrumental, "breadwinner" father of the past.

Some fathers of children with disabilities may reject their child and withdraw; some feel less competent and lower self-esteem; and some may experience considerable frustration as they confront the masculine injunctions they have learned to exercise in the face of powerful emotions. The issues then become, how might a father learn to be more accepting of his child and how can he come to terms with emotions that are not easily expressed or are manifested by excessive anger or withdrawal (Houser & Seligman, 1991; Greenspan & Wieder, 2003).

The following illustration reflects the type of family dynamics that may occur when a father is unable to come to terms with the circumstances brought about by the birth of his son:

> At about 2½ years of age, the Lewis family grew increasingly concerned about their son's symptoms. After a few futile attempts to secure a diagnosis, a psychologist they consulted provided them with a diagnosis, pervasive developmental disorder. Ann Lewis responded by learning as much as she could about the disorder. However, George reacted differently. He didn't read. He didn't search for answers. He didn't even talk to Ann about the diagnosis. He withdrew. He spent more and more time at work—he even brought work home at night to avoid facing his feelings about his son. He came home eight or nine o'clock, knowing that Michael would be in bed, to find Ann sleeping on the sofa. (Greenspan & Wieder, 2003, p. 354)

Thus, George's fears, anxiety, and depression led to his emotional and instrumental withdrawal, which, in turn, led to Ann's increased burden and anger. This dismal situation begs the question of what intervention efforts can be directed toward fathers to help them cope more successfully with their child.

The discussion group model proposed by Smith (1981), the support group format discussed by Seligman and Marshak (2003), as well as those discussed in Chapter 12 seem to provide the type of intervention that can help ameliorate some of the problems noted above. Individual and/or couples counseling can help parents sort out sources of conflict and stress and help reduce misunderstandings and faulty communication patterns. Another promising venture is the workshop format that has been developed at the University of Washington, which offers a manual specifying the methods of conducting groups for fathers.

Starting in 1978, fathers of young children with disabilities in Seattle, Washington were exposed to a group format that provides information and social support (Vadasy, Fewell, Greenberg, Desmond, & Meyer, 1986). Donald Meyer continues this work to this day by providing informative workshops throughout the United States. The basic structure was that fathers met twice monthly for 2 hours. They brought their child with them to sessions organized by two male facilitators, one a professional and one a father of a child with a disability. The meetings included activities in which fathers and children participated together, such as songs, dances, and games. Time was set aside for fathers to meet without their children so that they could discuss their concerns. Guests were invited to speak on topics selected by the fathers at some of the meetings. Mothers were often invited to attend the presentations, and special family meetings were scheduled at holidays and occasionally at other times. This format allowed fathers to acquire information, experience social support from other fathers, discuss feelings and practical concerns, and develop strong attachments to their child. Fathers' need for information about parenting is strong, and they prefer receiving information in parenting classes, in written form, or via telephone hotline (Summers et al., 2004).

The fathers' workshop manual, developed by the investigators at the University of Washington, describes in detail how to initiate a fathers' group, select leaders, and plan for the various components of the meetings. Since 1980, participating families have been the subjects of research on the program's impact on parents' stress levels and coping abilities.

Organizations serving children with disabilities should not neglect the fathers' involvement in the family and in programs promoted by agencies. Professionals need to make concerted efforts to establish partnerships with fathers (Friedman & Berkeley, 2002; Rump, 2002). Fathers have a need for information about their children's disability and about programs, services, and treatment that is equal to that of mothers (Darling & Baxter, 1996). Professionals need to create opportunities for paternal involvement by scheduling meetings that are convenient for both parents, sending home informative materials and newsletters addressed to both parents, and actively soliciting fathers' opinions about their child, their concerns, and their perceptions of the services provided.

Introducing a different perspective, Lillie (1993) asserted that fathers' lack of involvement with their children with disabilities can be attributed, in part, to (1) their inability to cope with such children, (2) the fact that the children are involved with female-dominated service systems, and (3) because historically fathers have been constrained by gender roles from providing direct child care. He believes that fathers are discouraged by service providers from providing direct child care, even though some fathers would welcome such involvement. To quote Lillie (1993), "Many fathers apparently want more involvement than they currently have but are constrained by 'gate keeping' roles of mothers and the structure of their children's programs" (p. 438). Lillie's observation suggests that social service agencies are not necessarily "father friendly." B. Gill (1997) noted that, "Without realizing it, mothers can drown fathers out. While harboring resentment because their partners are not helping them, they are in fact not making space for their participation." Furthermore, Gill added, "Fathers need to assert themselves and insist on being involved. Mothers should let fathers in and let them learn at their own pace to care for the child in their own way. Our children need both of us" (pp. 47–48).

These comments suggest that a firmly attached mother can inadvertently exclude the father's participation via her gate-keeping role. There may be a number of reasons for excluding fathers from their paternal rights and responsibilities in caring for their child. One may be the mother's anxiety related to the perception that she can be the only nurturer and caretaker due to a strong attachment to the child.

Social service agencies and the existence of certain family dynamics can lead to the exclusion of fathers. However, as described by Danny Presley (1995), fathers contribute to this problem as well:

> My wife and I have been to a few functions for parents of children with disabilities. For the most part, it is the mothers who attend these functions. So I began to wonder, where are the dads? After asking around I found that some of these men don't have anything to do with their special child. Some of them left when they found out about the disability.
>
> I find this downright shameful on their part. What's wrong with these guys? Is it shame? Guilt? Stupidity? Does it threaten their masculinity to admit it? I don't understand this at all. (p. 6)

Although it is important to urge fathers to become involved, it is equally important to be cognizant of cultural factors in developing programs with fathers in mind. For example, family privacy is a primary value in some cultures. Thus a discussion group format may be poorly suited for fathers from these cultures, who may be better served through natural systems of support (e.g., extended family, church) or by reading material such as newsletters, books, Internet information sites, and the like. Also, as Chapter 3 suggests, the roles of fathers vary across cultural groups, and service providers need to take these differences into account.

In summary, as a result of some modest research efforts, we know that some fathers experience adverse reactions to the birth of a child with a disability. Fathers who are coping poorly themselves tend to find it difficult to be supportive of their partners. When fathers experience stress and withdraw from their families, other family members (especially the mother) must take up the slack, resulting in family tensions. Furthermore, there is some evidence that fathers may cope better with a daughter than a son. A promising resource for fathers seems to be a discussion or support group format that can help them form more positive attachments to their young children with special needs, gain information, and discuss their common problems in a supportive context. Generally speaking, given the changes in fathers' roles, the existence of supportive groups, and the information available on the Internet, fathers should be in a better position to adapt to their children. It seems that most fathers do accommodate easily to their children with disabilities, whereas others have learned and grown from their experiences over time. However, a minority of these fathers struggle considerably with the reality of having a child with a disability. These fathers need to be encouraged, supported, and prompted to express their pain.

In closing, we reiterate that more research is needed on fathers to better understand their responses and coping behaviors to their sons and daughters with disabilities. Based on the information presented in this chapter, we offer the following observations:

- Service providers and agencies need to monitor how "father friendly" they are and to actively encourage paternal participation.
- Fathers as well as their family members and the professionals who serve them remain aware of male role injunctions, which often have a deleterious effect on them and their family.
- Communities and agencies should seriously consider developing discussion/support groups for fathers.
- It should be kept in mind that a poorly functioning father creates added stresses to the family unit.
- Interventions aimed at fathers must accommodate the family's cultural values and roles.

9

Effects on Siblings

In the late 1960s, in a sermon on equality, William Sloane Coffin said, "Am I my brother's keeper? No, I am my brother's brother." His concept was one that I instinctively understood and long for: A relationship of mutuality, based on respect, that neither diminished nor augmented either participant.

—MOORMAN (1992b, p. 47)

Similar to their parents, siblings share in the anticipation and excitement of a new child in the family. However, they also share in the grief, pain, and challenges that may accompany the birth of an infant with a disability. As we have seen, a considerable literature on family adaptation currently exists, which has primarily focused on the parents, with a particular emphasis on mothers. The research and personal accounts on siblings, however, suggest that, although many cope well, others may be "at risk" psychologically (Sharpe & Rossiter, 2002; McHugh, 1999; Orsmond & Seltzer, 2000; Safer, 2002; Lobato, 1990; Moorman, 1992b; Powell & Gallagher, 1993; Stoneman & Berman, 1993; Lardieri, Blacher, & Swanson, 2000).

The effect of a brother or sister with a disability on nondisabled siblings has emerged as a significant area of research and concern

(Ufner, 2004). In the first edition, we wrote that "we need considerably more research before we fully understand disabled and nondisabled brothers and sisters, their respective roles in the family, and the
reciprocal effects they have on each other (p. 111)." Based on prior
research and commentary, particularly since the mid-1980s, reasonable speculations can be made about sibling relationships.

This chapter explores the factors that appear to influence sibling
relationships. The first part of this chapter reviews sibling relationships in general. We then explore sibling relationships and adjustment
when one of them has a disability.

THE SIBLING BOND

Sibling relationships are usually the longest and most enduring of family relationships (Moen & Wethington, 1999). This long-term relationship makes it possible for two individuals to exert considerable influence over each other through longitudinal interactions. As Powell and
Gallagher (1993) noted, "Siblings provide a continuing relationship
from which there is no annulment" (p. 14). Different expectations for
siblings depend on culture, and age, birth order, and gender define
the roles and relationships siblings experience (Harry, Day, & Quist,
1998).

Sibling relationships are cyclical. In their pioneering book *The Sibling Bond*, Bank and Kahn (1997) observed that siblings follow a life
cycle of their own. They provide a constant source of companionship
for one another during the early childhood years. Ufner (2004) also
noted:

> From the time a baby enters the family, a special bond develops between
> the children. Older siblings take great pride in being the "big" brother or
> sister and help to care for younger ones. . . . The younger ones look up to
> the older brothers and sisters, seeking advice and assistance as they learn
> about the world. Siblings share household tasks and talk together about
> the world. They share secrets kept from their parents. Siblings protect
> one another, support one another, and ally themselves against parents.
> Siblings also see each other as competitors, teasers, and antagonists.
> (pp. 15–16)

During the school-age years, it is common for siblings to form relationships with others outside of the immediate family as they exercise the

social skills they have developed together. During adolescence, siblings manifest ambivalence about their mutual relationship, yet they still rely on each other as confidants, supports, and playmates. In adulthood, siblings tend to interact less often due to marriage and/or geographic distance. During this period, siblings provide long-distance support and encouragement as they embrace the vicissitudes of adult life.

In addition, as aunts and uncles they provide unique support networks for each other's children. And finally, in old age, when children move on to increased independence and spouses pass away, siblings continue to provide a social network for each other (Harris & Glasberg, 2003). During this later stage, sibling relationships often become reestablished or intensify in a manner similar to the first stages of their lives together.

The many changes in contemporary family life add to the importance of studying sibling relationships (Goldenberg & Goldenberg, 2003). Beilfus and Verbrugge (as cited in Ufner, 2004) report five patterns in sibling relationships: the caregiver relationship, the buddy relationship, the critical relationship, the rival relationship, and the casual relationship.

In short, sibling relationships, are intense, long term, cyclical, and complex. Professionals need to be particularly sensitive to the many facets of the siblings' experience. Siblings seem to share with their parents the loss that may accompany the birth of a child with a disability (Marsh, 1992). They may, however, be less vulnerable than their parents, who assume financial and caregiving responsibilities. In other ways, they are more vulnerable because of their age, which carries a special susceptibility to the stress and disruption that affect other family members. Some siblings may not be affected by, or they benefit from, this experience; other siblings simply do not fare well. Simple cause-and-effect explanations of the impact siblings have on each other are misleading. We agree with Stoneman and Berman (1993) when they observed that

> the sibling relationship is directly affected by specific characteristics of the individual siblings, by characteristics of the family in which the children live, and by the childrearing strategies used by the children's parents or primary caregiver. The childrearing strategies used by parents, in turn, are influenced by several factors, including characteristics of the parents and the emotional climate of the family and of the individual siblings. (p. 4)

In the following pages we examine the sibling relationship from both a research and an autobiographical perspective. Our plan is to explore the various factors mentioned in the literature that have a bearing on sibling response to a brother or sister with a disability.

THE NEED FOR INFORMATION

Families tend to be more empowered and better able to help their children when they have access to relevant information (Turnbull et al., 2006). However, parents may be reluctant to communicate with their nondisabled children about the child with the disability. As a result, siblings may have a limited understanding of their brother's or sister's condition. Generally speaking, there is a startling lack of information in these families about the disability, its manifestations, its implications, and its consequences. Misinformation or the lack of it confuses siblings in regard to several factors, such as feeling responsible for a particular condition, whether a disability is transmittable, what are the implications for the siblings' future, and the like. There may be several reasons parents choose to shield their concerns and emotions from their children. They may feel abnormal and shameful, and thus not want to burden their children, or believe that their anxieties should be hidden from their children because they are adult concerns (Harris & Glasberg, 2003).

The central concern about parents' lack of communication is the fantasies children create when ambiguity exists. When feelings and information are hidden, the mystery of a sibling's disability becomes rich fodder for imagination. As Harris and Glasberg (2003) contended, the inventions siblings manufacture can be more frightening than the actual disability.

Nondisabled children may imagine that they contributed to their sibling's disability or illness; minor infractions become major anxieties. For example, children under age 4 or 5 are egocentric and believe that things happen because of them. They may believe that their "bad" thoughts or actions (some minor indiscretion) caused their brother or sister's disability. "Preschoolers who have learned that one can 'catch' a cold by drinking from the same cup as someone who is sneezing and coughing may believe that they can 'catch' mental retardation" (Siegel & Silverstein, 1994, p. 68). Latency-age children (5–11) still believe in fairy tales and may conclude that their brother or sister with mental retardation will someday be normal. In regard to the subsequent years, McHugh (1999) observed that "later on, when we can understand more, we want information that is clear, structured, and definite. No vague simplistic answers" (p. 25). In all such instances age-appropriate information can help alleviate a child's anxieties and self-blame.

Simple explanations can ease feelings of resentment and jealousy. If the parents struggle with their emotions, they should feel assured that children can accept their sadness, mild and occasional depression, and anger when also being told about their feelings of love and concern. Harris and Glasberg (2003) offer the following advice:

> If you label your own emotions, and explain that they are linked to feelings of concern for your child but do not diminish your love for the child or for the other children, this may help ease siblings' concern about your emotional state. At the very least, your child will know that she is not the cause of your distress, and she can realistically label your feelings as due to other events in your life. (p. 86)

As noted, parents may not be willing or able to share information with their children. Turnbull et al. (2006) noted that parents have an especially difficult time discussing future plans with their nondisabled children. Such discussions generally center around care and responsibility for their child with a disability when parents are unable to provide such care. Children may harbor many questions about their special circumstances after the birth of a child with a disability, as listed by McHugh (1999):

> What's going on here? What happened to the new baby? Why are you always going to the hospital? Why didn't the new baby come home when Mommy did? Will I catch it? Did I do anything bad that made him sick? Why is everybody so sad, angry, and tired? Aren't you ever going to play with me the way you used to? Why do you push me away when I try to hug you? Why are you always telling me to be quiet? (p. 25)

A colleague of one of us (M. S.) had been told as a youngster that her sister suffered from asthma. In fact, her sister had cerebral palsy. Asthma was a more acceptable condition than cerebral palsy in a family where social appearances were paramount. When parents are unable (for whatever reason) to inform their children about their child's disability, siblings seek information on their own. Sometimes they search for information without knowing that they are doing so. Hazi (personal communication, 1992) described her own experience:

> In addition to taking two elective classes in special education, I volunteered to work as a tutor and aide. I worked with slower kids in teaching them to read and began to see learning problems at all levels. I volunteered at the child development center and saw small children who were "developmentally delayed" and learning to crawl. I also went to a local chapter of retarded citizens to stuff envelopes and stood on city street corners collecting money. I see now that these must have been early attempts to collect more information about Mary Louise's condition, information that I never got from my parents.

The type of information requested appears to be related to age (McHugh, 1999; Murphy, Paeschel, Duffy, & Brady, 1976). Cognitive abilities may place limits on understanding, especially for very young children. From ages 6–9, children asked questions about motor development and speech, discussed what their brothers and sisters could and could not do, and were interested in the medical and biological information presented to them. Concerns about the future became evident among the 10- to 12-year-old children, whereas the older adolescents showed concern about their own chances of bearing a child with a disability.

Informing a child about his or her sibling's disability falls to the parents. However, parents are not always well informed. "My parents never talked to me about Sally's illness. They couldn't have explained it to me even if they'd wanted to, for no one adequately explained it to them" (Moorman, 1992a, p. 42). Furthermore, the decision to withhold or shield them from the reality of the disability is more prevalent with children who have a mental illness (Ufner, 2004). Some parents decide to withhold the truth because of the cliché of protecting a younger child (Swados, 1991).

Siblings need a way to get information at various stages of their lives (Powell & Gallagher, 1993). They need a system that is responsive to their personal questions in addition to the generic, predetermined questions. Provision of information needs to be an ongoing process that reflects their age, maturity, and changing needs. Children at age 7 need information that is different from that sought out by an adolescent, young adult, or a 47-year-old sibling with questions about lifelong care and estate planning.

CAREGIVING

Excessive parental caregiving of the child with the disability or quasi-parenting can result in anger, resentment, and guilt, along with anxiety and depression, especially if it is combined with limited parental attention for the nondisabled children (Sharpe & Rossiter, 2002). A friend of one of us (M. S.), in her late 60s, mentioned that she still harbors angry and resentful feelings about her youth as a result of the attention her diabetic sister received from her parents. The friend expressed surprise that although her feelings felt very distant in time, they continued to evoke a strong negative reaction in her.

Depending on the disability or illness, the child with special needs may absorb a great deal of time, energy, and emotional resources. Before they are ready, siblings may be pressed into parental roles they are ill prepared to assume. *Parentification* is the term used for children who parent too early, and the danger is that such children lose their childhood (Siegel & Silverstein, 1994). The process of parentification can interfere with developmental stages important for emotional growth. As Siegel and Silverstein (1994) noted:

> In the egocentric preschool years (age 3 to 4), parentification prematurely pushes children into a more latency-aged stage of following rules that are needed to compensate for the difficulties imposed by having a developmentally disabled sibling who herself or himself has lingered too long in the egocentric stage. In the latency years, they are pushed into taking responsibilities like babysitting, a task usually given only to adolescents, who are regarded as having more fully formed capacities for judgement. As adolescents, parentified children are pushed into adulthood, and the normal stage of experimenting with different identities is cut short by the need to take on a specific adult role—that of caregiver, manager, and sometimes teacher—for the developmentally disabled sibling. (p. 114)

These authors suggested that when a child appears to be overly parentified, the following questions should be asked by parents and service providers:

1. To what extent has the child taken on family-related responsibilities he or she might not have if a sibling were not disabled?
2. Under what conditions were these responsibilities taken? (That is, how much choice did the child have?)

3. What responsibility gradually shifted onto this child out of convenience or necessity?
4. What has been the parents' response when the child refuses or is reluctant to take on responsibilities?
5. What has been the parents' response when the child has been helpful? Has he or she received praise, or have the efforts been taken for granted? (Siegel & Silverstein, 1994, p. 118)

A considerable amount of the literature on siblings focuses on the responsibilities children assume in a family as a result of having a brother or sister with a disability (Safer, 2002; Ufner, 2004; McHugh, 1999; Strohm, 2005). There is relatively little information on adult siblings and their experience of burden, guilt, and fear. Although some adult siblings live lives relatively free from excessive anxiety and fear, others do not:

> Whenever I tentatively imagined her [mother's] death, and myself returning to Virginia to take over Sally's care, I instantly thought of suicide. I was convinced I would have to give up my life; I just wasn't sure which way I would do it. (Moorman, 1992a, p. 44)

> We all have to worry. Who else is going to be there? I will have to worry and it will be my responsibility; I think about it all the time. I think about the person I am going to marry: When I meet someone, they are not going to just marry me, but they are going to have to love my brother and know he is going to be around all my life. (Fish, 1993)

One sibling said that "For many siblings, the responsibility for a brother or sister feels like a heavy burden. Indeed, when I allow myself to think about the future, the feelings can overwhelm me. For much of the time I tend to take a head-in-the-sand approach, knowing that I will take over the responsibility when I need to" (Strohm, 2005, p. 127).

McHugh (1999) believes that early caretaking responsibilities can lead to overfunctioning in marriage: "Unfortunately, many siblings who are caretakers think they can fix whatever is wrong with their partners. [One such woman] has always been drawn to men who needed fixing because she grew up with a brother with mental retardation" (p. 147).

It is difficult for adult siblings to accept their unique circumstances when they compare their lot to other adults who do not share this experience. Life with a sibling who has a disability may be even less comprehensible for children when they compare their family circumstances to others with nondisabled children:

> The whole situation is profoundly unfair. It is unfair that the family must live with schizophrenia, autism, blindness, or retardation while others do not. It is unfair that some children must function as adjunct parents even before they go to school, while others successfully avoid responsibilities of all sorts well into their second decade. The brothers and sisters of the handicapped child learn to cope with this unfairness, and with their own response to it, the sorrow and the anger. (Featherstone, 1980, p. 162)

Siblings may experience "survivor's guilt" due to their typical lives, which sharply contrast with those of ill or disabled children (Bank & Kahn, 1997; Siegel & Silverstein, 1994). Experiencing guilt for having escaped the fate of a disability can result in sabotaging one's efforts so that achievements do not surpass those of a brother or sister with a disability,

> like the man with a brother with mental retardation who was eligible to compete in the finals for the Olympic games as a squash player but fell and couldn't compete in the finals. He pointed out that unconsciously he was asking himself: "How come I don't have all those problems my brother has? How come I got away so easily? I can't win. I'm not going to win because look at my poor brother. I can't achieve what he can't achieve." (McHugh, 1999, p. 53)

Siblings can experience excessive caregiving responsibility depending upon the number of children in the family. In families where more children are available to help, there is more shared responsibility and less pressure on each sibling to excel in compensation for a brother or sister's disability. McHugh (1999) believes that additional children in the family dilutes the negative consequences of living with a sibling who has a disability. She quoted Ellen D'Amato, an educational psychologist, on this topic: "The situation is more difficult in families where there are just two children. The healthy sibling may feel intense responsibility in caretaking and also have the feeling that, I am the one who must achieve. I am the one who must be perfect. I must compensate for this child. When there are a number of siblings there may not be that sense of burden" (p. 85).

The gender of nondisabled brothers and sisters plays a significant part in the allocation of caregiving responsibilities. Female siblings are more subject to caregiving responsibilities than males and may thus be more prone to psychological maladjustment if these responsibilities are excessive. However, the relationship of gender and maladjustment has been questioned. One report asserted that some males fare more poorly than females and that sibling age, age spacing, and gender may interact in complex ways (Simeonsson & Bailey, 1986). Nevertheless, when it comes to caregiving, females probably do assume these roles more frequently than males, but perhaps this role assumption does not necessarily lead to problems. McHale and Gamble (1987) contended that problems should not be attributable to caregiving per se; rather, how children with disabilities behave when they are being cared for by their siblings may determine the degree of tension created. In addition, these authors reported from their research that children were more depressed, anxious, and had lower self-esteem when they were dissatisfied about how their parents treated them relative to the other children in the family. These findings held for siblings of both disabled and nondisabled brothers and sisters. Parental "fairness" is an important concern for siblings, in general.

Stoneman and Berman (1993) reported on a series of studies they and their colleagues conducted. They found that older siblings experienced increased conflict between them when they had greater child care demands. This finding applied only to child care responsibilities and not to household chores. Also, contrary to the expectation that younger siblings in caregiving roles will experience "role tension" characterized by anxiety and conflict (Farber, 1960a), younger nondisabled siblings who assumed more caregiving roles had less conflicted relations than did siblings with fewer responsibilities (Stoneman, Brody, Davis, Crapps, & Malone, 1991). Generally speaking, these researchers concluded that nondisabled siblings have more caregiving duties than other children who do not have a brother or sister with a disability, but that engaging in these activities does not necessarily, or by itself, result in negative outcomes.

In one of the few studies of college-age siblings, Grossman (1972) found that SES may be related to the amount of responsibility nondisabled siblings assume for a brother or sister. Financially secure families are better able to secure necessary help from sources outside the family. Parents who have fewer resources must rely more on resources within the family. Financial problems produce additional stress and can detract from general stability when excessive and unreasonable demands are placed on the family. In families worried and stressed primarily because of limited financial resources, a child with a disability is an added burden and may even be blamed as the source of the woes. Service providers need to be alert to the potential for abuse when the child is scapegoated and additional strains (e.g., financial) exist. Professionals need to make families aware of available financial resources and caregiving assistance programs.

After reviewing 51 published studies representing over 2,500 subjects (a meta-analysis) siblings of children with a chronic illness, Sharpe and Rossiter (2002) concluded that these siblings are "at some risk for negative effects." The authors pointed out that the most striking impression from the literature reviews is a lack of consensus. They quoted Cuskelly, who concluded that "to anyone reading the literature reporting research studies of the psychological adjustment of siblings of individuals with a disability, the overwhelming experience is one of contradiction and confusion" (Sharpe & Rossiter, 2002).

The willingness of siblings to accept care from, and give care to, each other can become a source of conflict during adolescence (Rolland, 2004). When becoming more independent from the family is an essential task, caregiving can result in increased anger and resentment. Heightened concern about one's appearance and public image can increase anxiety for siblings and embarrassment and humiliation for the child with a disability. Instead of increasing the caregiving of their nondisabled children because they increasingly trust their judgment, parents should realize the special vulnerabilities of adolescence. Moorman (1992a) reflected on her adolescent years with her sister, Sally, who has a mental illness:

> I saw her as a disturbance, an embarrassment. She seemed to speak in non sequiturs that caused conversations to jerk to an abrupt stop. She was overweight and ungainly. She had no friends. I was entering adolescence, and I wanted friends—neat friends. I was afraid that Sally's strangeness would get in the way of my social life. For me, Sally was a liability and I all but stopped speaking to her. If I could behave as if she were invisible, she might disappear.
>
> As a teenager, I earnestly pursued the fantasy that I was an only child. Denying Sally's very existence enabled me to concentrate on trying to make my own life seem as normal as possible, but it eventually took a toll. I couldn't bear to be alone, and I was often unable to concentrate. In my early teens, I began to have trouble studying, and, by the time I reached high school, I could barely keep up with my classes. I was often deeply depressed. (p. 42)

Siblings may be burdened by excessively high parental aspirations to compensate for parental disappointments and frustrations (Safer,

2002; Simon, 1997; Ufner, 2004). The responsibility for high achievement may fall to the nondisabled children, who may or may not be able to meet those expectations. Grossman's (1972) study of college-age students showed that pressure to achieve was especially high when the child with a disability was a son, whereas another study indicated that older, only daughters are prone to dual stresses (Cleveland & Miller, 1977): pressure to compensate for the parents' unfulfilled hopes while also assuming parent-surrogate responsibilities. McHugh (1999) elaborated as follows:

> The feeling that you must make it up to your parents for having a child who cannot achieve is a powerful force in the lives of many children growing up with a sibling with a disability, especially if the healthy sibling is the only other child. That force can indeed lead to great achievements, but there is often a price to be paid. (p. 23)

The issue of personal achievement seems particularly acute for siblings of children with mental illness. Simon (1997), whose older brother began hearing voices as a freshman in college and later committed suicide, and who has a sister with schizophrenia, authored the book *Mad House*. In this book Simon tells her own story and those of other siblings whom she interviewed. One interviewee said, "I had to be happy. I had to be successful. I had to be the good girl, because my parents had enough to worry about" (p. 45). In this regard, Marsh (1998) noted similarities between families with a mentally ill child and those in which a child has died. The remaining children may develop a "replacement child syndrome" wherein they attempt to compensate for the problems the ill child has caused. Simon (1997) pointed out that "ultimately, even those of us who had felt abandoned knew that our place in the family—tenuous though it seemed—depended on us fulfilling the role of the competent child, the one who did not need attention. And we, too, spent our energy trying to be what we should be" (p. 90).

From her review of the literature and her in-depth interviews of 11 siblings, Ufner (2004) concluded that "it appears that siblings dealing with a brother or sister with severe mental illness might have a different set of concerns than siblings with other disabilities" (p. iv). Some of the issues faced by the subjects in her study included relationship problems; fear of getting or their offspring becoming mentally ill; depression, alcoholism, and fear of acceptance from a prospective spouse; as well as anxieties about future responsibility for an ill brother or sister.

In the case of mental illness, siblings may present special challenges for future adjustment. Some of the potentially troublesome characteristics of mental illness include young-adult onset, unpredictability, genetic factors, stigma, and behavioral issues. We are struck by the recent publications of firsthand accounts of adult siblings and their experiences of living with a brother/sister with a mental illness (Safer, 2002; Simon, 1997; Moorman, 1992; Neugeboren, 1997). Safer, in her book *The Normal One*, offers her opinion that siblings of children with mental illness must overcome some significant issues, such as premature maturity, survivor's guilt, a compulsion to achieve, and the fear of contagion. These are not new revelations. Nevertheless, her presentation of these issues highlights the significant challenges to a successful adult life faced by siblings of children with mental illness. She contended that a child with a mental illness damages other siblings in the family:

> No one with an abnormal sibling has a normal childhood—every intact sibling is haunted by the fear of catching the disability—cheerful caretakers mature before their time—they feel tormented by the compulsion to compensate for their parents' disappointments by having no problems and making no demands—their success is always tainted by their siblings' failure, their future clouded by an untoward sense of obligation and responsibility. Their goal is to be as different from their sibling as possible. They live forever in the shadow of the one who does not function. (p. xviii).

In regard to the sense of obligation and responsibility and holding back opportunities for happiness, one sibling wrote:

> I became the perfect child to spare my parents more grief. I was forced to become responsible. In many ways it forced me to accomplish things in my life I might not have otherwise done. But I have spent my life trying to run away from this problem. Feeling guilty and helpless, the unending sorrow for not being able to help. I have not felt entitled to be happy most of my adult life. (Marsh, 1998, p. 270)

Generally speaking, mental illness in the family creates challenges that include: burden (Greenberg, Kim, & Greenley, 1997); frustration, embarrassment, sadness, anger (Friedrich, 1977); and grief, guilt, shame, and loss (Kristoffersen, Polit, & Mastard, 2000). This grim picture should be interpreted cautiously, keeping in mind such factors as how the family deals with the illness, the severity of the illness, the existence of social support, and the availability of appropriate services.

In instances in which a child needs lifelong care, supervision, or guidance, nondisabled brothers and sisters understandably look anxiously to the future. They wonder whether the responsibility their parents at present assume will fall to them later. They question whether they can cope with the decisions that need to be made in future years, in addition to worrying about whether they can physically, financially, or emotionally manage to care for their brother or sister. In an article on children's reflections about their sibling with mental illness, Lukens, Thorning, and Lohrer (2004) reported on a man in his 40s who stated: "I know I will have to take care of him and of course I will do that because he is my brother. So I have grown up being very serious when other people would be spending money going here and going there. I have just been very hard on myself." Another sibling said, "I get waves of fear about what will happen when my parents are gone" (pp. 493–494).

Inattention by a parent can be the source of confusion and hurt feelings for children. McHugh (1999) provided this example: "In those early years, I remember feeling that I had lost the mother I knew. She would look at me without seeing me. She didn't smile anymore. She always looked worried. I wanted my other mother back again" (p. 20).

Inattention to their nondisabled children, coupled with excessive concern over the one with a disability, may shield some parents from the problems their nondisabled child may be experiencing:

> She missed the signs of depression in me, her well and happy, outgoing and successful child, because I never revealed my suicidal thoughts and always appeared to have a new and plausible plan for my future. To the day she died, Mother was proud—no, thrilled—to introduce me as her daughter, as if to say, "See? I wasn't so bad, after all." She depended on me to clear her name, to show the world she was capable of being the mother of a healthy child. She didn't see that I was not so healthy inside—I was happy enough for her. "Peggy could always take care of herself," Mother liked to say, "I never had to worry about her." (Moorman, 1992a, p. 43)

Sibling responsibility for a brother or sister with a disability should thus be a major concern for parents as well as professionals.

The parents should be discussing the extent to which a sibling is expected to assume responsibility for a disabled family member is very important, yet difficult (Turnbull et al., 2006). How a sibling envisions the way he or she will manage life's future demands depends, in part, on whether there are vestiges of resentment and anger toward the parents. Professionals ought to help siblings consider how much responsibility should be assumed if there are other able family members. Counseling for confused or conflicted siblings is a recommended course of action (Safer, 2002; Max, 1985). In regard to counseling, Strohm (2005) wrote:

> Aims of individual counseling are to help siblings understand, accept, and express their reactions to having a brother or sister with a disability, to feel listened to, to learn ways of dealing with problems and to develop self-esteem. Some siblings need help in finding their own identity and working out goals for the future. (pp. 225, 226)

For some a central issue will be whether they can, without guilt, abandon the powerful burden of responsibility their parents may have placed upon them out of their own anxieties.

IDENTITY CONCERNS

As noted, young children may be concerned about "catching" the disability of a sibling. Featherstone (1980) noted that anxiety about possible contagion is exacerbated when siblings learn that the disability was caused by a contagious disease such as rubella or meningitis. In contrast to these childhood-related fears, older children who have siblings with mental illness fear becoming ill themselves during their adult years (Moorman, 1992a, 1992b; Simon, 1997). In Safer's (2002) words:

> Heredity is destiny, I warn myself, and I generalize its potential for harm. When anything goes wrong with my body, my moods, my work, or my social life, I search for signs of disaster. Everything seems tenuous; my footing is forever perilous. Anxiety does not rule me or paralyze me, and it has been tempered by years of therapy, but panic is still my reflexive response to uncertainty. (pp. 22–23)

And according to Rolland (1994), "A sibling's illness shatters children's myths that serious health problems and death happen when a person is old; they lose a sense of immunity. Siblings often develop fears or phobias that even the smallest symptoms may be serious" (p. 220). The fear of cancer runs high among siblings (Sourkes, 1987). Children need reassurance that there is little likelihood of getting the same disease, and they need to be told that the illness is not contagious. Siblings should be encouraged to pursue their own activities and relationships, which can help counteract the overidentification that occurs in some of these relationships.

Young siblings may have anxieties that they will become blind or deaf in the future (Moores, 2006). As noted above, siblings may believe that if a disability can happen to a brother or sister, then it can happen to them. Children also can develop somatic complaints in their attempts to gain attention from their parents (Luterman, 1979; Marion, 1981; Rolland, 2004; Sourkes, 1987). In siblings of hearing-impaired children, it is not uncommon for them to develop a pseudo-sensory deficit as an attention-getting behavior (Luterman, 1979). Furthermore, siblings of children with epilepsy have an inordinate fear that they will develop the disorder—a fear disproportionate to the possibility that they will indeed acquire epilepsy or another seizure disorder (Lechtenberg, 1984). Anxieties about getting ill or becoming disabled may take the form of sleep and appetite problems, headaches, or stomach pains. Somatic complaints can also serve another function in the family system. According to Rolland (1994):

> In some families somatic symptoms may become a dysfunctional way of expressing a need for attention. A well sibling may feel that physical complaints are the only valid form of currency that can compete with a chronic disorder. Often a sibling will protect parents by hiding his or her feelings or distracting them by acting out. Healthy children sometimes feel excluded from the family and different because they do not have physical symptoms. In response, they develop somatic complaints as a way to get attention. Frequently, this is not a conscious process, and may be resistant to change. (pp. 220–221)

The type or severity of disablement in children may bear a relationship to the identity problems of siblings. Tew and Lawrence (1975) concluded from their early study that siblings of children who were mildly disabled were most disturbed, followed by siblings of children who were severely and moderately disabled. It may be that identity confusion and the ability to differentiate self from brother or sister is a consequence of perceived similarities. In other words, the less disabled the sibling, the more likely issues of identity may surface.

Professionals can encourage siblings to express their identity concerns and their worries about contamination. Support or counseling groups with youngsters of similar ages are a useful adjunct to (or substitution for) individual counseling (Meyer & Vadasy, 1994; Seligman, 1993; Seligman & Marshak, 2003; Barrera, Chung, Greenberg, & Fleming, 2002). Siblings may feel different or odd because of their experiences and emotions but become less fearful in a group with others who share similar realities. The value of a support group for siblings is reflected in the following passage from Moorman (1992a):

> Some years later, I found the Sibling and Adult Children's Network, a branch of AMI [Alliance for the Mentally Ill]. There, everyone talked about what I had assumed were my own particular problems: dread of taking over, fear of having deeply troubled children, fear of relationships with lovers who might not understand or sympathize, inability to develop our own lives because we were expecting to have to drop them at a moment's notice to intervene in a crisis. When I aired my "secrets," which were commonplace in this group, I felt for the first time that I was with people who knew exactly what I was talking about. There was immense comfort in simply being in the room with my peers. (p. 44)

CAREERS

Life goals for siblings of children with disabilities may be affected. A child's career decision may be shaped by being a brother or sister with a disability. Nondisabled children are cognizant of others' reactions to their brother or sister, adding to their acute sensitivity to social relations. The continuous act of caring for a brother or sister with a disability, especially in a loving, attentive family, may become internalized to the extent that it influences career decisions in the direction of the helping professions (Meyer & Vadasy, 1994). Thibodeau (1988) reflected:

> I have found my upbringing to have been very positive, in spite of the emotional hardship that [my sister's] cystic fibrosis placed on the family. At the age of nine I perceived myself as being a vitally important participating member of the family. My parents encouraged me to assist in the care of my newborn sister and I learned to crush pills and mix them in applesauce, do postural drainage, and clean and fill the mist tent. Through this experience self-esteem was enhanced, responsibility was learned, and maturity was developed. Although I occasionally feel that I

grew up too fast, for the most part the experience gave me a personal insight and compassion that I carry with me in my practice as a pediatric specialist. (p. 22)

Strohm (2005) observed:

Many siblings of people with disabilities enter the caring professions. They have been influenced by their experiences in ways that develop their sense of social justice and social equity, resulting in a desire to support disadvantaged groups within the community. They generally understand and appreciate the differences between people [and] are able to show empathy and compassion. (p. 92)

Not all siblings have such a positive perspective. Safer (2002) noted:

One way normal siblings deal with their often hopeless desire to make a difference to their damaged sibling is to generalize it by joining a helping profession: they are overrepresented in the ranks of therapists, doctors, nurses, and advocates and educators of the disabled. Although a career as a symbolic caretaker meets the needs of many normal siblings, it can also represent an oppressive continuation of the role forced upon them as too responsible, prematurely mature children. Coming into your own may require leaving that profession as well as rejecting that role in private life. (pp. 152–153)

Farber (1959) and Cleveland and Miller (1977) found in their early studies that internalized helping norms have turned sibling career endeavors toward the improvement of humankind or at least toward life goals that require dedication and sacrifice. As noted, Strohm (2005) asserted that siblings have been influenced by their experiences, which leads to a heightened sense of social justice and equality and careers in fields where contributing to the welfare of others is a defining characteristic. Others, like Safer and McHugh, believe that siblings ought to be cautious about choosing a career out of a sense of guilt and obligation. Ultimately, siblings need to understand the forces that motivate them to select a career so that their choices will turn out to be gratifying.

Konstam et al. (1993) found that in a group of college-age children, those with brothers or sisters with disabilities were not more likely to consider a human service career than a group of young adults who did not have a sibling with a disability. This conclusion is supported in Meyer's (2005) *The Sibling Slam Book*, where few of the adolescents who responded to the question "What career choices sound good right now?" endorsed a helping profession. Of course, it is common for adolescents to declare career aspirations that are subject to change—and for some, frequent changes. McHugh (1999) reported that many of the siblings she interviewed for her book *Special Siblings* denied that their brother or sister with a disability had anything to do with their choice of a career.

The theoretical leap between the development of compassion, tolerance, and empathy and the selection of a particular career goal may be too ambitious. In fact, siblings who have developed such attitudes and who believe they have already made a significant contribution to a challenging life circumstance may seek out fulfillment in fields outside of the helping professions. In a small-scale study of siblings of children with hearing impairments, Israelite (1985) found that subjects indicated their desire to pursue careers that were unrelated to the human service professions.

Firm conclusions about the relationship between having a brother or sister with a disability and choosing a particular career path should be avoided due to the modest research base. There is, however, anecdotal information to speculate about the impact of a child with a disability on a sibling's career choice. If the experience of living with a brother or sister with a disability is a generally positive one, it is likely that compassion and empathy are natural outcomes that will be expressed through the nondisabled sibling's career choice (Strohm, 2005).

ANGER AND GUILT

Anger is a common emotion. Some handle the experience of anger better than others, whereas some deny that they experience anger at all. Siblings of children with disabilities may experience anger and guilt often and perhaps more intensely than siblings of nondisabled brothers or sisters (Ufner, 2004).

Anger may arise when a brother or sister with a disability is ridiculed or teased. Sometimes the anger is expressed in a very direct way: "I beat the crap out of this kid in the 6th grade because he was making fun of my little brother" (15-year-old boy, in Meyer, 2005, p. 82). And sometimes the pain is felt deeply: "When people call kids 'retards' a knife goes through my chest. I hate it because people are so arrogant when they say that" (15-year-old girl, in Meyer, 2005, p. 83).

As reflected in the following observation by Helen Featherstone in her classic book *A Difference in the Family* (1980), anger may arise in relation to numerous factors:

> Children feel angry at parents, at the disabled child, at the wider world, at God or fate, perhaps at all four. Some blame their mother and father for the disability itself (just as they blame them for any new baby). A handicap creates unusual needs; many children envy their brother or sister this special attention. And older children may rage secretly about the sometimes colossal sums of money spent on diagnosis and therapy—resources that might otherwise finance family comforts and college tuition. (p. 143)

More recently, Strohm (2005) discussed the inhibition of her anger as a child whose sibling was disabled: "As a child I felt much anger: at my sister for being the way she was; at my parents for the special treatment they gave her; at everyone else for staring and not understanding. This anger had to be hidden; there was nowhere to direct it, so it turned in on me. I became self-doubting and frustrated at my perceived inadequacies" (p. 47).

Finding it difficult to acknowledge his own anger, physician, author, and sibling Stuart Silverstein observed:

> We siblings are not supposed to feel angry and resentful. Such feelings imply selfishness and insensitivity. But in not acknowledging these feelings, we only feed into denial. Denial leaves you out of touch with your true feelings—you end up mistrusting your own intuition—and down the path to insecurity, low self-esteem, and depression. You are left a legacy of helplessness. (Siegel & Silverstein, 1994, p. 20)

Siblings may be placed in a difficult bind. Parents may demand that a child should care for and protect the brother or sister who has a disability. These demands clash with those of the child's playmates, who encourage shunning. The child's ambivalent feelings (anger, guilt, love, protectiveness) toward his or her sibling and resentment toward the parents for demanding that he or she love and take care of the sibling with a disability result in confusion, ambivalence, and anger.

Writing about his sister, Silverman (in Siegel & Silverman, 1994) described how her complaints about their brother Marc, who had autism, were dismissed by their burdened parents. This increased her sense of guilt and undermined her self-esteem:

My brother's worsening behavior coincided with Stacey's adolescence, and our parents had very little reserve left over to deal with her "emotional turmoil." Her complaints about his walking around in his underwear, his going to the bathroom with the door open, or his tearing up her clothes were deemed selfish. If she didn't "understand" she was immature and ungrateful for being normal. She was expected to adapt to his behavior accordingly, something that required a maturity beyond her years. She was to be a "little adult," denied the carefree days of childhood and adolescence. If you grow up with your needs and concerns trivialized by others, you begin to trivialize them yourself, automatically. It's a pattern that will follow you to adulthood. (pp. 13–14)

Strohm (2005) admitted, "As a child I felt anger or resentment if I upset my parents, or if I was having too good a time, I felt guilty. If I wanted my parents' attention, I felt guilty knowing that my sister needed it more. If I felt embarrassed by her, I also felt guilty" (p. 60).

Many factors contribute to anger—and the guilt that often follows in anger's wake. Professionals need to help siblings understand the source of their anger and to understand the universality of angry feelings.

Guilty feelings in the nondisabled sibling that he or she may have caused the disability and should be punished for it can lead to withdrawal, depression, suicidal thoughts, self-destructive and aggressive behavior, and declining school performance (Rolland, 2003). These feelings can be unwittingly reinforced by parents if a child is not allowed to express them. On this subject, McHugh (1999) wrote: "There are all kinds of guilt we siblings of people with disabilities torture ourselves with. My own particular brand of guilt comes from running away from my brother, pretending he didn't exist, blotting him out of my mind—or trying to" (p. 53). Parents may suppress their child's feelings by reassuring him or her too quickly. As noted earlier, parents sometimes believe that their child will be upset by talking about an illness/disability when, in fact, the child is already worried, anxious, and guilty and needs to express these emotions. By not allowing their children to reveal their feelings, parents may be attempting to protect themselves from their own anxiety-provoking thoughts.

Professionals should be sensitive to parents who discourage the open expression of feelings even as they (therapists) facilitate the expression of anger and guilt by their nondisabled children. It is also important to take note when parents are made anxious by their child's feelings and to communicate this observation to the parents sensitively. Again, sibling support groups are an excellent resource for coping with emotions such as guilt and anger. Encountering peers who share a particular life circumstance has powerful healing powers (Seligman & Marshak, 2003). However, the first line of action should be the family.

COMMUNICATION AND ISOLATION

Featherstone (1980) observed that the presence of a child with a disability in the family can inhibit communication, which, in turn, contributes to the isolation siblings experience. Siblings sense that certain topics are taboo and that "ugly" feelings are to remain hidden; they are thereby forced into a peculiar kind of loneliness—a sense of detachment from those to whom they typically feel closest. Family secrets or implicit rules forbidding the discussion of a problem force siblings constantly to pretend that circumstances are other than they seem.

The child with a disability is a total family concern. Sometimes decisions that bear on the disability are made without prior discussion with, or explanation to, siblings who may be affected by them. We therefore encourage open communication within the family to help reduce unpleasant side effects. Strohm (2005) points out the following negative consequence from constricted communication: "Without open communication within the family, everyone gets bound up in a cycle of protecting one another from real feelings. This only adds to the intensity of those feelings. It is difficult enough putting on a mask for the outside world without feeling it necessary to do so inside the family as well" (p. 165).

Communicating to children about their brother or sister's disability may be difficult, but it is also achievable. Powell and Gallagher (1993) offer the following communication guidelines to help the parent–child relationship:

1. Display active (not passive) listening.
2. Take the time.
3. Secure needed knowledge.
4. Be sincere and honest.
5. Respond in a comprehensive fashion.
6. Adopt an open attitude.
7. Provide balanced information.

8. Be aware of nonverbal communication.
9. Follow up earlier communication.

Michaelis (1980) noted that nondisabled siblings may resent that the brother or sister is "playing" when they themselves must work so hard doing school work. By explaining the educational methods used with the child and the skills that are being taught will help make it possible for the sibling to be supportive rather than critical and resentful. Also, young siblings may not understand that their brother or sister has certain cognitive limitations and as a result spends less time studying and participating in other learning activities.

Reactions from peers may further isolate siblings from their social group. Children who feel rejected by their peers and are ignored by their parents are youngsters at risk. Add excessive caregiving demands and the possibility of emotional problems looms in the future. Featherstone (1980) commented on the frustration and isolation siblings feel when they are unable to communicate with their brother or sister:

> [Siblings] yearn for a relationship of equals, for someone with whom they can play and tell secrets, someone who shares their child-view of an adult world. Even when the normal siblings perform some of these functions, they sometimes imagine the special relationship they might have with this brother if he were more accessible. The able-bodied member of a two-child family may feel very much alone. (p. 159)

FOR BETTER OR WORSE

Early research and clinical reports suggested that siblings of children with disabilities are children at risk. More recently, others have concurred with this conclusion (Safer, 2002; Thompson & Gustafson, 1996; Barrera et al., 2002). Several factors that contribute to emotional problems include the number of children in the family, sibling age and gender, parental reaction to the child with a disability, and the like. Other potential contributing factors have already been mentioned in this chapter. These and other variables have also been noted in several reviews of the literature (e.g., Boyce & Barnett, 1991; Lobato, 1990; Marsh, 1992; Powell & Gallagher, 1993; Stoneman & Berman, 1993; Turnbull et al., 2006).

Research and personal accounts by siblings with brothers or sisters who are mentally ill reported generally negative outcomes. (Moorman, 1992a, 1992b; Safer, 2002; Marsh, 1998; Poznanski, 1969, San Martino & Newman, 1974; Trevino, 1979; Ufner, 2004). An early study by Poznanski reported that psychiatrists treat more siblings than children with disabilities themselves. Other researchers reported a higher incidence of negative outcomes due to emotional and behavioral problems (Fishman, Wolf, Ellison, & Freeman, 2000). Hannah and Midlarsky (1999) did not find more behavioral and emotional problems. Trevino (1979) contended that children who have a disability as well as behavioral problems are children at risk and can benefit from counseling. For Strohm (2005), Safer (2002), and Simon (1997) guilt provides the foundation for subsequent difficulties siblings are likely to experience. Personal accounts attest to the fact that guilt is a common emotion for siblings (McHugh, 2003; Strohm, 2005). As noted earlier, siblings who are ill informed about the nature of their brother or sister's condition seem to be at risk for experiencing somatic complaints and excessive guilt and anger (Rolland, 2003). Other negative effects include embarrassment, pressure to achieve, guilt, and isolation (Turnbull et al., 2006). Another study found that siblings have a higher incidence of behavioral and emotional problems (Fishman et al., 2000). However, Turnbull et al. (2006) stated, "positive and negative reactions occur simultaneously" (p. 39). Thus, we can hold in great esteem the same person with whom we are also angry and disappointed.

Featherstone (1980), from personal experience and in recounting the experiences of others, and Grossman (1972) and Kibert (1986), from their research on brothers and sisters in college, take a more cautious view of the effects on siblings. They contended that a child with a disability in the family may have differential outcomes with respect to the nondisabled sibling's subsequent adjustment and coping: little impact, negative impact, or positive outcome. Farber's (1959, 1960a) pioneering research tends to support the same conclusion, as does other research. Klein (1972), Schreiber and Feeley (1965), Lobato (1990), Thompson and Gustafson (1996), and Grakliker, Fishler, and Koch (1962) did not find any adverse effects reported by the siblings interviewed in their studies; nor did McHale, Sloan, and Simeonsson (1986) in their study of siblings of brothers and sisters with autism and intellectual disability. This study is noteworthy because it had 90 carefully selected subjects and included a matched control group. The statistical differences between groups were not significant, however, children with brothers or sisters with a disability had more variable experiences, with some children reporting very positive and some describing very negative relationships with their brothers or sisters (McHale et al., 1986). These researchers noted that children who reported difficult relationships worried about the future, perceived parental favoritism toward the child with a disability, and experienced rejecting feelings toward their brother or sister. The children with a better outlook viewed their parents and peers as reacting positively to their brother or sister, and they had a better understanding of the disability.

In another well-conducted study, siblings of children with a chronic illness were reported to be well adjusted (Tritt & Esses, 1988). However, the siblings of the ill children were perceived by their parents as having more behavioral problems, such as withdrawal and shyness. This finding raises the issue of the differential perception of the siblings regarding their own experience versus those of their parents.

A study using a matched control group found that siblings of children with disabilities displayed the same level of self-concept, behavioral problems, and social competence as the control group children (Dyson, 1989). In support of Dyson's study, others reported fewer behavioral problems and more empathy in siblings of children with disabilities than in those without (Carr, 1988; Cuskelly & Gunn, 2003). Self-esteem and self-efficacy have been studied with mixed results. McHale and Gamble (1987) reported lower self-esteem and self-efficacy in those with disabled brothers or sisters compared to those without. Other research found no differences between the sibling groups (Grisom & Borkowski, 2002; Van Riper, 2000; Hannah & Midlarsky, 1999). In the Dyson (1989) study, there were some differences between the study groups: Siblings of children with disabilities were less active in extracurricular activities; brothers between the ages of 7 and 11 showed fewer fantasizing, deviant, and isolated behaviors; and for the age range of 12–15, brothers were less aggressive and hyperactive and tended to have fewer behavioral problems than children of brothers or sisters who did not have disabilities. Further, type of disability was associated with adjustment; specifically, siblings of brothers or sisters with mental disabilities showed better behavioral adjustment, higher self-esteem, and more social competence than siblings of children with physical or sensory disabilities or siblings of children with milder disabling conditions. This finding runs counter to more recent research on siblings of brothers or sisters with mental illness (Ufner, 2004).

Also, in Dyson's (1989) research, the older the child with a disability, the greater the number of behavioral problems exhibited by the siblings, and the larger the age gap, the better the sibling's adjustment. Furthermore, the larger the family and the higher the mother's education, the more social competence a sibling showed. Of particular interest in this study was the finding of variability in adjustment in both groups of children, suggesting that there are individual differences in adjustment among children, whether they reside with a brother or sister who has a disability or not.

Siegel and Silverstein (1994) reported that the less depressed and emotionally troubled the mother, the better off are the children. Bank and Kahn (1997) observed that adjustment can be affected by the age and developmental stage of the nondisabled sibling. Also, in chronic illness, the chronicity of a medical condition determines whether the sibling must cope with a time-limited or more chronic situation. Furthermore, the stigmatizing aspects of a child's condition should also be considered in evaluating sibling adjustment (Marsh, 1998; Marshak & Seligman, 1993). In a public situation, a well-behaved youngster with an invisible disability will be less noticed than a drooling, bent figure in a wheelchair.

From an empirical point of view, the question of whether siblings are not affected, are helped, or are harmed by the presence of a brother or sister with a disability remains as open to speculation as it was in the earlier editions of this book (Ufner, 2004; Turnbull et al., 2006). The data have not yet established the prevalence of adjustment problems in siblings of a disabled brother or sister compared with those in families where there is no disability. The variables discussed in this chapter that interact with, and subsequently lead to, adjustment difficulties are many and combine in complex ways.

Some contributors to the professional literature are pessimistic about the effects of a child with a disability on siblings, while others are remarkably optimistic. In reviewing some of the research, commentary, and accounts about siblings, we could be left with the impression that largely negative effects are the norm. This is simply not true. Some would argue that a common adversity tends to mobilize positive efforts on behalf of the nondisabled child.

Simeonsson and Bailey (1986) noted that siblings who have been actively involved in the management of their brother or sister tend to be well adjusted. It is difficult to integrate this observation with the studies that caution against excessive caregiving. It seems that shared family caregiving and responsibility along with attention to, and the expression of affection to, *all* children in the family promotes a healthy, caring environment.

In the few sibling studies of college-age students, Grossman (1972) and Kibert (1986) reported on their subjects' relationships with their brother or sister with intellectual disability: "The ones who benefitted appeared to us to be more tolerant, more compassionate, more knowing about prejudice" (Grossman, 1972, p. 84).

After discussion of brothers and sisters of children with disabilities and their adaptation to this special circumstance, Featherstone (1980) remarked:

> I have focused, up until now, on the difficulties that the able-bodied child faces. These problems are real enough, and assume major importance in the lives of some children. Nonetheless, the sheer length of my discussion creates a misleading gloomy impression. It may suggest that for the brothers and sisters of the disabled the developmental path is strewn with frightful hazards, that all but the most skillful parents can expect to see their "normal" children bruised irreparably by the experience of family living. The truth is quite otherwise. (p. 163)

After their extensive review of parental and sibling adjustment to chronic illness, Thompson and Gustafson (1996) wrote: "It is now known that parents and siblings [have] increased risks for adjustment difficulties. It is also known that good adaptation and adjustment is possible. Thus, what is most impressive are individual differences in adjustment. Consequently, the question of interest becomes delineating the processes that are differentially associated with adjustment" (p. 176).

We believe that Lobato's comprehensive review of the literature in 1990 continues to reflect the state of sibling adjustment in this edition:

> To many parents of young children, it may seem as though the child's illness or disability will do nothing but harm to the other children. However, this is actually quite far from the truth. As young siblings mature, evidence is clear that they usually do not have more problems than other children. In fact, many siblings show areas of great social and psychological strength. Their relationships with and behavior toward one another also tend to be more nurturing and positive than between many other sibling pairs. (p. 60)

The "Sibshop" model, created by Don Meyer, is alive and well. Meyer and his colleagues conduct Sibshops, or workshops for siblings of individuals with a disability, across the nation. After the workshops, community agencies should have the expertise to conduct meetings for siblings. These meetings provide support, guidance, and information for siblings in their quest to come to terms with the issues and concerns they have. For more information on Sibshops the reader can go to www.siblingsupport.org.

From this review of the literature, we believe that insights about sibling adjustment has come some distance from the first edition of *Ordinary Families, Special Children*. The literature does provide some guidance for families, professionals, and siblings, who should heed the admonition that sibling adjustment is dependent on numerous variables and that simple answers based one or two characteristics can be misleading. The impact of a child with a disability may be "for better or for worse" and may depend on various mediating factors.

▪10▪

Effects on Grandparents

Intergenerational relationships affect contemporary family life. Yet much of the literature has focused on the nuclear family, with little mention of the extended family. The influences of previous generations are important to the understanding of the nuclear family. The grandparent–grandchild relationship has the potential for affecting the development of children in a way that is different from other relationships (Baranowski, 1982; Kornhaber, 2002). This relationship is considerably different from those of previous decades. The number of three-generation households is declining, which puts grandparents in settings outside the nuclear family (Gardner, Sherman, Mobley, Brown, & Schutter, 1994). Also, adults live longer and spend more time in the grandparenting role than those in previous generations. Such changes serve to redefine the nature of grandparenting.

The traditional perspective of a grandparent as a domineering, controlling family matriarch or patriarch has given way to a more positive view. Grandparents now view their roles as being less associated with power and more related to warmth, indulgence, and pleasure without responsibility (Wilcoxon, 1987). Contemporary roles, then, seem to be multidimensional and generally supportive (Kornhaber, 2002). Kornhaber and Woodward (as cited in Wilcoxon, 1987) identified the following grandparent roles:

1. Historian: A link with the cultural and familial past
2. Role model: An example of older adulthood
3. Mentor: A wise adult experienced in life transitions
4. Wizard: A master of storytelling to foster imagination and creativity
5. Nurturer/great parent: An ultimate support person for family crises and transitions

Kornhaber (2002) adds that such roles as hero and spiritual guide bring emotional and spiritual qualities to the grandchild and grandparent relationship. According to Kornhaber, the spiritual dimension refers to such qualities as love, reverence, compassion, gentleness, faith, and kindness. Parents are also often seen in a hero role, but grandparents, with their broader range of experience, offer a different dimension "that is a bit more connected to the mythic" (p. 17). Given the reality that public heroes are often involved in scandals or aggressive and inappropriate behavior, there is a dearth of heroic figures in a child's life. Grandparents can also promote tolerance toward others, such as those of other races, religions, and for those with disabilities. Teaching and companionship as well as serving as a therapeutic agent are additional roles served (Gardner et al., 1994).

Some years ago, eminent theorist and clinician Murray Bowen (1978), positive relationships between generations can add to a family's well-being:

> One of the most effective automatic mechanisms for reducing the overall level of anxiety in a family is a relatively "open" relationship system in the extended family. Any successful effort that goes toward improving the frequency and quality of emotional contact with the extended family will predictably improve the family's level of adjustment and reduce symptoms in the nuclear family. (pp. 537–538)

Becoming a grandparent confers a special status on a person. Grandparents witness the emergence of a new generation, which allows them the satisfaction of seeing their grandchild take on new and fulfilling roles—a source of considerable pride. Grandchildren provide a new "lease on life" for grandparents.

Grandparents assume their status earlier in their lives and will continue in this role for longer periods than in previous generations (Meyer & Vadasy, 1986; Gardner et al., 1994; Kornhaber, 2002). The grandparent role can be assumed in the late 30s, 40s, or 50s, younger than grandparents in the recent past. Also, increased life expectancy means that some people will assume grandparent roles for almost half their lives.

Many grandparents live within 30 minutes of their grandchild, making regular contact between nuclear and extended family a reality. An earlier survey reported that almost half of U.S. grandparents see a grandchild every day (Harris & Associates, 1975), although a more recent American Association of Retired Persons (AARP) survey reported that only 33% of grandparents reside near enough to a grandchild to see him or her once or twice a week (as cited in Kornhaber, 2002). This finding reflects the increased mobility of families as well as greater geographical distance between extended family. Although it isn't always easy, Kornhaber suggested that grandparents keep regular contact with the grandchild and arrange their lives to provide as much one-on-one attention as possible. These objectives are certainly easier to achieve when there is a sound relationship between generations.

Between the years 1980 and 1990, the number of children in the United States residing with their grandparents or other relatives increased by 44% (Cox, 2003). Almost 4 million grandparents in 1997 were raising their grandchildren with the majority of 2.3 million being grandmothers (Lugaila, 1998). Grandparents who raise grandchildren tend to be poor, and receive public assistance, and are less likely to have health insurance (Casper & Bryson, 1998, as cited in Cox, 2003). State laws protecting grandparents' rights to continue their relationships with their grandchildren (after divorce) demonstrate how seriously grandparents regard their roles and how important this relationship is to them.

About 1.4 million children lived in households headed by grandparents in 1999 (Force, Botsford, Pisano, & Holbert, 2000). This new responsibility has resulted primarily from an increase in single parenthood. In some instances, grandparents care for their grandchildren while the parent works or goes to school. They also become caregivers when their children become addicted to drugs, are incarcerated, have children out of wedlock, are guilty of child abuse or neglect, divorce, become unemployed, or die (Downey, 1995). In a New York study of 164 grandparents who provided primary care for their grandchildren with disabilities, 96% were women and 80% were African American (Janicky, McCallin, Grant-Griffin, & Kolomer, 2000). In this study, approximately three-fourths of the grandparents reported that school problems, developmental delays, and difficult behavior presented challenges for them. They also noted:

- Caregiving was an all-consuming role in their lives.
- They experienced uncertainty because of the difficulty in accessing formal and informal supports.
- They were anxious about remaining alive long enough to provide care for their grandchildren into adulthood. (Janicky et al., 2000, p. 49)

Some of these grandparents who "inherit" a grandchild become surrogate parents of typical children, whereas others assume parenting roles of children who have chronic health problems or disabilities (Force, Botsford, Pisano, & Holbert, 2000). Also, the number of grandparents who become caretakers for grandchildren has increased substantially over the last decade (Janicky et al., 2000).

Grandparents caring for a grandchild with a disability (in some cases they care for more than one child) may need special attention. They tend to have greater needs for help from schools, as well as a greater need for transportation and speech therapy services (Force et al., 2000). Strikingly, only about 10% of the grandparents who were raising a grandchild with a disability had contact with an agency providing disability services. It is important for agencies to be aware of grandparents raising a grandchild with a disability and their special needs. Attention to African Americans caretakers is particularly critical.

Considering these various circumstances and roles, how might a grandparent be expected to react when confronted with a grandchild who has a disability? What meanings do grandparents attach to this experience? How do grandparents cope with the grandchild? With their adult child? With their son- or daughter-in-law?

GRANDPARENTS AND CHILDHOOD DISABILITY

As one grandmother put it some years ago:

> There is a very special magic between grandparents and grandchildren. There is a joy, a delight, an unencumbered relationship. The responsibility of parenthood is over. Grandparents have an opportunity to sample the mysteries and watch with awe the unfolding of a new personality. This new unique human being is a stranger, but is hauntingly familiar. He is the link between our past and the future. But what happens when this link, this claim to immortality, is born less than perfect? What is the relationship then between grandparent and grandchild? (McPhee, 1982, p. 13)

The remainder of this chapter attempts to address the questions posed by McPhee. Just like the parents, when a child with special needs is born, grandparents must face the likely disappointment of their grandchild with special needs and ponder the relationship between this child and themselves (Turnbull et al., 2006). They must also reflect on their relationship with their own children and how they will interact with this newly constituted family of which they are a part.

A compelling case can be made for grandparent involvement in the nuclear family when there is a child with a disability. Indeed, research in the area of family stress provides evidence that social support (e.g. grandparents) provides a buffer that contributes to coping with life's challenges (Trute, 2003). Based on data from survey research and interactive interviews with grandparents and parents of children with disabilities, Green (2001) reported the following findings:

1. More than other relatives, friends, or neighbors, grandparents are a common source of assistance.
2. Other sources of support are increased when grandparents are involved.
3. Grandparent support has a more salutary influence on a positive emotional outlook for the family than other sources of help; it also contributes to less emotional exhaustion.
4. A normalized attitude and a sense of pride are realized when grandparents are involved. When grandparents exert their "bragging rights," the parents are reassured. Grandparents viewing their grandchild as "just a normal kid," in spite of the child's disability, has a powerful impact.
5. Parents feel that they need to manage information and the emotional responses of grandparents who have not bonded with their grandchild.
6. Due to their needs and age, grandparents worry that their children won't ask for help when they need it.

Just like the parents, grandparents can harbor guilt feelings that last a lifetime:

My mother called to see how things went. I told her what they [the doctors] said, and she told me it was crazy, they were crazy, and she would never accept it. She hung up on me. She wouldn't talk to me. It took my mother years, and she has finally accepted it. I found out later my mother always blamed herself. My mother only recently told me that she feels that God punished her because she was always a very proud, vain person. Because she was that way, God was teaching her a lesson and bringing her down a notch. She still feels that guilt. I was totally stunned. I never knew she carried that all those years. (Marsh, 1998, p. 173)

Grandparents may feel so distraught by the grandchild with a disability that they reject the child or blame the parents. Lavin (2001) speculated that adults who blame others often feel that they are responsible for contributing to the disability. She further noted that some grandparents are uncomfortable caring for a grandchild with a disability or chronic illness. And some feel isolated because there are few others with whom to identify. However, there are now a modest number of available resources to help them connect with others who are facing a similar situation. The emergence of support groups for the extended family members is discussed later in this chapter.

An event that reassures grandparents—that the future will be carried on by a grandchild—instead introduces uncertainty about what the future holds for the family. The birth of a grandchild with a disability evokes strong emotions (Meyer & Vadasy, 1986; Naseef, 2001b). Grandparents experience a dual hurt, not only for the grandchild, but also for their son or daughter, whom they may see as burdened for life (Marsh, 1992; Turnbull et al., 2006).

Grandparents have a difficult time when a grandchild with a disability is born. Like the parents, the grandparents have lost a dream. The birth of a grandchild with a disability can set into motion a set of worries:

I was expecting a perfect child but instead we got a permanent loss. A lot of tears were shed. My main concern was for my daughter. How was this going to affect her and her husband? I hadn't planned on this kind of life for her. I kept thinking, "how could this be happening?" We hadn't had a problem like this in our family and I wondered where it came from. Then I worried about the prognosis for my other daughters' children. (Lavin, 2001, p. 33)

Another grandparent said:

Because I was raised valuing achievement and intelligence, it was especially difficult for me to have a grandchild with Down's Syndrome. But I learned a lot from Casey. She's taught me that one doesn't have to be brilliant and perfect to be valuable. Accepting her has made me easier on myself. I'm eternally grateful for Casey. (Lavin, 2001, p. 34)

The grandparents' wish for their adult children's happiness is shattered as they see their offspring preparing to cope with a family crisis that won't go away and cannot be easily remedied. To avoid the pain of reality, grandparents may deny a grandchild's problem ("There's nothing wrong with her"), trivialize it ("He will grow out of it"), or have fantasies of unrealistic cures (Meyer & Vadasy, 1986). Grandparents who deny the existence of a child's special needs and those who reject the child can prove difficult burdens to the parents who are attempting to cope with the crisis (Naseef, 2001b; Hornby & Ashworth, 1994). The parents must attend to their own pain and are compelled to cope with their own parents' or in-laws' reactions. Generally speaking, strong negative reactions from extended family members can lead to triangulation and cutoff between and within generations (Walsh, 1989). Grandparents siding with one or the other parent can lead to triangles that harm family functioning. An example of triangulation is when a grandmother sides with her daughter around the issue of whether her grandchild, who is deaf, should be schooled in a segregated setting that promotes signing as a means of communication. The father favors another educational setting and communica tion approach that supports aural learning as opposed to signing. The father is the odd man out in this triangle. A less conflicted approach would be one in which the parents discussed the pros and cons of the available choices and then made a decision, asking the grandparent to support their choice.

We do not know a great deal about how grandparents react to the birth of a grandchild with a disability, and most of the information available comes from clinical sources rather than from research (Green, 2001). Grandparents appear to experience a mourning period following the loss of the idealized grandchild that they had expected (Marsh, 1992; Lavin, 2001; Turnbull et al., 2006). Just as the parents experience the "death" of the expected healthy child, so too may the grandparents feel a great loss and mourn for the grandchild they had wished for. Many negotiate similar stages as the parents: denial, grief, anger, detachment, and eventually acceptance. Reporting on the reactions of grandparents who attended the grandparent workshops at the University of Washington, Vadasy, Fewell, and Meyer (1986) noted that their initial reactions were most often sadness (67%), shock (38%), and anger (33%). Although 43% reported that they continued to feel sad long after they first learned of their grandchild's disability, 57% eventually expressed acceptance. (Of course, sadness and acceptance also can coexist in a parent or grandparent.)

Earlier we alluded to the guilt some grandparents feel. In this regard Lavin (2001) stated that a grandparent may experience guilt if a child's condition has its roots in the grandparent's side of the family. According to Lavin, grandparents take time to become acclimated to their new identities and roles. Like the parents, they may be saddened and disappointed. Before the birth of the child, grandparents imagined their future with less responsibility and more fun than they experienced when their children were born. Faced with opposite circumstances, some of them will "act irresponsibly, be unsupportive, and generally cause hurt feelings" (Lavin, 2001, p. 35). There is a difference between disappointment, sadness, and immaturity. Disappointment and sadness are expected; immaturity is not and can contribute to family conflicts.

As noted earlier, grandparents may be coping with their own health issues and may find that having a grandchild with a disability or chronic health issues to be too much to bear. In such cases the parents should consider enlisting them for emotional support, if they are able, and less for instrumental help (e.g., babysitting, taking the child to a medical appointment). Being fixers (see Chapter 8), if is probably not surprising that grandfathers tend to respond more with instrumental than emotional support (Baranowski & Schilmoeller, 1999). Also, parents of children with disabilities say they receive less practical help with everyday tasks than parents of children without disabilities, according to Heller, Hsich, and Rowitz (2000). Both groups, however, receive the same amount of emotional support. One might hypothesize that grandparents coping with health issues find it easier to be emotionally supportive. Grandfathers often engage in activities and caretaking with their grandchild, in addition to (later) loaning or giving money. However, grandfathers are likely to be more diverse than what Baranowski and Schilmoeller suggest. It is likely that practical support is also experienced as emotional support by both the grandchildren and the parents. Thus this distinction may be artificial to some extent. For many grandparents, being emotionally supportive and playing with their grandchild is healthy and helpful for both parties. And, indeed, emotional support can be the most sustaining form of support.

In Frisco's (2002) survey of 37 grandparents, 25% experienced depression/sadness and 22% felt helpless. In the stage theories discussed in Chapter 2, depression/sadness and helplessness are common first reactions to the birth situation. Frisco's survey research does not answer the question of whether these emotions were temporary or chronic—an important question in an effort to understand reactions beyond the birth situation.

Grandparents may be mourning at the same time the parents are grieving. During the stressful initial period of discovery, both parents and grandparents may be experiencing great loss and grief; they may, therefore, be unable to be supportive of one other, but that generally changes over time. According to Green (2001), in responding to their own grief and negative emotions, grandparents can impede positive relationships with their grandchild and other family members. One pattern that can emerge is one of open hostility, as when the paternal grandmother expresses her resentment toward her daughter-in-law. The hurling back and forth of accusations between family members heightens the sense of crisis. The mother, already guilty about the birth, can feel even more burdened when she is accused by an in-law of destroying her husband's life. At a time when the mother needs support, she is instead confronted with hostility. The husband, in turn, is placed in a difficult position, feeling that he needs to be supportive of both his mother and his wife, while coping with his own pain, which is often unexpressed. During this period of conflict, children may view the mounting tensions between their parents and their grandparents with considerable apprehension. The other children in the family may be confused about how they should respond to the new addition to the family. In short, hostility between the parents and the extended family may, if not reduced or resolved, become a major source of continuing intergenerational conflict.

According to Gardner et al. (1994), grandparents' poor adjustment may be related to their difficulty in identifying gratifying roles to assume. They may be "viewed as unsupportive, uninformed, ineffective, and meddlesome by their overburdened child" (p. 186). These authors also stated that the grandparents' attempts to be helpful may be thwarted by the ambiguous messages from the adult child regarding his or her own grief. The researchers further stated that the grandparents' failure to adjust to their grandchild can "dramatically weaken the family unit as a whole" (Gardner et al., 1994, p. 187).

In regard to the similar or dissimilar adjustment of parents and grandparents, Siegel (1996, 2003), an author and researcher in the field of autism, contended that grandparents tend to adjust better than the child's parents to this situation:

Maybe it is because older people come from a generation in which less educated people were more common. The idea that their autistic grandson might never graduate from high school, or learn to read or write, and maybe "just" be able to be a gardener, may be acceptable to them. Grandparents take the diagnosis of autism less "personally" than parents, who are more often flooded with waves of conflicting emotions of grief, shame, and guilt. Maybe grandparents can be more objective because they don't feel they'll have to worry what will happen to the child when he's an adult or when *his* parents are too old to care for him. (1996, p. 154)

The intergenerational family relationship that is discussed most in the literature is that between the mother and the child's paternal grandmother (Farber & Ryckman, 1965; Kahana & Kahana, 1970; Lavin, 2001). Paternal grandmothers have been known to blame the mother for the child's disability:

The mother and mother-in law relationship was seen as often being a locus of hostility, with the mother-in-law holding her daughter-in-law responsible for bringing the "burden" of a child with a disability to the family. Recent research suggests that grandmothers of children with disabilities tend to respond to the daughters in more of a "teacher/therapist relationship" than is the case in families with children without disabilities. (Trute, 2003, p. 120)

Findler (2000) reported that mothers rated maternal grandmothers (i.e., their own mothers) as the most important family member to supply both emotional and instrumental support. In his study of 64 parents, Trute (2003) reported a higher sense of well-being and less parenting stress when mothers of children with disabilities experienced support from their own mothers. For the father, the support from his mother is the most beneficial. Trute (2003) speculated that a mother's conflict with her mother-in-law is related to intergenerational problems, as it is in any family. Weisbren (1980) also found that the father's relationship with his parents was more important than all other support sources. Weisbren noted that fathers who perceived their parents as highly supportive engaged in more activities with their child, felt more positive about their child, and were better able or more willing to plan for the future than fathers who had unsupportive parents. She further found that mothers who perceive their in-laws as supportive also feel more positive about their child. This research suggests that grandparents may have considerable influence on how parents respond to their child with a disability.

Although resentment, guilt, and anger can be destructive, such feelings should be viewed in context. Negative emotions should probably be expected, especially early on, and do not necessarily lead to a crisis. To discourage family members from expressing their pain through anger or disappointment is to encourage its expression in subtle ways; then, these major underlying issues, which are never directly confronted, may affect the lives of family members in more camouflaged ways. At any rate, just as professionals must understand and accept the parents' anger, so too must they accept similar feelings from grandparents. One grandmother commented:

> Anger and hostility can be destructive forces to live with. Will anger and hostility be all this child will ever mean to me? I wondered. I suffered for him—for what he might have been, should have been. I resented what his birth had done to my lovely daughter.
>
> I cried a lot and prayed a lot and yelled at God a lot. Then, I said, "So be it. You're sorry for yourself, but look at that child. Just look at him. Not what he might have been, but what he is. Grow up, lady." (McPhee, 1982, p. 14)

Most grandparents looked forward to the time when their own parental role would cease (Kornhaber, 2002). The birth of a child with a disability can suddenly thrust them back in time, causing them to resume a role they thought had been fulfilled, Click (1986) spoke to this issue years ago:

> When my own kids were little the chaos just all seemed to go with the territory—spilled milk, scattered cereal, orange peels behind the couch, lost socks, wall-to-wall toys. I cleaned it up a dozen times a day without a second thought. Now, just bending over sometimes sparks that second thought! We don't have the peace and quiet we sometimes think we'd like to have. Sometimes I find myself thinking, "I served my time at this! What am I doing here?" (1986, p. 3)

One grandparent, who was thrust into a parent role due to the parents' drug addiction, remarked, "I feel I've been cheated. I'm not ready for the rocking chair, but if I want to go out with friends, I can't. I feel like something has been stolen from me" (Minkler & Roe, 1993, p. 60).

By their reactions and lack of support, grandparents can be a source of conflict to the nuclear family coping with childhood disability (Turnbull et al., 2006; Hornby & Ashworth, 1994). The grandparents' sense of vulnerability, the loss they experience, the ambiguity the situation holds for them, their denial and lack of acceptance can indeed be burdensome for the family. In this regard, Hornby and Ashworth (1994) reported that, in their small-scale study of 25 parents, the perceived level of support from grandparents was low. A quarter of the grandparents were considered to have added to the parents' burdens and almost a third of the parents expressed a wish for more support from grandparents.

As noted by Kornhaber (2002), just like parents, grandparents make mistakes. He contended that grandparents are at a disadvantage when they fail to (1) understand their role, (2) not support the parents, (3) recognize their unique perspective, (4) make time available for their grandchildren, (5) work to maintain a positive relationship with the family, and (6) respect the rights of the parents to make their own mistakes and learn from them. In regard to the last point grandparents need to acknowledge that their grandchildren already have parents. However, for most families of a child with special needs who have living extended family, the situation is more positive. Indeed, as Vadasy and Fewell (1986) reported, mothers of deaf–blind children ranked their own parents high on their list of supports. An important indicator of positive intergenerational relationships that augur well for the family's future is an ongoing historical pattern of close and supportive relationships between parents and their parents.

Grandparent contributions to the nuclear family can be many and varied. Some professionals conceive of grandparents as valuable resources for their grandchildren and the family (Lavin, 2001; Green, 2001; Lawrence-Webb, Okundaye, & Hafner, 2003). However, as with fathers, not all professionals consider grandparents a resource. Professionals and policy makers often overlook the contributions of the family's informal network, including grandparents (Findler & Taubman, 2003). In their questionnaire study of 81 social workers, these researchers found that social workers rarely involved grandparents as a resource. They also found that the social workers showed little interest in getting professional training to learn more about how grandparents could benefit their children and grandchildren with disabilities. Other sources of support (e.g., sisters, professionals, friends) were considered to be more important. Findler and Taubman urged professionals to view grandparents as important resources in families of children with disabilities.

Grandparents have much to offer in advising about child care, providing access to community resources, and sharing coping strategies that helped them in the past (Kornhaber, 2002). They also may have more time available to assist with shopping, errands, and child care, and can provide respite for the parents from the daily chore of caring for the child. Respite services are scarce in some communities, making this an essential contribution. Grandparents may be able to provide the family with access to services within the community through their contacts with others. Through the grandparents' resources, the family might gain access to child care, special equipment, and other types of support. In their study of 120 mothers of children with moderate to profound intellectual disabilities, Heller and colleagues (2000) reported that grandparents:

- Helped with childcare (45%).
- Gave advice and encouragement (40%).
- Helped with household chores (16%).
- Provided financial assistance (15%).

These above percentages can be interpreted in different ways; as an indication of significant grandparent support or as a disappointing finding that many grandparents appeared to withhold their involvement and support. And finally, as noted above, as a consequence of divorce, substance abuse, violence, and chronic illness or disability, grandparents sometimes serve as parents to children with disabilities (Lawrence-Webb et al., 2003; Simpson, 1996).

In lower SES families, grandparents may be an important source of material support. A family described in Chapter 3, for example, lived in a house owned by the grandparents (who themselves lived across the street) and received financial assistance from them. For families like this one, material help may be the most important form of support that grandparents provide.

For many families, however, the most important type of help from the extended family may be emotional support (Trute, 2003). For grandparents who live some distance from the nuclear family, emotional support is achievable whereas instrumental help, other than financial assistance, may be impossible. The support of grandparents during the initial diagnostic phase and throughout the child's development adds immeasurably to the parents' ability to come to grips with the demands of raising a child with special needs.

Grandparents can thus be a source of emotional support and instrumental assistance; but as noted above, they can also add to the family's burden when they do not accept their grandchild and fail to be supportive. As noted elsewhere in this volume, a central concept in the family therapy literature is that of boundaries. For families to function optimally, they need to consider the negative effects of rigid and enmeshed boundaries, which contribute to conflict and stress.

Boundaries between the nuclear family and the extended family need to be carefully drawn. Boundaries are influenced by the family's history of interaction and by its culture and nationality. Boundary issues can be related to how grandparents respond to their adult child's parenting style. It can become problematic when there are differing methods of childrearing, when grandparents do not respect their adult child's role as a parent, and when grandparents overextend their role in their grandchild's life (Kornhaber, 2002). Ideally there should be a balance between being overinvolved or underinvolved.

Generally speaking, grandparents who become too involved with the grandchild may be considered by the parents as "out-parenting" them (Lavin, 2001). When this situation occurs, the parents feel as if they have lost control of their children, and their parenting confidence may suffer. It is helpful for grandparents to keep in mind that their adult children are the primary source of parenting. Instead of taking over, it is best for grandparents to ask the parents how they can help, allowing the parents to assume the parenting role. By the same token, the adult children can tell their parents how they can best help. The key is to keep communication open so that if the adult children feel that their parents are overly intrusive, they can say so. By the same token, if the grandparents feel excluded, they should communicate their feeling of being left out. At the outset it is a good idea that both the nuclear and extended family members agree to strive for an open expression of feelings.

Another challenge is when there are two sets of grandparents vying for involvement or when one set lives close to the nuclear family and the other is some distance away. Unless there are preexisting issues between the parents and the grandparents, the same idea of open and frequent communication is a good rule to follow. In her book, Lavin (2001) offered good advice on how parents and grandparents can help each other during this challenging time.

An important question is how can professionals help those grandparents who wish to be involved and useful, as well as those who are struggling with their negative or ambivalent feelings and, thus find it difficult to come to terms with the family crisis? The grandparents' sense of threat or burden exacerbates stress in the family. Several models and programs have been offered to help grandparents gain essential information and come to terms with their reactions. These resources are discussed in the next section.

SUPPORT GROUPS

Support groups have a long history. Joseph Pratt (1907), a physician, prescribed support groups for his tuberculosis patients to help with their feelings of discouragement and depression. There are currently hundreds of support groups in existence for people with a variety of circumstances and conditions (Seligman & Marshak, 2003). The interest in support groups for persons with an illness or disability and for family members has been encouraged by the surge of studies linking emotional factors to health outcome (Spira, 1997).

Specific groups for those with an illness or disability provide opportunities to address social and emotional issues often intensified by a disability (Seligman & Marshak, 2003). In such groups members can share information, are comforted by seeing that others are confronted by the same or similar challenges, gain hope, inspiration, and encouragement, and are bolstered by being helpful to others, instead of always being the recipient of help.

We believe that, for the most part, grandparents enhance the coping abilities of the entire family. Others support this view as well (Green, 2001; Seligman, 2001; Kornhaber, 2002; Trute, 2003; Turnbull et al., 2006). George (1988) advocated a support group model whereby grandparents of grandchildren with disabilities exchange information and feelings with other grandparents who are confronting a similar crisis. In such groups, grandparents benefit through mutual support and increased knowledge about children with disability and about grandparent–nuclear family dynamics. They become better able to provide support to the parents, thereby alleviating stress. Moreover, the child benefits greatly from the increased acceptance by his or her grandparents.

Another resource for grandparents is the Internet, where support and information are really available.

Research indicates that grandparents want to be better informed about available therapies for their grandchild, want to know more about the child's disability, and want to have some idea of the child's potential (Vadasy, Fewell, et al., 1986; Kornhaber, 2002; Frisco, 2002). Grandparents also wonder whether they are doing the right things for the grandchild and express anxiety about the future. A support group model can help grandparents and their adult children cope with the crisis and concerns of childhood disability.

Grandparents are important resources, and their involvement in the life of the child with the disability benefits them as well as the nuclear family. We believe that grandparents are an unrecognized and underutilized resource, even though some grandparents struggle with their reactions to the grandchild and may actually exacerbate stress in the family. Professionals should make an effort to look to extended family members as a resource and consider their potential contributions to the family. In addition, that the adult children should be appreciative of, and helpful to, their parents, remembering that this relationship is bidirectional. Turnbull et al. (2006) provide direction for enhancing extended family interactions:

- Provide parents with information to help them better understand the needs and reactions of extended-family members.
- Provide information about exceptionality, the needs of children, and the needs of families that parents can give to extended-family members.
- Encourage the development of grandparent or extended-family-member support groups.
- Encourage extended-family participation in IEP conferences, classroom visits, school events, and family support programs.
- Provide library materials and resources for extended-family members. (p. 43)

We would like to conclude this chapter by quoting from Arthur Kornhaber (2002), a national expert on grandparenting and the author of a definitive book on the subject, *The Grandparent Guide.*

Everyone involved with the child's care—from doctors to parents—needs to understand how to access the helping and healing power of grandparents. No matter what the problem is, the normal healthy part of any child with special needs wants to love and be loved, to grow, to learn, to have freedom, and to have fun. Although the parents have the primary responsibility for following medical regimens and giving direct care, grandparents can supplement their efforts. (p. 185)

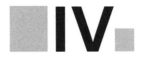

IV.

APPROACHES
TO INTERVENTION

■11■

Professional–Family Interaction

Working toward Partnership

Ask any five parents of visually impaired children how they first learned their child had vision problems and you will get five different horror stories. ... We parents try to be grateful that professionals pay any attention to the imperfect children we have produced, but we cannot avoid feelings of betrayal and anger when we are the recipients of misinformation or of the kind of callous treatment that ignores parental expertise.

—STOTLAND (1984, p. 69)

When I placed Matthew into a strange woman's arms on his first day in the infant program, I didn't know what she hoped to accomplish with my 4-week-old baby. ... As the weeks and months passed, I sensed my baby's growing attachment to his teacher and his response to her obvious delight whenever he accomplished a new feat. I, too, unconsciously formed my attachment to her. ... Professionals who work with families in the early months of the child's life can have a profound influence on parents. A mother may hear the first hopeful words about her child from the teacher or therapist. And those words and assurances can become the basis of strong attachments, acknowledged or unrealized, between parents and program staff.

—MOELLER (1986, pp. 151–152)

Professionals can evoke strong feelings, both positive and negative, in their interactions with parents. During the early months of the child's life especially, both parents and professionals are highly vulnerable: The professional is charged with conveying the "bad news" of a child's disability to parents but is also in a position to offer badly needed information, hope, and support. The parent, on the other hand, is the recipient of the news about the child and looks to the professional as an expert who can provide answers to the many questions raised by the diagnosis. The reactions of professionals during these early months can form the basis for parents' future trust.

In this chapter, we explore the views that professionals and parents have of each other and examine some of the sources of those views. We also look at the parent–professional encounter from a sociological perspective, as an interaction situation. Finally, we discuss the need for a parent–professional partnership and explore some of the new roles available to both parents and professionals in their quest for improved services for children and families. Most of the literature in this area deals with physicians and educators; however, our discussion may apply equally well to counselors, clinical sociologists, social workers, psychologists, and other professionals.

PROFESSIONALS AND PARENTS: HOW DO THEY VIEW EACH OTHER?

Parents' Predispositions toward Professionals

Long before they become the parents of children with disabilities, individuals have various beliefs about, and attitudes toward, professionals. They have interacted with physicians, nurses, teachers, and possibly therapists, counselors, or social workers in different contexts; they have also been exposed to media images of these professionals. As a result, when their children are born, they have expectations about professional behavior that may or may not be fulfilled by the actual professionals with whom they come into contact. As one mother wrote, "The last thing I wanted was a home visitor. . . . I thought Public Health Nurses were for people who beat their kids and drink too much" (Judge, 1987, p. 20).

Professional Dominance

The most common image associated with physicians and other professionals in our society has been one of *professional dominance* (Freidson, 1970). By virtue of their education and high status in the community, professionals, especially physicians, have been expected to play a dominant role in their interactions with clients or patients. Dominance generally includes elements of paternalism and control: The professional determines "what is best" for the client and provides only as much information to him or her as is necessary for the clinical management of the case. To maintain their dominance, some professionals discourage parents from obtaining information on their own: "[The doctor] wants you to get the rest of the information from the specialist, the genetics counselor. Before leaving, he advises you against going to the library to do your own research" (Pelham, 2001, p. 24). Sometimes parent knowledge is even met with resentment, as this parent's comment suggests: "One administrator admitted that her staff didn't like me because I 'knew too much.' Funny, I'd never held that against them" (Clark et al., 1996, p. 17).

Parents who have been exposed to the idea of professional dominance may view physicians and other professionals with respect, even awe, and submit to their recommendations without question. In other cases, they may resent professional control of their lives. As we show later, submission to professional authority is becoming less common in society today. Along with increasing consumer empowerment, trends toward increasing bureaucratization in medicine have eroded physician autonomy. Also, as Chapter 3 has shown, subcultural values and beliefs play an important role in shaping parents' views of, and behavior toward, professionals.

Studies (Seligman, 2000) indicate that parents may be more positively predisposed toward teachers than toward other professionals. On the other hand, as Seligman has noted, parents' perceptions of teachers may be colored by negative experiences *they* had in school. In addition, teachers spend many hours with their pupils and may be regarded as being in competition with parents for their children's time, attention, respect, or affection. Lortie (as cited in Seligman, 1979) also suggested that parents may resent a teacher's control over their children when the teacher's values are different from those of the parents. Some parents have found that early intervention professionals are more willing to work in partnership with them than the educational professionals encountered later in their children's lives: "Our experiences with the educational system have been mostly negative. Birth-to-three (B-3) was wonderful, but in the public schools, the attitude changes from one of 'Parent knows child best' to 'teacher will tell you how to care for your child' " (Hickman, 2000, p. 168). Other parents have reported positive experiences with teachers who exceeded their professional duties by becoming advocates for their children:

Michael's teacher came to the house the whole summer before he started
school and worked with him. Her telephone line is always open, every
night, if you have any questions. . . . She fights the system she works with
from within, which makes it twice as hard to let them screw the parents
over. I am scared to death for next year, because she is moving to another
school system. But I think I can take them on. (Hickman, 2000, p. 169)

A number of studies has indicated that professional dominance,
in general, may be declining somewhat in today's society as part of a
trend toward greater consumer control in the marketplace. Betz and
O'Connell (1983) suggested that the sense of trust is diminished as the
physician–patient relationship becomes more specialized, impersonal,
and shortlived as a result of population mobility, professionalization,
managed care, and bureaucratization. Haug and Lavin (1983) suggested further that "in the dialectic of power relations, the increasing
monopolization of medical knowledge and medical practice could
only call forth a countervailing force in the form of patient consumerism" (p. 16).

Rodwin (1994) argued that the Patients' Rights, Women's Health,
and Disability Rights Movements fostered consumerism over professional dominance. However, he noted that the shift away from professional control is still incomplete. Pescosolido, Tuch, and Martin (2001)
noted similarly that although confidence in physicians has decreased
somewhat since 1976, over 90% of the respondents in their study were
still confident. Some social class differences were found, with higher
SES respondents reporting less confidence than those of lower social
status. They concluded that although professional dominance is declining somewhat, the decline varies among groups, and professional control is still an important factor in the health care system today.

Prior to their child's birth, then, parents are likely to have been
exposed to both professional dominance and consumerism. Shortly
after the birth and initial diagnosis, they are likely to defer to the
expertise of the professional. As indicated in Chapter 4, parents are
typically in a state of anomie when they first realize that their child
may have a disability. Because they are ill prepared for the birth of a
child with an impairment, they are likely to rely heavily on the advice
of the professionals they encounter at that time. In a recent study
involving life-and-death decisions, Brinchmann et al. (reported in
Tripp & McGregor, 2006) found that the majority of parents in their
sample "respected the expertise of the doctor." Later, especially in
cases in which professionals are not able to provide appropriate infor-

mation and guidance, parents' awareness of consumerism may lead them to challenge professional authority. Such changes in attitude and behavior toward professionals are discussed later in this chapter.

The Professional Role as an Ideal Type

Professional dominance is one of several images of professionals common in society today. Parsons (1951) classically described the role of the professional as being characterized by the traits of achievement, universalism, functional specificity, and affective neutrality. Although real professionals only approximate these traits to greater or lesser degrees, the public image of the ideal–typical professional may be a composite of all of them.

The professional role is achieved rather than ascribed; that is, to become a professional, one must successfully complete a program of education and training. Professionals who work with families of children with disabilities have *chosen* that specialty. Unlike the parent who has given birth to a child with a disability, the professional works in this field because of interest, altruism, monetary or other reward, or convenience. Parents may resent the professional, who deals with their problems only during working hours, while they deal with them 24 hours a day.

Parents are appreciative of physicians who are willing to exceed conventional role expectations:

> He's an excellent doctor. If there's anything I need, . . . I call him. Even if it's two o'clock in the morning. I call him at home. I've done that plenty of times. B always gets sick on the weekend. And I hate to call him on his time off, but sometimes, you have to do it. (mother of child with severe disabilities, interviewed by Jon Darling, personal communication, August 25, 2005)

The professional role is also universalistic; that is, the professional is expected to be fair. Ideally, all children will receive treatment of the same quality. In reality, though, many parents discover that their children with disabilities are *not* treated like their nondisabled children. These parental reports are illustrative:

> [Our pediatrician] seemed to feel that Brian was an unnecessary burden. . . . He didn't take my complaints seriously. . . . I feel that Brian's sore throat is just as important as [my nondisabled daughter's] sore throat.

> Our pediatrician . . . says, "She's retarded, and there's nothing you can
> do about it. You're wasting your time going to specialists." He blames all
> of her [medical] problems on retardation instead of treating them.
> (Darling, 1979, pp. 151–152)

Such experiences may eventually result in parental challenges to professional authority. As we show later in the chapter, newer training
programs for physicians and other professionals are resulting in fewer
such experiences today than in the past.

In addition, even when professionals practice universalism (treating all children in a like manner), they may engender anger in parents,
whose relationship to their child is particularistic. For parents, *this*
child is important and may have special needs that warrant extra time
and attention from the professional.

The professional role is also functionally specific and continues to
become increasingly more specialized. Parents expect teachers to be
experts in the field of education but do not expect them to be experts
in the field of medicine as well. Teachers, physicians, therapists, and
other professionals who work with children and families all have their
own areas of expertise. Parents, however, are not always aware of the
distinctions among disciplines and may not be sure whether a question about feeding skills, for example, would be more appropriately
asked of a pediatrician, speech therapist, occupational therapist, or
teacher. Parents generally appreciate professionals who show an interest in aspects of a child that might be outside their area of expertise,
as this parent's report suggests:

> The neurologist we see has been seeing Cassie since she was 24 hours
> old. We have a wonderful relationship. He has always been supportive of
> me. If I'm upset with something new that has developed, no matter what
> area of her disability it affects, he always takes the time to boost my spir-
> its up and make me more confident in how I'm doing with her.
> (Hickman, 2000, p. 197)

Parents are also interested in the whole child. They see their children playing many roles—child, grandchild, playmate, pupil—as well as
"child with a disability." Most parents appreciate physicians who take
the time to inquire about how their child is doing in school or teachers
who show an interest in their child's medical problems. Likewise, they
may come to resent professionals who do not show an interest in the
whole child. As one father remarked, "The pediatrician . . . would
keep him alive but he wasn't interested in Brian as a *person*" (Darling,

1979, p. 152). Similarly, one mother writes, "I even lost my name. Professionals called me 'Mom.' Some referred to my daughter as the 'handicapped child.' What happened to our identity as people?" (Tillman, 2001, p. 154). As one parent suggested, "I think all children should be valued for who they are and not what they can or cannot do. Every child is a treasure and deserves to be valued and respected" (Clark et al., 1996, p. 26).

Finally, professionals are expected to be affectively neutral and not become emotionally involved with their clients. Again, the professional role is the antithesis of the parental role in this regard, and regardless of ideal–typical role expectations, many parents appreciate professionals who do become attached to their children. Matthew's mother, quoted at the beginning of the chapter, described a strong bond between her infant program teacher, her child, and herself. Because of the frequency and intensity of contact, parents are more likely to develop such a bond with teachers and therapists in a home-based program than with physicians seen only during brief clinic or office visits.

The Need to Be Aware of Parental Expectations

Professionals who work with families, then, should be aware that parents have preconceived notions about the nature of the professional role. The degree to which professionals are able to meet parents' expectations may determine the nature of the relationship they will have with a family. Parents' expectations are shaped by the views of the larger society and, as Chapter 3 has shown, by their subculture as well. Attitudes toward professionals differ among the various social classes, and parents may react differently as well to professionals who are of different ethnic groups. An awareness of these differing parental perceptions and expectations can help professionals improve the services they provide to families.

Professionals' Predispositions toward Children with Disabilities and Their Families

Stigmatizing Attitudes

Families with children who have disabilities come into contact with a variety of professionals. Some of these professionals, such as pediatric physical therapists, have chosen their specialty because they want to work with this population. Other professionals, such as pediatricians or teachers in regular classrooms, may not enjoy working with children who have disabilities at all. As one pediatrician said: "I don't enjoy it. . . . I don't really enjoy a really handicapped child who comes in drooling, can't walk, and so forth. . . . Medicine is geared to the perfect human body. Something you can't do anything about challenges the doctor and reminds him of his own inabilities" (Darling, 1979, p. 215).

Like others in society, these professionals have been exposed to stigmatizing attitudes toward individuals with disabilities. A number of studies (e.g., Gething, 1992) have shown that health professionals, like others in society, tend to devalue this population. Most professionals have not had any direct experience with individuals with disabilities either in their training or in their personal lives. As a result, they may not be able to understand the positive aspects of relationships between parents and children with disabilities. They may also feel inadequate in their ability to work with such families. These concerns are evident in this pediatrician's comments:

> There are personal hang-ups. You go home and see three beautiful, perfect children; then you see this "dud." You can relate more easily to those with three beautiful perfect kids. . . . If somebody comes in with a cerebral palsy or a Down's, I'm not comfortable. . . . My inadequacy to the task bothers me. . . . I liked problems as a resident but I can't say that I enjoy sick kids anymore. It's hard to find much happiness in this area. The subject of deformed children is depressing. . . . As far as having a Mongoloid child, I can't come up with anything good it does. There's nothing fun or pleasant. It's somebody's tragedy. I can find good things in practically anything—even dying—but birth defects are roaring tragedies. (Darling, 1979, pp. 214–215)

With newer training programs, such attitudes may be less common today than in the past, especially among recently trained physicians.

Professionals may have more negative views of families than families have of themselves. One study (Blackard & Barsch, 1982) found significant differences between parents' and professionals' responses to a questionnaire about the impact of the child on the family. As compared with parents' responses, the professionals tended to overestimate the negative impact of the child on family relationships. The professionals overestimated the extent to which parents reported community rejection and lack of support and underestimated parents' ability to use appropriate teaching and behavior management techniques. A study by Sloper and Turner (1991) also showed how professionals overestimate the negative impact of a child with a disability on the family.

Middleton (1999) noted that many children with disabilities would not wish to eliminate their impairments if given the opportunity. Like the adults with disability pride discussed in Chapter 6, they had no desire to be "normal." Rousso (1985) suggested that professionals without disabilities have difficulty identifying with clients who have disabilities because they would not wish to be disabled themselves:

> When, as professionals, we find ourselves feeling too tragic, too despairing about our disabled patients' lives . . . we need to look at our own attitudes and our own history regarding disability. We may be imagining how our lives would be if we were suddenly disabled. . . . But keep in mind that congenitally disabled people are not newly disabled. . . .
>
> Being disabled and being intact at the same time is an extremely difficult notion for nondisabled people to make sense of. I keep thinking of my mother's words: "Why wouldn't you want to walk straight?" Even now, it is hard to explain that I may have wanted to walk straight, but I did not want to lose my sense of self in the process. . . . Fostering self-esteem in our congenitally disabled children and clients means helping them reconnect and reclaim these scattered pieces of their identities and once again feel whole, as they deserve. (p. 12)

In the well-publicized "Baby Doe" cases of the late 20th century, physicians' negative attitudes may have contributed to their recommending against treatment in some cases ("Protection of Handicapped Newborns," 1986). When such decisions are made shortly after a child's birth, most parents, like most physicians, have been exposed only to society's stigmatizing attitudes toward people with disabilities. They have not had any of the positive experiences reported by families who have lived with disability for any length of time. In addition, parents are vulnerable in the immediate postpartum period and likely to accept the advice of an authority figure or expert. A physician's recommendation, then, about whether or not an infant with a disability should receive lifesaving treatment may strongly influence the parents' decision. Consequently, physicians and other professionals who may be involved in these situations have an obligation to be as fully informed as possible about the consequences—*both positive and negative*—of such decisions for families.

Some studies have suggested that parents are more likely than professionals to favor lifesaving treatment in the case of medically unstable infants. Streiner, Saigal, Burrows, Stoskopf, and Rosenbaum (2001) reported that parents of extremely premature infants were more likely than professionals to favor intervention to save the child. Similarly, a study in Newfoundland (Lee, Penner, & Cox, 1991) found that most parents favored, whereas most nurses objected to, the treatment of very low-birth-weight infants. However, parents' views do not always carry the same weight as those of professionals in the decision-making process. In a study of a neonatal intensive care nursery, Anspach (1993) found that parents were consulted only after professionals had already reached a decision. She wrote: "Members of the nursery staff refer to this process as 'presenting a united front.' This practice is said to protect the parents from being confused by conflicting opinions" (p. 92). Similarly, Heimer (1999) found that medical professionals exercised control over the decision-making situation.

Professionals' preexisting beliefs and attitudes also may influence their treatment recommendations later in a child's life. In one study (Gillman, Heyman, & Swain, 2000), professionals who had negative assumptions about the quality of life of individuals with intellectual disabilities were less likely to recommend psychological services or certain medical tests to those individuals. Professionals need to be aware that their predispositions may result in discriminatory practices.

Apart from a child's disability, professionals may have negative attitudes toward parents because of their ethnicity, race, gender, or social class. Like others in society, professionals may have stereotypical views of various minority groups and have difficulty relating to families from those groups. Some strategies for assisting professionals in relating to those who are "different" are suggested in Chapter 3.

The nature of a child's impairment may also affect the attitudes of professionals toward the family. Some professionals may have more negative views of intellectual disability than of physical disability, for example. Certain impairments appear to be more stigmatizing than others. Wasow and Wikler (1983) found, for example, that professionals tended to react more positively toward parents of children with intellectual disability than toward parents of children with mental illness. Whereas parents of children with intellectual disability were viewed as part of the treatment team, parents of children with mental illness were seen as part of the problem, even though chronic mental illness is recognized to be largely organic in etiology. With respect to mental illness, such views may be changing thanks to newer "CASSP" (Child and Adolescent Service System Program) models (Cohen & Lavach, 1995). The attitudes of professionals noted by Wasow and Wikler are an example of victim blaming, which is discussed further in the next section.

The Clinical Perspective: Blaming the Victim

In addition to their exposure to stigmatizing attitudes in everyday life, professionals, especially those out of school for more than 20 years, may in fact have been *trained* to have negative views of individuals with disabilities and their families as part of their professional education. As one of us (Seligman, 2000) noted, much of the early professional literature in this field characterized both children with disabilities and their parents as deficient.

In the past, some social workers, psychologists, and other professionals were trained in a psychoanalytic perspective, which located the source of human problems within the psyche of the client (or the client's parents) rather than in the structure of the social system. When seen from this perspective, parents' concerns about their children were interpreted as indications of parental pathology. In much of the literature, this pathology was traced to parental guilt over having given birth to an "imperfect" child (e.g., Forrer, 1959; Powell, 1975; Zuk, 1959). When such an interpretive framework is used, expressions of parental love may be defined as "idealization," and treating a child as normal may be seen as "denial." Regardless of whether parents apparently accept or reject their children, their actions are believed, in either case, to be based on guilt.

Within this perspective, when parents are unable to cope, their failure is blamed on a supposed neurotic inability to accept the child. Real systems-based needs for financial aid, help with child care, or medical or educational services tend to be discounted and attributed to parental inadequacy rather than to a lack of societal resources. Although some parents certainly do have neurotic tendencies, the victim-blaming model is inadequate to explain the many problems faced by parents of children with disabilities. Because society is structured largely to meet the needs of people without disabilities, goods and services for those with disabilities are often difficult, if not impossible, to find. Many older textbooks stressed guilt-based theories of parental behavior, and as a result, professionals often completed their education with the belief that parents of children with disabilities are responsible for their own problems.

Gliedman and Roth (1980) argued that the nature of the parent–professional encounter encourages the professional to see the parent, in addition to the child, as the patient. They suggested that parents are expected to play the classic "sick role," that is, to be passive, cooperative, and in agreement with the decisions of the "experts." When parents disagree, they are sometimes treated like recalcitrant children, and efforts are made to convert them to the "correct" position. Victim blaming and professional dominance can combine to render the parent powerless. "As for the parent . . . he [or she] finds himself [or herself] in a double bind: either submit to professional dominance (and be operationally defined as a patient) or stand up for one's rights and risk being labeled emotionally maladjusted (and therefore patient-like)" (Gliedman & Roth, 1980, p. 150). Such views are sometimes perpetuated when young professionals learn them from their older colleagues.

As a result of their training and experience, then, professionals may come to adopt a "clinical" perspective. Mercer (1965) suggested that this perspective has the following components:

- The development of a diagnostic nomenclature.
- The creation of diagnostic instruments.
- The professionalization of the diagnostic function.
- [The] assumption that the official definition is somehow the "right" definition. If persons in other social systems, especially the family, do not concur with official findings, . . . the clinical perspective assumes that they are either unenlightened or are evidencing psychological denial.
- Finally, . . . social action tends to center upon changing the individual. . . . Seldom considered [is] the alternative . . . of . . . modifying the norms of the social system or of attempting to locate the individual in the structure of social systems which will not perceive his [or her] behavior as pathological. (pp. 18–20)

Mercer proposed an alternative *social system perspective*, which "attempts to see the definition of an individual's behavior as a function of the values of the social system within which he [or she] is being evaluated" (p. 20).

The clinical perspective has persisted in services to families of children with disabilities for a number of reasons, including professional socialization, transdisciplinary understanding, rewards for the clinician, ease of intervention, and the maintenance of professional dominance. Each of these is considered in turn.

PROFESSIONAL SOCIALIZATION

As indicated earlier, the clinical perspective has been a part of professional training in schools of medicine, education, and social work, as well as in courses in psychology and other related fields. Courses in sociology or a social system perspective have not always been included in curricula used in training professionals in these fields, although such curricula have been changing in recent years to include such courses.

TRANSDISCIPLINARY UNDERSTANDING

Most intervention programs in medical and educational settings employ a team of professionals. A variety of individuals, including a pediatrician, speech therapist, physical therapist, occupational therapist, and social worker, for example, may work together to provide services to each child and family. All of these professionals may share the clinical perspective as a result of their training and consequently have been able to communicate with one another fairly easily. Although the instruments of each specialty vary, they all use some sort of assessment tool to measure the child's or family's dysfunction and then develop a course of remediation involving changing the child or family to meet professionally defined goals. More recently, team members have been trained in a systems-oriented perspective in a variety of disciplines (Darling & Baxter, 1996; Darling & Peter, 1994), and intervention strategies are changing as a result. Chapter 13 presents one model for these strategies.

REWARDS FOR THE CLINICIAN

The clinical perspective tends to quantify its concepts. Children can be placed at a specific point along a developmental scale; even family coping skills can be quantified. As a result, progress in a treatment program can be readily measured. When a child or family makes measurable progress, the professional feels rewarded. Social systems variables (e.g., the availability of financial resources) are not as easy to control, and methods for their measurement are not widely taught in professional schools.

EASE OF INTERVENTION

A consideration of all of the systems within which a family interacts complicates the intervention process. Treating the family in isolation is easier for the clinician and allows for more variables to be controlled. The system of categorical labels associated with the clinical perspective also facilitates intervention. Once a family is labeled, a known treatment method can be applied. Recent trends in managed care have reinforced the necessity for labels by only funding services deemed appropriate for a particular diagnosis category.

MAINTENANCE OF PROFESSIONAL DOMINANCE

If they recognized the family's perspective as valid, professionals would have to yield some of their dominance. Many clinicians believe that their dominant status is justified because of their education and clinical experience (e.g., Goodman, 1994; Coulter, 1997).

In some cases, professionals may actually fear parents because of the threat they pose to the professionals' dominance. Lortie (as cited in Seligman, 1979) noted that teachers, in particular, experience a sense of vulnerability because of parents' rights in the educational realm. Other professionals, such as physicians (the increase of malpractice suits notwithstanding), may feel more secure, but those in private practice must always be sensitive to the need to please the client.

Limitations of the Clinical Perspective

The clinical perspective is limited in its value as a holistic approach to the treatment of children and their families. By extracting the child and family from their situational context and evaluating them with professionally constructed instruments, the clinician may be attaching meanings to their situation that are different from those attached to it by the family members themselves. When clinicians place children and families in diagnostic categories, they lose some of the uniqueness of any particular family. When the child and family are the primary focus of attention, social-system-created problems—the causes of which are external to the family system—may be overlooked.

The interaction between parents and professionals is only one of many interaction situations encountered by families. While their child is in a treatment program, parents continue to interact with relatives, friends, strangers, and other kinds of professionals. In some cases, the demands of a program may even conflict with the family's pursuit of a normalized lifestyle in other areas. The professional in such a program cannot understand a family's failure to cooperate without an understanding of that family's competing needs. The following quote from the mother of four teenagers with disabilities illustrates the gap that sometimes exists between parent and professional:

> I'm seeing [a new psychologist] now. He's kind of giving me the blame for the way I am: "It's your fault you feel the way you do about things." I don't *want* to feel this way. . . . He says, "You create your own problems." My problem is that I have four handicapped children, and that has nothing to do with the fact that I had an unhappy childhood. . . . I'm nervous because I have reason to be nervous. . . . That very night we were supposed to go someplace, and the van at the CP Center broke down, so suddenly we had four kids to worry about. . . . We had to change our plans. . . . That's the problem with these professionals. . . . They have a job. . . . They don't live with the parents 24 hours a day. What sounds nice at the office just doesn't work in real life. (Darling, 1979, pp. 179–180)

Similarly, a parent of a three-year-old wrote:

> Our first county health nurse . . . was not very helpful. . . . She was not very understanding of our situation and hated my questioning her on anything. Her mentality was, "Lots of people have three children" (and that is a direct quote). It was then I realized she didn't have a clue about my daily struggles raising triplets: children the same age at three different developmental ages, feeding, sleeping, breathing issues, etc. (Hickman, 2000, p. 193)

Parents' priorities may be different from those of professionals, and, as a result, professionals often have little success when they try to intervene in these cases. As one professional who became a parent remarked, "Before I had Peter I gave out [physical therapy] programs that would have taken all day. I don't know when I expected mothers to change diapers, sort laundry, or buy groceries" (Featherstone, 1980, p. 57).

The following anecdote illustrates another pitfall of the clinical perspective: "One parent . . . told me of her initial clinic visit where the social worker assured her that guilt in a parent was natural and that she shouldn't feel bad about it. . . . Stunned, she allowed the social worker to go on at some length before informing her that the child, in fact, was adopted" (Pieper, as cited in Darling & Darling, 1982, p. viii).

Although this anecdote may not be typical, professionals can overlook important individual and contextual differences by making parents and children fit into clinical categories. Each family's situation is unique and derives from that family's particular place in society. A preconceived diagnostic nomenclature tends to prevent the clinician from seeing the client in a new or creative way.

When families are seen outside of their situational context in a school, clinic, or treatment center, the cause of their problems is more likely to be sought within the family itself. When the family's situation is not completely understood, parents' neurotic symptoms may be attributed to their inability to cope with the child rather than to some external cause. As earlier chapters have shown, however, such symptoms are as likely to result from lack of social support or community resources as from the child's disability. Parents are expected to *accept* and *adjust* to their situation, and the professional role is perceived as one of helping parents cope. This view assumes that the situation of most families cannot or should not be changed.

In fact, sometimes the situation *can* be changed. The child can be placed in a more appropriate program; respite care can be provided; financial aid may be available. (See Chapter 13 for additional systems-based interventions.) Parenting a child with a disability is expensive and exhausting, because society does not have sufficient resources available to help ease the burden for parents. Society's lack of resources is not the parents' fault. Learning to cope may not be a more appropriate response than learning techniques to bring about social change. In an early study of 50 Australian families who did not have access to any kind of program for their children with intellectual disability, Schonell and Watts (1956) found that the parents were "almost desperate." After a training center was established in the city, however, the parents' "neurotic symptoms" virtually disappeared (Schonell & Rorke, 1960).

Gliedman and Roth (1980) remind us that professionals exist to serve their clients:

> The parents' rights over the child take precedence over the professional's personal moral views. To put it bluntly, the professional exists to further the parent's vision of the handicapped child's future. Should the professional disagree, he [or she] has every right to try to *persuade* the parent to adopt a different view. . . . But except in the most extreme cases of parental incompetence and brutality, such as child abuse, the professional has

no right to use his [or her] immense moral and practical power to intimidate or to manipulate the parent. (p. 145)

As noted earlier, newer approaches in this field have taken a social system, rather than clinical, perspective. Changing service models are discussed more fully later in the chapter.

THE PARENT–PROFESSIONAL ENCOUNTER: ROLE TAKING AND ROLE PLAYING

Both parents and professionals, then, bring preconceived ideas and views with them when they interact for the first time. Because of their differing life experiences, parents and professionals tend to view children with disabilities differently. The parenting experience is a powerful means of socialization and, as earlier chapters have shown, may shape parents' perceptions and definitions in unique ways. A professional who is not a parent cannot readily "understand" parenthood in the same way as a parent. The divergent views of parents and professionals sometimes result in strained interaction between them. As Freidson (1961) classically wrote, "the separate worlds of experience and reference of the layman and the professional worker are always in potential conflict with each other" (p. 175).

The Setting

Although some intervention programs operate in the homes of the families they serve, many parent–professional encounters take place in clinics, hospitals, offices, schools, and treatment centers, which are natural habitats for professionals but not for parents. Many parents are intimidated by such settings. They may recall prior experiences in schools or hospitals that made them feel uncomfortable during their own childhood or at some other time in their lives. They may also feel powerless because the setting is professionally controlled. Large treatment facilities also tend to have a bureaucratic atmosphere, which depersonalizes families and their problems.

Presentation of Self

In his classic work, Goffman (1959) showed how people attempt to create images of themselves in the course of interaction with others. Individuals act in a manner they believe will convey a desired impression. Parents and professionals also engage in self-presentation in their interactions with each other.

One of us (R. B. D.) once made an unscheduled home visit to a family in her early intervention program to find the usually neat and clean home in complete disarray. Toys were strewn about the floor, and dirty dishes filled the kitchen. The mother was extremely embarrassed and uneasy throughout the visit. R. B. D. realized, as a result of this experience, that all of her previous scheduled visits had been preceded by much house cleaning and preparation by the family. Activities such as cleaning the house, dressing the child for the visit, and reporting about having worked on therapeutic or educational programs are all forms of self-presentation. Parents' awareness of such presentation is variable. As the following parental statement suggests, some parents may deliberately and consciously attempt to convey a certain impression to the professional:

> I was conscious of the need to make these doctors identify with us as strongly and as quickly as possible. . . . I made sure that Julian and I dressed in a way that we imagined the doctor's family might dress. We were meticulous about showing up for appointments, at least 15 minutes early, to prove that we were concerned, responsible parents. We paid our bills promptly at the end of each visit. I tried to elicit personal comments from the doctor by referring to topics that might interest him. . . . Finally, I worked with David to make sure he was a cooperative and likable patient. (Stotland, 1984, p. 72)

The need to have the professional see them as "good" parents may be very stressful to some.

Professionals also engage in self-presentation in their interactions with parents. They may want to be perceived as authority figures, friends, or sympathetic listeners. Self-presentation is learned in the course of professional training and experience. Professionals should try to become more aware of the images they are creating and of those they wish to create.

Role Taking

The concept of *role-taking ability*, which derives from symbolic interaction theory in sociology, describes the ability to see a situation from another person's perspective in the course of interaction with that person. As the above discussion has indicated, our definitions of any situation are products of our unique life experiences. As a result, professionals may have difficulty "taking the role" of the parent, and parents likewise may have difficulty understanding the professional's point of view. This difficulty is summarized by Dembo (1984): "The professionals frequently appear to be insensitive to the parents because the professionals' position and values as outsiders stand in opposition to the position and values of the parents as insiders" (p. 93). When people in a particular situation are not easily able to take the role of the other, interaction based on mutual understanding becomes impossible.

The Diagnostic Encounter

The literature has suggested that the situation in which parents are first informed of a child's disability has often been characterized by the poor role taking of professionals. Quine and Rutter (1994) reported that 58% of the parents they surveyed were dissatisfied with their physicians' communication of diagnostic information. As Chapter 4 indicated, until fairly recently professionals tended to delay in providing such information to parents because they did not want to be the bearers of "bad news." Many physicians also incorrectly believed that parents did not want to receive this information shortly after a child's birth (see Darling, 1979, for pediatricians' statements expressing this belief). Studies (Berg, Gilderdale, & Way, 1969; Carr, 1970; Drillien & Wilkinson, 1964; Gayton & Walker, 1974; McMichael, 1971; Quine & Pahl, 1986) have indicated, however, that most parents *do* want diagnostic information as soon as possible.

Parents' reactions to lack of information resulting from poor role taking by professionals are illustrated by this mother's story:

> On our third visit, the neurologist said, "I think I know what's wrong with your son but I'm not going to tell you because I don't want to frighten you." Well, I think that's about the worst thing anyone could say. . . . We didn't go back to him. . . . We insisted that [our pediatrician] refer us to _____ Children's Hospital. He said, "He's little. Why don't you wait—you don't need to take him there yet." I have a feeling that he knew what the diagnosis was going to be and he didn't really think that we needed to know yet. . . . The chief of pediatrics at _____ Children's Hospital told us he was retarded. . . . That was the first person we talked to that we really felt we could trust. . . . Everyone was pablum-feeding us, and we wanted the truth. (Story related to R. B. D.

in 1978 by the parent of a 6-year-old child with intellectual disability and cerebral palsy)

In addition to their desire for information, studies have suggested that parents also value emotional empathy during the diagnostic encounter. One study of parents of children with cleft lip/palate (Byrnes, Berk, Cooper, & Marazita, 2003) found that the parents wanted professionals to show more caring and to show more of their own feelings during the informing interview. Another study (Krahn, Hallum, & Kime, 1993) mentioned the importance of physical contact with the child. Halpern (1984, p. 171) summarized some of the recommendations of a number of studies regarding effectiveness in the diagnostic situation:

- Communicate in clear, simple, straightforward language.
- Be willing to spend extra time with the parents.
- Present strengths, positive attributes of the child before communicating the diagnosis of disability.
- Be aware of one's own feelings and attitudes.
- Take parents' own evaluation of their child seriously.
- Offer specific advice on next steps.
- Offer information on prognosis honestly, with a caveat of the difficulty of prediction.
- Show respect for the child and family.

During the last 25 years or so, programs have been developed in medical schools to aid physicians in the experience of role taking during the diagnostic encounter (see Darling & Peter, 1994, for descriptions of some of these). These programs include such activities as role-play exercises and spending time with families. McDonald, Carson, Palmer, and Slay (1982) found, perhaps because of such programs, that 88% of physicians surveyed stated that they presented diagnostic information to both parents immediately after birth. Gill and Maynard (1995) suggested that professionals today still do not generally present diagnostic information outright; rather they present small amounts of information at a time, waiting for reactions from parents before proceeding. By taking the role of the parent, they are able to adjust their statements to take parents' expectations into account. Interactions between physicians and parents in the diagnostic situation are discussed further in the section on role playing below.

Other Encounters

Examples of poor role taking can also be found in later encounters between parents and professionals, after a diagnosis has been established. Studies of the doctor–patient relationship, in general, have indicated that misconceptions of patients' needs for information are common. Waitzkin (1985) found, for example, in an analysis of 336 outpatient encounters, that physicians overestimated the time they spent in giving information and underestimated patients' desires for information.

One suggestion for improving the assimilation of information during parent–professional encounters has been the use of a tape recorder. During an electronic mail exchange on this subject, some physicians expressed concern with liability issues and with the self-censoring that sometimes occurs when statements are being recorded. However, the advantages of this method to families might encourage some practitioners at least to offer a recording option to their patients or clients. One physician wrote:

> One I remember best was a young couple with . . . a poor prognosis and some difficult therapeutic choices including amputation. . . . They asked for my permission [to tape] and then we talked for more than thirty minutes. At subsequent [and non-taped] visits they noted how helpful the taped session had been as they listened to it many times prior to making a decision regarding further treatment. (A posting on the *Children with Special Health Needs Listserv,* June 27, 1995)

Another area of misperception involves parents' psychosocial concerns and needs for emotional support. One study of mothers seeking care in private pediatric offices (Hickson, Altemeier, & O'Connor, 1983) found that only 30% of the mothers were most worried about their child's physical health; the others were more concerned with parenting, behavioral, developmental, or psychosocial issues. Yet most parent–physician communication involved only health issues. Mothers were not aware that pediatricians could help them with these concerns, or they believed that pediatricians were not interested in helping them. Pediatricians, on the other hand, assumed incorrectly that mothers who did not raise such issues were not concerned about them. Lack of physician interest was also a barrier to communication, leading some mothers to "cloak psychosocial worries in physical terms to gain the attention of the physician" (Hickson et al., 1983, p. 623). In another study (Cadman et al., as cited in Bailey & Simeonsson, 1984), clinicians rated interactions within the family as the most important outcomes of intervention, whereas families rated these as next to least important.

One study (Liptak & Revel, as cited in Institute for Health & Disability, 1999) found a considerable mismatch regarding service priorities between parents and physicians. The parents' first priority—community resources—was ranked only 14th by the physicians. The physicians also largely underestimated the importance of recreational opportunities and summer camps. This finding is reminiscent of one from a study of human service professionals and their clients (Darling, Hager, Stockdale, & Heckert, 2002), which found that professionals tended to emphasize needs for therapeutic services to solve "problems," whereas clients were more concerned about universal human needs such as finding time for recreation and access to public libraries. Because professionals see only one aspect of their clients' lives (their "problem"), they tend to perceive their clients as more needy (and pathological) than the clients perceive themselves.

Role Playing

The concept of role playing used here derives from symbolic interaction theory and includes all of the verbal and nonverbal activity in which an individual engages. The behavior, or role playing, of parents and professionals is based on their role-taking ability. They will act in a manner they believe will evoke the desired response on the part of the other. Role playing is based not only on preexisting perceptions but also on what actually happens in the course of a conversation. Both parents and professionals constantly adjust their behavior as they engage in an ongoing process of redefining the situation.

With regard to the parent–professional encounter, Gliedman and Roth (1980) classically wrote: "Most people adjust their behavior unconsciously to reflect the prevailing structural asymmetries in a relationship" (p. 170). When parents perceive a difference in status between themselves and professionals, they may defer to the expertise of the professional and not express some of their questions or concerns. As Strong (1979) noted in a study of two hospital outpatient departments:

> Many parents disagreed strongly with the doctors' verdict at one time or another. Nevertheless all but a handful made no direct challenge to their

authority. Most maintained an outward pose of agreement with what they were told, even though they might say rather different things to ancillary staff such as therapists or social workers. (p. 87)

Studies in the medical sociology literature reveal a rather high rate of noncompliance with doctors' orders among patients who do not openly express any disagreement while they are in the doctors' offices.

Noncompliance with medical advice appears to be related, at least in part, to lack of satisfaction during the parent–physician encounter. Francis, Korsch, and Morris (1968) found, in a study of outpatient visits to a children's hospital, that the extent to which parents' expectations were not met, the lack of warmth in the physician–parent relation, and the failure to receive a diagnostic explanation were key factors in noncompliance. Compliance was significantly related to parents' satisfaction. More recently, Leiter and Krauss (in press) found that parents who met resistance when requesting additional special education services were more likely to be dissatisfied with the services they received.

Professional dominance of the parent–professional encounter also varies in response to the degree of professional uncertainty present in the situation. In a classic study, Fox (1959) found that in a situation of medical uncertainty, patients had a more collegial relationship with their physicians. Many childhood impairments fall within the realm of "physician uncertainty." Diagnosis of intellectual disability is very difficult, if not impossible, in very young children with cerebral palsy and other motor disabilities or sensory impairments, such as blindness or deafness. Subtler conditions, such as learning disabilities, are also difficult to diagnose at young ages.

In a classic study, Davis (1960) noted a distinction between *clinical* and *functional* uncertainty, the former a "real" phenomenon and the latter a patient management technique. Davis found that in the case of paralytic polio convalescence, treatment staff tended to be evasive with parents, avoiding the truth even after clinical uncertainty had disappeared. Such avoidance served to prevent emotional confrontations with parents. Functional uncertainty is also apparent in this statement from the medical report (in 1986) of a child with severe brain damage in one of our (R. B. D.'s) programs: "I have discussed the above results with John's parents but have not emphasized his very poor developmental outlook. I feel it is more humane and would be easier for them to accept this child if they observe and come to understand his slow progress for themselves." Similarly, in a study of a neonatal intensive care unit, Sosnowitz (1984) noted that "the staff wanted a chance to observe how the parents would react to the crisis. When the staff was unable to predict the parents' reactions, they usually gave just enough information to keep the parents involved" (p. 396).

Functional uncertainty is especially characteristic of the diagnostic encounter. As noted earlier, physicians sometimes delay in providing complete diagnostic information to parents because they believe that parents "are not ready" to hear the truth. Such delays also have the function of avoiding an emotional confrontation. As one of us has noted elsewhere (e.g., Darling, 1979, 1994), physicians may use one or more of four stalling strategies to delay the sharing of diagnostic or prognostic information: avoidance (simply not telling), hinting ("listening longer than necessary to the child's heart"), mystification (using professional jargon or technical terms unfamiliar to laypersons), and passing the buck (making a referral to another professional). As earlier chapters have shown, these techniques can increase rather than alleviate parental anxiety. Svarstad and Lipton (1977) found that parents who received specific, clear, and frank communication were better able to accept a diagnosis of intellectual disability in their children than those who received vague or evasive information.

The expectations attached to parent roles can also be a potential source of conflict between parents and professionals. In many intervention programs, parents are expected to play the role of teacher with their children and are trained for this role by program professionals. As Farber and Lewis (1975) and others argued, however, some parents may not *want* to play a pedagogical role, and "such parental training subordinates the uniquely personalized component of the parent–child relationship" (p. 40). In order to be effective in their interactions with families, professionals must develop realistic role expectations for parents that are compatible with parents' expectations for themselves.

When parents were asked directly to offer advice to medical professionals that would improve the parent–professional relationship, these are some of the recommendations that were offered:

- Really *listen* to the parents and respect their knowledge. Despite your advanced degrees, the parents are the experts on their own child.
- Be a person. There are things in life to discuss with that family other than the syndrome. Be their friend. Always remember that it is the family who has to live together 24 hours a day.

- Deliver awful diagnoses in a compassionate manner; to you, our kid may be a number, but to us our kid is our life.
- Appreciate [the child] as a person and believe in what she can accomplish.
- Tell the parents all the information you know about a topic. . . . The better informed we are the better we are able to determine the type and extent of treatment we want for our children. (Hickman, 2000, pp. 266–268)

THE EMERGENCE
OF A PARENT–PROFESSIONAL PARTNERSHIP:
NEWER ROLES FOR PARENTS AND PROFESSIONALS

Although parent and professional roles have historically been in conflict, some initiatives have emerged that are helping to bring them closer together. The human service sector has undergone some significant changes during the past few decades. In the past, the helping professions were based on a *status inequality model*, reminiscent of the clinical approach discussed earlier, which tended to value the practitioner's perspective more than the client's; as a result, recommended interventions did not always appropriately address client concerns. More recently, a *partnership* model (Darling, 2000) has become the norm in a variety of human service fields. Similar approaches have been called "strengths-based," "client-centered," "family-centered," or "empowerment" models. In these approaches, the client's point of view is valued and even serves as the basis for service delivery. Chapter 13 explores this shift in perspectives in social work, psychology, education, health care, and other fields.

Interactions between professionals and parents of children with disabilities are beginning to reflect this shift. For example, in a study of parents in Great Britain, Case (2001) found that a "high degree of negative interaction . . . is no longer inevitable." In his sample, "parental expertise [was] increasingly acknowledged within a consumer-type relationship model" (p. 850). However, evidence exists as well of the persistence of the status inequality model. In another study, Case (2000) found that professionals continue to control the parent–professional relationship and that parents express concerns and fears about professional dominance and neglect of parental knowledge.

New Roles for Parents: The Emergence of Parent Activism

Ayer (1984) and others suggested that the failure of professionals to meet family needs has resulted in self-help activities by families. Although most parents begin by acquiescing to professional authority, many come to play an *entrepreneurial* role (Darling, 1979, 1988) in order to secure needed services. This role includes (1) seeking information, (2) seeking control, and (3) challenging authority.

As noted earlier in this chapter, parents of children with disabilities, like others in society, have been socialized to accept professional dominance. However, the consumerist movement has been growing, and parents have become more aware of the possibility of challenging professional authority. Parents' disillusionment with professionals may begin shortly after a child's birth, when professionals fail to provide desired diagnostic or treatment information or deny parents' control over their child's management and care. Parents may come to resent their role as helpless bystanders:

> We were always going back and forth to _____ Children's Hospital. . . . It was a constantly pulling away. We could never be a family. . . . It was always, "We have to go to the hospital." We had to go to doctors, doctors, doctors. . . . We could never get to know our child. . . . We got to the point where we hated doctors, we hated _____ Children's Hospital. (Darling, 1979, p. 154)

On the other hand, some professionals willingly share information with, and seek advice from, parents:

> The most important aspect of the doctor's presentation was that he involved us as equals in the decision-making process. . . . By involving us in the process and by giving us his professional opinion as an opinion, he returned to us our parental rights of making the important decision that would affect our child's life. *We were in control,* but we were no longer alone. (Stotland, 1984, p. 72; emphasis added)

> The staff at the early intervention center knew we wanted Aric to attend a regular kindergarten class. . . . They gave us ideas to get him into the setting. They never took control out of our hands, and we always did the steps ourselves. They were there as a resource and support. The staff at the early intervention center helped me to gel the vision. But it didn't take the Family and Child Learning Center to show me promise [in Aric]; I could see that when he was born. (Leifield & Murray, 1995, pp. 246–247)

As noted in earlier chapters, the more parents interact with their children, the more committed they become to their children's welfare. The emotional bond that develops between parent and child is a strong catalyst to parental activism. Pizzo (1983) suggested that the bond "energizes" parent advocacy:

> The most universal shared experience we have as parents is the struggle to protect children and to get them the resources they need to develop well. Listening to parent activists describe their work, one soon learns that their organizational activities are not radically different from the basic task we undertake as parents. In self-help and advocacy, parents take the intimate, nurturing vigilance needed for effective child-rearing into a social and political domain. (p. 19)

When parents encounter difficulties in meeting their children's needs, they are likely to continue to search for appropriate services and helpful professionals. Negative experiences with professionals can be a catalyst for further action. Pizzo (1983) argued that parent advocacy derives from "acute, painful experiences," and Haug and Lavin (1983) reported that the most important variable in consumerist challenges to medical authority is the *experience of medical error.* Such an experience erodes trust in professional authority and may provide the needed turning point to launch parents on a career of activism.

Parents of children with disabilities are more likely than many other people to encounter medical error or errors in professional judgment. Because of the frequency and intensity of their contacts with the many professionals involved in their children's care, they have more opportunities to encounter professional failure. Haug and Lavin (1983) suggested that "chronic patients, who live with their conditions for long stretches of time, often learn by their own experience which therapies are helpful and which are not" (p. 33). The mother of a child with multiple medical issues explained her actions:

> There is so much confusion. Each doctor tells me something different. . . . I wish they would talk to each other. I have requested that all communication between doctors be carbon copied to me, in the hopes of deciphering what is being said. . . . I have purchased some medical dictionaries so I can better understand the terminology and discuss Michael's condition with my doctors on a more realistic level. I'm starting to wonder if perhaps Michael doesn't need to see some other specialists. . . . I keep asking my cardiologist, and he finally responds, "It's your

dime. If you want to see one, go ahead." I want to trust him, but at the same time I don't feel that he is taking Michael's condition seriously enough. . . . I refuse to simply wait for him to die. (Spano, 1994, pp. 38–39)

Through their children's medical treatment or educational programs, most parents meet other parents of children with disabilities, with whom they exchange stories and thereby learn that their problems are shared. They also learn about the possibilities for activism and advocacy through the relationships they develop in support groups and disability organizations. When they interact with others, parents learn about techniques that have worked and come to realize that authority can be successfully challenged.

Pizzo (1983) noted that many parents become involved in self-help groups after seeing something in the media. In addition to general newspapers, magazines, and television programs, specialized publications are targeted specifically at parents of children with disabilities. The *Exceptional Parent* magazine, for example, prints success stories about and by parents who have actively challenged professional authority. Such stories may inspire other parents to pursue more or better services for their own children.

In addition to opportunities to learn from experience and the informal socialization offered by parent groups, more formalized training in assertiveness and advocacy is available to parents. A number of books and manuals has been published that familiarize parents with their legal rights and teach strategies for interacting with professionals and bringing about social change (e.g., Biklen, 1974; Dickman & Gordon, 1985). An online course (Minnesota Governor's Council on Development Disabilities, 2003) is also available.

As noted in Chapter 5, the goal of most parent advocacy and activism is to promote opportunities for "normalization" for their own or others' children. Although some activists continue to subscribe to a medical model and seek better services in order to improve their child's functioning, an increasing number of parents today espouse at least some tenets of the social model, which seeks social, rather than individual, change. This mother's explanation for her activism is illustrative:

What we're looking at doing is building a playground so that typical children will be challenged and children with disabilities will be able to play. What we're trying to get across to people is we don't want pity for our kids. . . . When the environment is the thing that creates the handicap, you have to change the environment. (personal communication, November 6, 2003)

Not all advocacy is successful. As Swain and Walker (2003) and others noted, parents' ability to get what they want for their children may be limited by the professionally controlled choices available to them. Funding for services is typically controlled by government agencies and the professionals who represent them. Although parent advocacy may impact decisions about service creation and allocation, limits may exist. For example, parents may learn of a physical therapist located far from their home who employs techniques not available locally, but the local funding agency may be unable to afford the costs involved in transporting the child such a long distance. Whether the child, in fact, "needs" the services of the distant therapist cannot be determined from existing statutes regarding entitlement, resulting in court challenges in some cases. The issue of service rationing in an environment of limited resources is currently being debated in the health care field.

Leiter (2004) identified other barriers to parents' use of their rights:

- *Professional socialization.* Professionals may not have been trained in partnership models.
- *Professional power.* Resources are controlled by professionals.
- *Parent–professional intimacy.* Some professionals come to be regarded "like family" and sources of support and friendship, making challenges to their authority difficult.
- *Limited awareness of rights.*
- *Parental/family constraints.* Parents' own disabilities, employment, or family responsibilities may limit their ability to advocate for their children.

Nonetheless, increasing parent awareness of rights and methods for acting on those rights is an important step toward the creation of a true parent–professional partnership. Parents and professionals must work together to meet the needs of children with disabilities. Moreover, as Judge (1997) has shown, family empowerment results in a greater sense of control, eliminating the anomie that plagues so many families of children with disabilities, especially during the early years.

New Roles for Professionals: Advocacy and a Social System Perspective

Developing Role-Taking Ability

In order to be truly effective, the professional must learn to take the role of the parent. The professional exists to help families achieve their goals. To serve that purpose, the professional must understand, as well as possible, the *family's* definition of what its members want and need and must adopt a social system perspective.

Professional awareness of the point of view of families has certainly been increasing in recent years, as evidenced by a growing body of literature in professional journals and books about the family experience. Professional training programs use videotapes, trained parents, adults with disabilities, and other methods for making professionals more aware of parent perceptions (e.g., Bailey et al., 1986; Darling & Peter, 1994; Guralnick, Bennett, Heiser, & Richardson, 1987; Wells, Byron, McMullen, & Birchall, 2002). Newer programs for medical students and residents (Cooley, 1994; DiVenere, 1994; Lewis & Greenstein, 1994) have involved them in the lives of families in various ways, and the field of early intervention has moved toward a family-centered approach in both legislation and practice (Darling, 1989; Darling & Darling, 1992). In addition, medical school curricula have begun to include communication skills training (e.g., Yedidia et al., 2003) to help students learn to build relationships with patients.

As noted earlier, the helping professions in general have been rapidly shifting during the past few decades from a clinical perspective to a partnership model, in which the client's perspective is highly valued by the professional. The recent proliferation of service models involving home visits and family centers attests to the growing acceptance of a system-based, partnership paradigm. The special expertise of professionals has always been recognized; the special expertise of clients (in understanding their own life situations) is now being recognized as well. Some professionals have not been comfortable with the shift from professional dominance to partnership; most, however, are discovering that the newer, community-based, family-centered models are working because they enable families to participate in their "treatment" in a meaningful way.

Partnership is important because neither the professional nor the parent alone has all the expertise necessary to assure that children receive what they need. Wesley, Buysse, and Tyndall (1997) have shown, for example, that professionals have knowledge about the existing service system that parents lack. On the other hand, the parents in their study were better able than the professionals to describe the "ideal" service system. Hamre-Nietupski et al. (1988) and others have noted that parental advocacy is more successful when parents work in partnership with professionals, because the status and expertise of professionals tend to lend credibility to the parents' requests. Professionals, of course, also have a wealth of knowledge based on their training and experience, whereas parents are clearly the experts regarding the "whole" child, the family's lifestyle and culture, and the child's needs in relation to their vision of their child's future.

Blue-Banning et al. (2004) discussed the dimensions of successful family–professional partnerships as including communication (positive, understandable, respectful); commitment (to the child and family); equality (a sense of equity in decision making); skills (team members' competence); trust (in the reliability and honesty of each partner); and respect (between partners). They found that the agreement between parents and professionals regarding what constitutes positive behavior was "fairly remarkable." One difference in emphasis was the parents' focus on commitment; the professionals expressed reservations about doing "too much" for families rather than empowering families to act in their own behalf. In Chapter 13 we illustrate the application of a partnership model in actual intervention situations.

In order to become more effective in taking the role of family members, professionals must explore their own attitudes, accept their own limitations, and try to share some of the experiences of the families they are trying to help. Some practical exercises for increasing role-taking ability are suggested below (adapted from Darling & Darling, 1982, pp. 184–189):

1. *Write a sociological autobiography.* Think about your own background and the experiences that have shaped your attitudes. Try to remember your earliest experiences with children or adults with disabilities. Do you recall any individuals with disabilities in your family, your neighborhood, your school, your church, or your Scout troop? What did you think of them? How did you feel in their presence? What did your parents, friends, and other significant people tell you about them?

How have your other group affiliations shaped your attitudes toward disabilities? Do your religious values affect your attitudes? Did your social-class background stress hard work, achievement, and "getting ahead" and deprecate those who were dependent on others for a livelihood? How has your gender-role socialization affected your attitudes? Did you learn that men are supposed to be physically and emotionally strong or that women are supposed to be physically attractive?

Think about the strangers with disabilities you have seen in public places or on television and those about whom you have read in books or magazines. Have you watched telethons on behalf of various disabilities? As a child, did you read *A Christmas Carol, The Prince and the Pauper,* or *Heidi?* Have you seen televised faith healings or read any of the publications of the Christian Science church?

Have you ever deliberately avoided interacting with a person with a disability? Have you walked away from an opportunity to help a person with blindness? Have you avoided a friendship with a neighbor who has a child with Down syndrome? Why do you think you acted the way you did in these situations?

Make a list of all of your group affiliations and experiences with disability and examine how each has affected your attitudes toward people with disabilities. Use your list to write an autobiography that traces your experiences and shows how they shaped your present attitudes.

2. *Design and conduct in-depth interviews with (a) one or more adolescents or adults with disabilities and (b) one or more parents of children with disabilities.* Get to know someone with a disability. Make a list of questions that will serve as the basis for an in-depth conversation so that your respondents tell you how they feel about their disability. Do they welcome questions about their disability? What kinds of questions are upsetting or offensive? What kinds of questions are helpful?

In interviewing parents, questions should include the following topics: (1) their expectations prior to their child's birth (e.g., did they want their unborn son to be a football player or a doctor?); (2) their experiences during labor and delivery (did they suspect that "something was wrong" with the baby?); (3) their reactions to the first information that their child had an impairment (how were they told? how did they feel?); (4) their attitudes toward professionals (which professionals have been helpful to them and why?); (5) their feelings about their children (what negative and positive effects have they had on their lives?); (6) their experiences with friends, relatives, and strangers (have grandparents been supportive?; how do people react to their children in restaurants, shopping malls?); (7) their perceptions of their child's effect on family relationships (has their marriage been strengthened or weakened?; how have siblings reacted?); and (8) their expectations and hopes for the future (what do they think/hope will happen to their children when they grow up?)

Students and others not currently involved professionally with people with disabilities can usually find respondents in parent groups affiliated with hospitals, clinics, preschool programs, or organizations such as the Arc or the United Cerebral Palsy Association. Adults with disabilities may be located through associations such as Centers for Independent Living; advocacy or activist groups such as Not Dead Yet; mainstream disability organizations such as the Easter Seal Society or the Spina Bifida Association of America; workshops, such as those operated by Goodwill Industries; or group homes and other community-based housing facilities for people with disabilities. Organized groups for students with disabilities can be found on some college campuses. Participation in such interviews must always be voluntary.

These interviews are not intended to provide a complete picture of the lives of individuals with disabilities, and you must be careful not to generalize from your respondents to others with similar impairments. Individuals with disabilities are just as different from one another as individuals without disabilities. This exercise is only intended to make you more aware of how *one person* or *a few people* feel about their situation.

3. *Observe a special situation.* You may want to spend some time observing any or all of the following: Meetings of an association of parents of children with disabilities or of an adult activist group; a preschool center for children with disabilities; a special education class in the public schools (or a classroom that includes students with disabilities); a vocational training program for adults with intellectual disability; a support group for adolescents or adults with disabilities; a group home for adults with physical or intellectual disabilities; a day program for adults with intellectual disabilities.

4. *Read some personal accounts written by parents of children with disabilities.* The following is a small sample of such books. Many others are available as well:

Berube, M. (1998). *Life as we know it: A father, a family, and an exceptional child.* New York: Vintage Books.
Park, C. C. (2001). *Exiting nirvana: A daughter's life with autism.* Boston: Little, Brown.
Pieper, E. (1977). *Sticks and stones.* Syracuse, NY: Human Policy Press.

5. *Read some literature written from the parents' perspective.* Magazines and newsletters written for parents provide insight into the parents' point of view. See, for example, *The Exceptional Parent*, a magazine written especially for the parents of children with special needs. Newsletters such as those of the National Down Syndrome Society, the Spina Bifida Association of America, and United Cerebral Palsy Associations are also valuable.

6. *Participate in awareness-promoting activities.* Accompany a child with an obvious disability to a shopping mall, restaurant, or other public place. Watch the reactions of waitresses, store clerks, and other customers.

7. *Evaluate your goals.* Why have you decided to enter the helping professions? Why have you chosen a field that brings you into contact with families that have children with disabilities? Make a list of your professional goals. Evaluate each of your goals in terms of its potentially beneficial or negative effect on the families you serve.

Professionals as Advocates

Traditionally, helping professionals worked to change their *clients*, to cure them, to improve their functional abilities, to make them more comfortable, to aid them in adjusting to their situation. In recent years, we have learned that changing the "client" is not always enough. Sometimes, the family's *social situation* needs to be changed. Because society is designed primarily to meet the needs of those without disabilities, structural barriers exist that prevent those with disabilities from achieving full integration. These barriers include the following:

- Physical barriers, such as curbs, stairs, and narrow doorways
- Cultural barriers, such as stigma and "ableism"
- Social barriers, such as lack of needed services or accommodations

These barriers cannot be eliminated without social change to produce access, public awareness, and resources to meet the needs of families whose children have disabilities.

Advocacy involves working to bring about social change. Is advocacy an appropriate part of the professional role? This question was addressed by a number of writings in the 1970s and 1980s. Adams (1973) argued that professional advocacy poses ethical dilemmas.

The professional must decide whether to support the rights of the individual or the rights of society when the two are in conflict. Kurtz (1977) noted that advocacy may produce role conflict, involving the professional's agency of employment, as well as parents, children, and others who may be deprived of services; and Frith (1981) stated that "it is becoming increasingly difficult for professionals in the field [of special education] to assume the role of child advocate, while simultaneously attempting to support their employing agency" (p. 487).

Two professional organizations, the Council for Exceptional Children and the Ad Hoc Committee on Advocacy of the National Association of Social Workers, have taken the position that, in the case of advocacy dilemmas, the professional *should act as an advocate for the client.* The Council for Exceptional Children (1981) issued the following statement:

> The Council for Exceptional Children firmly believes that the role of the professional as an employee should not conflict with the professional's advocate role. Rather, these roles should complement each other. . . . Failing to assume responsibility [as an advocate], the professional can only play the role of participant in whatever injustice may befall the child. (pp. 492–493)

Today, many human service workers assume that advocacy is part of their job.

When they become advocates for vulnerable families, professionals become partners with families in working toward social change. Professionals should certainly not usurp advocacy roles that families can play themselves; however, even the most "empowered" families sometimes need help in negotiating a system that was not created with their needs in mind. Unlike the professional dominance that characterized parent–professional interaction in the past, today's parent–professional partnerships are marked by equality and mutual respect. Although we must continue to help families adjust to situations that cannot be changed, we cannot continue to blame families for their problems when society *can* be changed. Social action rather than passive adjustment may be the hallmark of parent–professional interaction in the future. Together, professionals and families can work to eliminate the physical, cultural, and social barriers that prevent families from attaining the best possible quality of life.

The next two chapters suggest some concrete ways that professionals can help families. Chapter 12 employs a micro-level perspective (changing the family system) and reviews counseling techniques that respect the family's perspective and empower families to optimize their life situations. Chapter 13 uses a sociological perspective (changing the social system) and illustrates the application of family-centered principles in the development and implementation of service plans. Both chapters reflect the systems approach that has been advocated throughout this book.

■12■

Perspectives and Approaches for Working with Families

Various approaches to working with families of children with disabilities in order to improve the functioning of the family system are explored in this chapter. The perspectives and approaches that are discussed are primarily designed to promote healthy family relationships; however, some of the approaches used to achieve this goal are not necessarily family interventions per se. Individual, marital, or support group counseling approaches can be used with the intention of helping the family system. The systems approach advocated in this book is central to both theoretical and treatment aspects of families, in that when disability or chronic illness occurs, it affects all family members. Therefore, when working with family members, it is essential, we believe, to maintain a family systems mindset irrespective of the approach employed.

Some professionals in the helping professions embrace a pathology orientation and assume that the birth of a child with special needs would necessarily result in pathology in a family's functioning. When families neither need nor desire intervention, some approaches may be more intrusive than helpful. Some families *do*, however, need psychotherapy or counseling for individuals as well as couples and family counseling. Overly anxious or depressed parents or those with significant family conflict can benefit from psychotherapeutic treatment.

This chapter presents an overview of existing interventions along with references for further reading. Some of the strategies require extensive knowledge and training. Some therapeutic approaches are beyond the scope of some professionals. In such instances, referrals to other professionals should be considered. We begin our discussion by examining the characteristics of effective helpers.

EFFECTIVE HELPERS
AND THE HELPER–FAMILY RELATIONSHIP

Effective helpers have certain qualities, skills, and values, and persons who lack these should not work with families of children with disabilities. We believe that Ross's assertion is as germane now as it was in 1964:

> A student may be able to develop these [characteristics] in the course of closely supervised experience but some people lack these qualities in sufficient measure and these should probably not enter a profession whose central task is helping other people. No amount of exhortation can make a rejecting person accepting, a frigid person warm, or a narrow-minded person understanding. Those charged with the selection, education and training of new members of the helping professions will need to keep in mind that the presence or absence of certain personality characteristics make the difference between a truly helpful professional and one who leaves a trace of misery and confusion in the wake of his activities. (pp. 75–76)

The following are essential skills of professionals who work with families:

1. *Positive regard*: Helpers should communicate acceptance of family members as worthwhile persons, regardless of who they are or what they say or do.
2. *Empathy*: Professionals must be able to communicate that they feel and understand the family's concerns from their point of view.
3. *Concreteness*: Professionals should respond accurately, clearly, specifically, and immediately to family members.
4. *Warmth*: Professionals should show their concern through verbal and nonverbal expression. We can sense when someone is warm and accepting—or cold and distant.

Gladding (2000) added the following attributes:

- A natural interest in people
- An ability to find listening stimulating
- Comfort in dealing with a wide range of emotions
- An ability to sustain emotional closeness
- A sense of humor

Turnbull and colleagues (2006) added the following recommendations for professionals:

- Be friendly.
- Listen carefully.
- Be clear.
- Honor cultural diversity.
- Affirm strengths.
- Treat families with dignity.

Another essential characteristic for the professional helper is self-awareness (Sommers-Flanagan & Sommers-Flanagan, 1993). An awareness of one's attitudes toward persons with disabilities, persons from other cultures, as well as toward families of children with disabilities is essential (Marshak & Seligman, 1993; Turnbull et al., 2006). Negative attitudes become manifest in behaviors that communicate coldness, distance, abruptness, and rejection. Such behaviors, in turn, can contribute to feelings of guilt, depression, and shame in family members. Therefore, professionals need to examine their attitudes carefully so that they do not interfere with efforts to be helpful to families.

Research regarding the quality of relationships families experience with professionals is discouraging (Darling, 1991; Darling & Peter, 1994). Indeed, Naseef (2001b) referred to the parent–professional relationship as "a perilous partnership." As noted in the last chapter, parents of children with disabilities are often dissatisfied by their experiences with professionals. Years ago, Telford and Sawrey (1977) quoted a mother who characterized her contacts with professionals as "a masterful combination of dishonesty, condescension, misinformation and bad manners" (p. 143). Parents are sometimes considered a nuisance rather than a resource and are frequently criticized, analyzed, or made to feel responsible for their child's problems. Furthermore, it is not unusual to hear of parents described as lazy, stupid, demanding, greedy, conniving, or angry and defensive (Rubin & Quinn-Curran, 1983).

The parents of 84 school-age children with cerebral palsy were interviewed in regard to their experiences in dealing with health professionals (McKay & Hensey, 1990). Seventy percent of these parents were dissatisfied with some aspect of their contacts during the initial period of diagnosis. A large percentage (58%) of dissatisfaction was related to a lack of explanation by physicians, by having their concerns dismissed, and by having to make repeated visits before the child's condition was recognized. Other concerns had to do with how the parents were informed about their child's disability and a lack of understanding of the practical difficulties the parents faced. These issues are discussed further in Chapter 4.

Holden and Lewine (as cited in Bernheim & Lehman, 1985) found in their research that there are high levels of dissatisfaction with mental health services. Families reported that professionals increased their feelings of guilt, confusion, and frustration. Seventy four percent were dissatisfied with the services received, for reasons including lack of information about diagnosis and treatment, vague and evasive responses, professional avoidance of labeling the illness (which increased families' confusion), lack of support during critical periods, lack of help in locating community resources, and little or no advice about how to cope with their child's symptoms or problem behaviors.

It is generally believed that parent–professional relationships have improved in recent years (Darling & Peter, 1994; Marsh, 1992; Chapter 11, this volume). However, the professional community is currently experiencing massive changes in systems of service delivery that are affecting the quality of existing services. These changes, rooted in mandates to reduce medical and other service charges, are resulting in confusion, added burden, and frustration for professionals. One might expect that as stress increases, relationships between professionals and their patients will be less satisfactory.

The very proliferation of specialists sometimes complicates rather than clarifies issues. Support and assistance should be free from petty professional jealousies that may cause one group to attempt to keep another from giving help. Another source of difficulty is to be found in the anxieties the child's disability may arouse in the professional. Parents may have visited numerous professionals but remain poorly informed about the nature and implications of their child's disability. This problem is not due to their resistance to facts but rather the failure of the professionals to inform the family adequately. A parent's lack of knowledge about a child's disability may sometimes be attributed to the professional's anxiety and withdrawal from the family. Yet information, communicated in a human and honest manner can eliminate misunderstanding and reduce anxieties (Frankland, 2001).

Another reason for the family's confusion or lack of information may be the professional's use of jargon, which can render communication difficult. Professionals need to be concrete (yet not condescending) and be sensitive to nonverbal cues that suggest that they are not being understood. In regard to medical professionals, it has been jokingly suggested that medical terms were invented to keep patients from understanding what medical providers do (McDaniel, 1995). When a professional believes a message is misunderstood, he or she can say, "I'm not sure if I made myself understood. If it didn't make sense to you, I'd be happy to try again." The use of professional jargon does not generate respect; it causes distance and implies aloofness and insensitivity, and as Chapter 4 suggested, can increase feelings of anomie.

The timing of professional interventions is a key barometer of the success of relationships between professionals and families. Professionals need to be sensitive to a family's receptiveness to a particular approach or communication. For example, parents may not be ready to explore their feelings about their child and what the disability means to them when they are confronted with the practical implications of the child's diagnosis and need to know what services are available to help with immediate problems. On the other hand, when parents need to sort out their feelings, professionals, threatened by affective disclosures, should not hide behind a laundry list of agencies and services and avoid discussing emotional responses. The timing of an intervention determines whether family members truly hear what is being said; it also affects their level of trust in the professional and their perception of his or her expertise.

Although we acknowledge that family members can contribute to tension between themselves and professionals, we would argue that professionals must shoulder most of the responsibility. To be respectful listeners we believe that professionals should (1) gain a thorough understanding of family systems theory, especially the dynamics within families of children with disabilities; (2) have effective interpersonal skills; and (3) acquire extensive experience in working with families of children with disabilities or chronic illness.

BARRIERS TO EFFECTIVE HELPING

In any type of helping endeavor it is imperative that professionals interpret parents' circumstances from *their* point of view. This means that the professional must listen to them carefully. Empathic listeners have an ability to put their own biases and opinions aside as they try to understand what is being said and felt. As Turnbull and colleagues (2006) stated, "When you truly seek to understand the other person before stating your own perspectives, you will find yourself in a listening mode, you will hear the family's 'language' and you will incorporate it into your communication with them" (p. 142). Family members intuitively know when they are in the presence of an empathic helper because they feel understood and valued.

Although it is a poor excuse for negative behavior, professionals in medical, educational, and social service occupations are often burdened by the nature of their work and the demands placed on them, (Naseef, 2001b). Professionals in stressful occupations are often fatigued psychologically and physically and are thus hard-pressed to interact comfortably and productively with family members. If we wish to help promote healthier family–professional relationships, we must create less stressful job environments for professionals, who typically begin their careers with energy, high goals, and positive expectations and attitudes.

Preoccupation with personal concerns is another barrier to listening (Friend & Cook, 2002). Novice professionals often "think ahead," thereby making it difficult to empathize with the client. Preoccupation with personal problems also tends to distract from careful listening. Because the lives of professionals may sometimes be challenging, like those of the people they serve, it is not surprising that occasional personal concerns can interfere with one's effectiveness. Whereas occasional preoccupation is not a serious problem, chronic distractions can result in communication impasses. Strong feelings about the family member(s) with whom one is working can be a major barrier to effective listening and rapport building. Angry or anxious feelings toward someone we are trying to help generally limit our ability to be helpful. In regard to physicians, Darling (1979) provided compelling evidence that some medical practitioners view families with at least some degree of personal discomfort. In this regard, Naseef (2001b) observed:

> From my own experience as well as the testimonies of countless other parents, professionals lacking in feeling and hope, who seem to be just

doing their jobs, provoke sharp resentment. It is rare to meet a parent who doesn't have a horror story or two about a doctor or the educational system. On the other hand, professionals who are compassionate and hopeful and who take a special interest in the family are remembered kindly and effusively praised. (p. 173)

Being distracted by phone calls or interruptions from secretaries and other colleagues makes it more difficult to be attentive and empathic (Friend & Cook, 2002). Such behavior conveys a lack of concern and respect as well as inattentiveness to family members. Families should be given a predetermined period of time all to themselves. Phone calls, a colleague "just wanting a word," or interruptions of any kind (unless they are emergencies) are considered discourteous. We might reflect on how we feel when our conversation with someone is marked by a series of cell phone conversations.

THE FAMILY'S NEED FOR COUNSELING

We have indicated the challenges with which families must contend in the face of disability, although we acknowledge that many families adapt remarkably well. We have discussed how a major event to one family member reverberates throughout the family unit, leading us to emphasize the wisdom of a systems perspective. The family must come to terms with its destiny—that of frustrated expectations and, possibly, thwarted life goals. Depending on the nature and severity of the child's disability, his or her capacity to achieve independence may be limited and therefore not allow family members to live out a family life cycle comparable to other families.

Ambivalent emotions, such as love and hate, joy and sorrow, elation and depression, are common among family members. There is also guilt, anger and frustration in dealing with a complex and difficult service delivery system (Upshur, 1991; Marshak & Prezant, 1999). There are concerns about the future—about a child's educational opportunities and vocational alternatives as well as prospects for independence. In addition, families will need to confront the stigmatizing attitudes of others in professional, educational, social, and public contexts.

As noted in Chapter 5, for some parents, financial burdens may be the major problem. Medication, special equipment, physical therapy, speech therapy, physician visits, and perhaps counseling sessions all reflect potential sources of financial drain. Severe financial problems due to low paying jobs or poverty can, in themselves, create great strain within the family system.

Fatigue can lead to burnout and derives from the many tasks parents must assume, such as feeding, toileting, and managing disruptive behavior. Fatigued and burned-out family members need support from professionals to help explore the demand characteristics of the child and family dynamics that may have contributed to this state of affairs. Teachers and other professionals can also help families obtain needed services, such as respite care, to help relieve stress and to allow time away from the challenges at home (Turnbull et al., 2006).

Family members may become clinically depressed, or just occasionally dispirited. Certified professionals can help family members accept the fact that their distress is a reasonable response to a difficult situation. Depressed family members, however, can benefit from psychotherapy and perhaps even medication in some cases. It is important to distinguish between clinical depression and temporary and mild "blues" and make appropriate referrals when it seems that a serious form of depression is present.

Guilt, anger, and other problems such as marital discord can be addressed by a professional psychotherapist. Furthermore, professionals should be alert to problems that may develop in more peripherally involved family members, such as siblings or grandparents.

INDIVIDUAL INTERVENTIONS

Parents are on the front lines in locating educational, medical, and psychosocial services to help them address the challenges that occur as a result of childhood disability. In trying to negotiate the maze of service delivery systems, parents may behave in a way that can result in negative outcomes. In this regard, Naseef (2001b) argued that learning how to channel anger into effective assertive behavior is essential to the family's welfare. Naseef described the range of responses from passive, assertive, to aggressive problem-solving styles.

Passive problem solving allows others to set the agenda, leaving family members to follow without questions or challenges. The family allows others to do what they want, and not what they believe is best. People who engage in passive styles avoid conflict and allow others to dominate, which usually results in disappointment. Taking a one-day-at-a-time approach is considered a passive appraisal approach as reflected in the following statement:

> I try not to worry about where Eric will get a job after he graduates from high school. I try not to think about what his adult life will be. It works best for me to just take a day at a time. There is no use getting all upset over something that is years away. (Poston & Turnbull, 2004, p. 97)

Aggressive parents stand up to others and do not take others' opinions or feelings into account. They believe that their position is superior and attack and try to intimidate others. Their ultimate goal is to get their way. An unwanted by-product of this aggressive style is that the other party becomes more defensive, angry, and less sympathetic to the aggressor.

Assertive parents act in ways that reinforce their child's rights. They express strong opinions and emotions without intimidating others. Their position is carefully articulated, they do not attack, and they remain open to others' opinions. Services, rights, and wishes are discussed without extreme anger and with openness to input. In the end parents need to state where they stand without being aggressive or passive. However, as noted in Chapter 3, interactional styles vary by culture and social class. In some groups, passivity, especially in interactions with professionals, is the norm. Professionals need to respect these diverse styles.

Opirhory and Peters Model

Although it was developed some years ago, Opirhory and Peters (1982) described a useful and still relevant guide to interventions with parents of newborns with disabilities. As noted earlier, stage theory holds that parents generally follow a fairly predictable series of emotions and actions after a child's diagnosis has been communicated. These authors contended that the sequence of phases is useful in providing general benchmarks for considering appropriate interventions. (As noted in earlier chapters, stage theory is not universally accepted.)

During the *denial* stage, professionals should gently provide an honest evaluation of the situation the parents are confronting. They should simply describe the child objectively and indicate the care that is needed. They should not remove the parents' hopes or interfere with their coping style unless it is inappropriate or dysfunctional for the family.

During the *anger* stage, professionals must provide an open and permissive atmosphere in which that parents can vent their anger and pain. They must be accepting of the parents' criticism, even if it is directed toward them, without personalizing their observations or defending other professionals or themselves. It is important to keep in mind that anger reflects the parents' anxiety in the face of a situation that will significantly change their lives. They should be mindful, too, that some parents have been treated so badly by professionals that their anger and frustration derive from thoroughly objective circumstances.

During the *bargaining* phase, parents feel that they can reverse their child's condition by engaging in certain redemptive activities. At this point professionals should point out the child's positive characteristics, encourage involvement, and remain optimistic without giving any guarantees about the child's prognosis or potential progress. While parents continue to establish a warm and loving relationship with their child, they nonetheless should be encouraged to balance their lives with personally fulfilling goals and activities.

Mild or severe mood swings characterize the *depression* stage. Again, the professional needs to be able to distinguish between clinical depression and milder forms of dysphoria. Mild, situational, and time-limited depression is common and is likely to emerge at various points in the child's development. Parents need to be reassured that what they are experiencing is normal. They should not be criticized or made to feel that they have a major psychological problem when they experience occasional mood changes.

The professional should continue to reinforce the positive aspects of the parent–child relationship during the *acceptance* stage. Parents become more realistic, less emotional, and more oriented to solving problems during this stage. The need for professional help and support is unlikely to be crucial, although problems can emerge when the child reaches certain developmental milestones.

Laborde and Seligman Model

The model Laborde and Seligman (1991) proposed is comprised of three somewhat distinct counseling interventions: educative, personal advocacy, and facilitative counseling. *Educative counseling* is appropriate when families need information about their child's disability. This approach is based on the premise that families know little about disability until they are confronted by it in their own child. As Chapter 4 shows, parents' need for information tends to be stronger than their need for support early in the infancy period, although both are important. At the point of diagnosis educative counseling can be used to inform parents, to lessen their sense of confusion and ambiguity, and to decrease the stress that is partially a result of not knowing essential information and how to access help.

One of the greatest unmet needs of families of children with special needs is access to information. This is especially problematic for parents from culturally and linguistically diverse cultures (Zoints, Zoints, Harrison, & Bellinger, 2003; Shapiro, Monzo, Rueda, Gomez, & Blacher, 2004). Families want user-friendly, relevant, easily accessible, research-based information (Ruef & Turnbull, 2001).

In addition to being informed about their child's disability, its etiology and prognosis, family members need to know about available services, reading materials germane to their situation, and specialized equipment for their child. Family members should know about their legal rights to service or education as well as about parent organizations, self-help groups, and local professionals who can help with problems of a more psychological nature.

Educative counseling is not just for family members of newborns. Information and guidance communicated in a concrete way are needed at all stages of the child's development as the disabling condition stabilizes, worsens, or improves. Professionals such as social workers, rehabilitation counselors, and psychologists are often in a position to help family members gain access to community resources after the initial hospital stay.

Psychotherapy is not a substitute for practical help when such help is needed. Elsewhere in this volume we cited Australian research reporting that the parents studied were "almost desperate" in their plea for help until a training center for children with intellectual disability was established in their community. As a consequence of this resource, parents reported being much happier and more relaxed, and their "neurotic symptoms" virtually disappeared.

Personal advocacy counseling is another element in Laborde and Seligman's (1991) model. We have already established that families need guidance in finding relevant information and in locating appropriate services. We also believe that parents should normally be their own case managers or service coordinators. Parents are, after all, the logical choice to serve as chief coordinators and evaluators of service, with the *assistance* of a competent professional.

Advocacy means "speaking out and taking action in pursuit of a cause. Advocacy is problem oriented; it identifies the nature of a problem, the barriers to solving it, the resources available for solving it, and the action to be taken" (Turnbull et al., 2006, p. 153). Advocacy issues often arise in educational settings. A national survey of over 500 parents of children in special education revealed the following:

- Forty-five percent of the parents surveyed believe that their child's special education program needs improvement or is failing their children.
- Thirty-five percent said the program is doing a poor job when it comes to being a useful source of information about disability-related issues.
- Thirty-five percent said it was frustrating to get the special education services for their children.
- Thirty-three percent rated their child's school as doing a fair to poor job in giving their child the help they need (Johnson, Duffett, Farkas, & Wilson, 2002, cited in Turnbull et al., 2006).

The professional acts as a broker of services by assisting the parents in formulating a clear idea of which needs they wish to have met and in deciding where to receive services. With information on hand, the professional can help the family members develop a plan of action for obtaining needed assistance.

Advocacy counseling is designed to help parents experience a sense of control over events in their own lives and their children's lives. Family members are encouraged to ask questions of their service providers, to question a provider's responses to inquiries, to seek out second opinions, and to request services they need and are entitled to receive. In short, parents are given the support and "permission" to obtain the professional help they need without guilt or feeling that they do not have the right to ask questions. Family members are encouraged to seek out professionals who are knowledgeable and candid yet compassionate, and to feel confident enough to dismiss professionals who do not meet these requirements.

The third and final component of Laborde and Seligman's model is *facilitative counseling*, wherein a professional helps a family member accept or change distressing thoughts, feelings, or behaviors in the context of a trusting relationship.

As noted previously, parents experience a plethora of contradictory emotions when they first learn their child has a disability. It can be helpful to the parents to acknowledge that their dreams and plans for their child may be severely shaken. The professional needs to accept these distressing feelings and not encourage family members to deny or repress them. Family members require time to overcome their grief, and the most helpful professional behavior is to be accepting and available yet not intrusive.

When the parents are prepared to move on, they can be helped to see that they can still, to a large degree, live normal, productive, and comfortable lives. Professionals should encourage the necessary parent–child bonding while also encouraging family members to pursue their own interests and aspirations.

Parents sometimes blame themselves for their child's disability, but they are rarely the cause (fetal alcohol syndrome and disabilities resulting from physical abuse of the mother during pregnancy are two exceptions). Professional need to help parents understand that their child's condition is not their doing.

Unable to shed their guilt feelings, some parents begin an endless and unproductive search for the cause of their child's disorder or for a "cure." Parents may base their feelings on perceived "misdeeds," or they may focus on behaviors or even "bad" thoughts that occurred during pregnancy. Professionals need to listen and not pass off such ruminations as silly or unimportant.

Parents may also wish to "make up" for supposed past indiscretions by overprotecting their child or holding the child back from activities that can facilitate his or her growth and independence. Professionals can help parents explore their guilt, understand its negative effect on the family, and curb their overprotective behavior. At the very least, the professional needs to understand that as an overprotective bond develops between a parent and child, the other parent and other children are generally adversely affected. The boundaries of the parent–child relationship may become so impermeable that other family members feel abandoned and look to other sources for affiliation and gratification.

Professionals can help parents separate their confused feelings of anger about becoming the parent of a child with a disability from their generally positive feelings toward their child. It is helpful that parents find appropriate outlets for expressing anger and feelings of rejection so that they are not inappropriately directed toward their child with a disability, the other children, or each other.

Family members who deeply love their child may find aspects of the child's condition or behavior difficult to accept. Also, feelings of rejection, like other emotions, are cyclical—they come and go. It is important for professionals to help family members realize that feelings of anger and occasional or limited rejection are normal and that their expression is acceptable.

Professionals can also help parents cope with their feelings of shame, which involve the expectation of ridicule or criticism from others. It is not uncommon for families to confront community and public attitudes and behaviors that are negative. A useful contribution from professionals is to help family members locate self-help groups, which can reduce feelings of isolation and demonstrate how others cope with negative public attitudes. It is particularly important that families of children with disabilities reduce their contact with professionals who hold negative attitudes. Furthermore, professionals can help family members consider strategies that facilitate involvement in activities from which they may have withdrawn, such as family outings, sporting events, movies, and associating with friends (Marshak & Seligman, 1993).

The denial of a child's disability is a defense mechanism that operates on an unconscious level to ward off excessive anxiety. The mere idea of being the parent of a child with a disability is so anxiety provoking that they deny the reality of their child's disability. Parents fight unconsciously to keep their pain hidden from their own awareness. Intransigent denial is one of the more difficult coping mechanisms for the professional to address. A reasonable approach would be to accept the parents' view of their child while gently, when appropriate, pointing out where the child may need special help. A general rule is to never force parents to cast aside a defense mechanism that is rigidly held. The abrupt unveiling of what is being kept from conscious awareness can have a negative effect and only deepen the denial. Also, it is not unusual for parents to seek out appropriate interventions for their child while simultaneously denying the disability. Some parents are able to provide for and love their child while holding on to the unrealistic hope that the child will make dramatic improvements. For most parents, the reality of their child's situation becomes clearer over time. It is advisable to be cautious about assuming that parents who do not accept a professional's diagnosis are in denial. Some diagnoses are, in fact, not correct or appropriate.

Guilt and rejection and can lead to shopping for a more encouraging diagnosis. Denial can be caused by the threat the disability presents to the family, but alternatively it can reflect a realistic appraisal of the situation due to the nature of the disability and/or the quality of professional care available.

Facilitative counseling must also attend to concerns that surface— or resurface—as the child approaches various milestones, such as beginning or completing school. Professionals should not be alarmed if parents need to cover "old territory" at different times of their child's development. As noted in earlier chapters, key periods that may trigger the family's anxiety include the following:

1. When parents first learn about or suspect that their child has a disability.
2. At about age 5 or 6, when a decision must be reached regarding the child's education.
3. When the time has arrived for the child to leave school.
4. When the parents become older and possibly unable to care for the child.

As the child grows into adolescence and young adulthood, parents may have a difficult time giving up their child, either to a residential treatment setting or to independent living (Marshak et al., 1999). For a number of reasons parents may be so invested in their child that they find it exceedingly difficult to let go. Allowing a child to be more independent is especially difficult for overprotective or enmeshed parents who view their son's or daughter's growing independence with apprehension. As the child differentiates from his or her parents and begins to live a more independent life, the professionals can remind parents that independence is in the best interest of the child and that contact between them and their child will not cease. Furthermore, some attempt should be made to help parents who are uneasy about this stage of the family's life cycle, understand why their child's emerging independence is so anxiety provoking.

In working with families, Turnbull et al. (2006) asserted that professionals must respect families by honoring cultural diversity affirming strengths, and treating families with dignity. It is essential that in developing relationships and partnerships with families, multicultural factors and personal preferences to be taken into account (Kalyanpur & Harry, 1999). Parents value professionals who mention their child's strengths and do not dwell on weakness, as evidenced by this parent's statement: "I often think [school staff should] do one-on-one [meetings] instead of with five people, telling me Susie can't do this, and Susie can't do that, and Susie can't this, and Susie can't that. And I am thinking, what about 'Susie *can* do this and Susie *can* do that'?" (Lake & Billingsley, 2000, p. 245).

Although children with disabilities differ from their nondisabled peers, they are alike in other ways—a point to keep in mind when working with family members. By focusing on similarities rather than on differences, parents can view their child in a more normal fashion. For example, parents of an adolescent who is physically disabled can note how typical it is for their child to enjoy rock music, show an interest in the opposite sex, display occasional moodiness, and be more secretive. Also, some children with disabilities show unique characteristics or abilities that can be highlighted.

By concentrating on normal aspects of childhood disability, the professional must be careful not to inadvertently reinforce denial. A denying family will not be aided by a professional who *unrealistically* concentrates on a child's normative qualities.

An appreciation for the existence of ambivalence is important for professionals who work with families. It may be difficult to understand that positive and negative emotions exist at the same time. For example, families may want help but be unable to ask for it; they may request advice but not follow through on it when it is given; they may agree to certain plans but fail to carry them out; and then there are those who tell us one thing but manifest the opposite by their behavior.

Ambivalent behavior can be puzzling and even annoying for some professionals, even though it is a family common phenomenon. An appreciation of this behavior along with a greater tolerance of it can be developed by understanding the unconscious motivation that lies behind behavior. What family members verbalize may be what they believe on a conscious level, but what they *do* is often motivated by unconscious needs that become manifest in the ambivalent behavior they display. It is the professional's task, then, to help family members understand their contradictory behavior—which, incidentally, may be as enigmatic to them as it is to the professional.

BEHAVIORAL PARENT TRAINING

For some families, the presenting behavioral problems of their children are so severe and disruptive that parent training is a particularly useful intervention. Behavioral parent training (BPT) has been used extensively (Baker, 1989; Harris & Glasberg, 2003; Kaiser & Fox, 1986; Siegel, 2003) and has been the subject of numerous studies (Marsh, 1992; Carr et al., 1999; Peck-Peterson, Derby, Berg, & Horner, 2002). BPT has specific applications and tends to be used and recommended by professionals with a strong behavioral bent. Parents have been trained successfully to modify diverse behavioral problems and to teach such adaptive abilities as chewing and feeding skills, motor imitation, self-help skills, appropriate play behaviors and social interaction with parents, articulation and vocabulary skills, and compliance behavior (Kaiser & Fox, 1986).

A drawback with the BPT model is that some families fail to acquire or maintain newly learned skills. Reasons for parental noncompliance include parents' lack of time to do the training, lack of spousal support, limited materials for teaching, not being convinced of its efficacy, and lack of confidence. The presence of disruptive life events, such as death, divorce, illness, or substance abuse in the family and other reasons BPT is unsuccessful. Marsh (1992) believes that parent training can be a narrow approach to facilitating family adaptation in that it fails to embrace the whole family and the intricate dynamics that characterize family functioning. Also, for some families and in some cultures, the "parent as teacher" role is not an appropriate model. Many parents who experience other major stressors are so preoccupied by survival activities that they do not have time to be their children's teachers or therapists.

The move to have parents assume a teaching role was initiated and promoted during the 1960s, 1970s, and 1980s. To be successful in this role parents had to learn many skills, which took away from other necessary functions. According to Turnbull et al. (2006), some parents found teaching their children to be satisfying but for others, it produced guilt and stress. Therefore, this role should be reserved for the most motivated parents, who find teaching gratifying and for whom it would not interfere with other parental roles and functions.

Professionals should also consider the situation of parents who must follow the prescriptions of the special education teacher, the speech therapist, the hearing specialist, the vision specialist, the physical therapist, and the doctor. Such assignments or "homework," if not monitored by a professional, can overwhelm a family and create additional stress.

COGNITIVE APPROACHES

Cognitive approaches to helping individuals achieve realistic perceptions of their circumstances have a fairly long and distinguished history (Gladding, 2000; Simos, 2002; Mennuti, Freeman, & Christner, 2005). It has been easier to conduct research on this method than on other therapeutic approaches, such as psychoanalysis, because cognitive therapy, like behavioral approaches, deals with measurable outcomes rather than unconscious processes. Cognitive therapy, which is designed to calm emotions by uncovering and disputing destructive perceptions and self-talk, can be applied readily to families of children with disabilities (Turnbull et al., 1993). "Often the thoughts that clients report are so extreme that it is hard to believe that intelligent, capable, well-educated individuals could believe such things without there being some 'deep' reason behind it" (Freeman, Pretzer, Fleming, & Simon, 2004, p. 4).

For example, parents may believe that having a child with a disability means that they will no longer be able to experience joy in their lives. A sibling may conclude that no one will like her or choose her as a mate because of her brother with Down syndrome. Such beliefs are subject to change under the guidance of a capable cognitive therapist.

GROUP FORMATS

We believe that groups for family members represent an important option for help, as noted previously, and we want to include an expanded discussion on this topic in this chapter. Group approaches are indeed being used with increased frequency with family members of children who have disabilities.

Until World War II, when the necessity to treat war casualties overwhelmed available resources, group interventions were considered a lesser form of therapeutic help. Group formats were considered more efficient, in that they could serve more people, but less effective in outcome than existing individual therapies. This early view of groups has changed dramatically (Yalom & Leszcz, 2005; Gladding, 2000; Berg, Landreth, & Fall, 2006). Although therapeutic groups are now considered an efficient modality, the central rationale for their use is that, for many persons experiencing a variety of problems, including those with disabilities and their family members, they are more effective.

The decision to recommend group or individual counseling needs to be carefully considered by the professional. The suggestion that parents consider some type of group should be based on the following considerations:

- Parents feel relatively comfortable in a group context.
- They are basically mature and emotionally stable, but their functioning is temporarily impaired.
- They are not overly self-absorbed and monopolistic.
- They have pronounced yet well-controlled feelings of hostility.

- They are not overly controlling, masochistic, or passive–aggressive, and do not have psychotic tendencies.
- They have a modicum of empathy for others, and they are open to others' opinions and guidance.

Group formats vary greatly in that they may be open or closed in membership, gender, or disability; homogeneous or heterogeneous; small or large; professional or member led. Group purposes may differ in that they may be educational or therapeutic (although some would argue that educational groups are also therapeutic), designed to help parents cope immediately after diagnosis or to consider living and working arrangements and problems of their postschool children, or designed to help siblings and extended family members cope.

The major distinction in terms of purpose is between providing education and information or therapy (Seligman & Marshak, 2003; Seligman, 1993; Gladding, 2000). *Educative* groups focus on providing families with information about their child's disability as well as training in effective coping and parenting skills. Educationally oriented groups also serve to inform families about their legal rights and benefits, where to obtain needed services, where to access special equipment, and the like. In these groups, parents learn from one another, from the leader, and from guest speakers. It is assumed that family problems arise from deficiencies in skills or information and that families function adaptively to meet their own needs when provided with accurate and relevant information.

Some groups are homogeneous and are composed of parents with children who have a particular impairment. As long as the child's condition falls within a recognized diagnostic category—for example, autism—parents are free to join. However, some groups may be composed of parents with children from a subcategory of a major disorder, for example, Down syndrome (a form of intellectual disability). Lundgren and Morrison (2003) cautioned professionals to inform parents of what is to take place and how the meetings are conducted. Informed parents are more likely to attend and to be less anxious about the initial meeting. This is especially important for parents from nonmainstream or minority cultures.

Between six and eight weekly 2-hour evening sessions is ideal (Hornby, 1994a, 2000). Fewer than six sessions does not allow enough time to cover the relevant material and to benefit from the therapeutic process. More than eight sessions may be too great a commitment of time and too tiring. Furthermore, parent dropout tends to occur more often when meetings are spaced more than a week apart. Evening meetings are preferred so that both parents can attend. According to Hornby, the 2-hour time period is ideal for a presentation followed by discussion and parent interaction.

The following guest speakers are recommended:

- A physician to explain the disability and the medical implications of the condition.
- A physical therapist to discuss exercise and strengthening regimens.
- A mental health worker to help with problems of child management and assist parents in understanding their emotional reactions.
- An attorney to elaborate on legal aspects, guardianship, and parent rights, as well as to help interpret relevant legislation.
- A local or state politician to discuss community/state policies regarding disability issues and enlist support for important disability-related legislation.

A pioneer in developing and conducting parent groups and workshops in Great Britain and New Zealand, Hornby (1994a) described a typical 2-hour meeting:

> 7:30–7:45 P.M. *Socializing.* Tea and coffee are served while parents talk informally with professionals and each other.

> 7:45–8:05 P.M. *Lecture presentation.* A 20-minute lecture on a topic of concern to the parents is presented by a professional.

> 8:05–9:15 P.M. *Small group discussion.* Parents are divided into small groups in order to participate in discussion. Opportunity is provided for discussion of the applications of the lecture content to specific problems brought forward by parents. Parents are encouraged to express and explore any problems, concerns, or feelings regarding their children with disabilities.

> 9:15–9:30 P.M. *Summary, handouts, and homework.* The large group is reformed so that issues raised in small group discussions can be summarized and shared, homework tasks explained, and handouts summarizing the content of lectures distributed.

These groups can be even further expanded to incorporate needs that emerge from the group. For example, it may be advantageous to have open-ended sessions after the more structured program to allow

parents to express feelings, achieve closure, and terminate the friendships they have developed in the group. There are always some members who continue relationships begun in the group, thereby adding
to their support network.

As noted, support groups can either be led by professionals or by
members, the latter either with or without professional consultation
available (Seligman & Marshak, 2003). Support groups can benefit
their members in several ways:

- The identification with others who are experiencing similar
  problems
- The 24-hour availability of group members to assist during critical periods
- The development of a network of friends to help reduce isolation
- The lack of costly fees

Also, such groups offer long-term support, an opportunity to develop
skills and coping mechanisms, a forum to share concerns and problems, and a sense of belonging.

Agee, Innocenti, and Boyce (1995) reported on a study designed
to assess whether a group for parents who were involved in an early
intervention program helped reduce stress. Half of the parents in the
early intervention program were asked to participate in a parent group
that was chiefly educationally oriented. The parents participated in
groups of 8–12 members and met for 90- to 120-minute sessions one
time a week for 15 or 16 weeks. The results showed that both "highly
stressed" and "typically stressed" parents experienced significantly
lower levels of stress than parents who were not in the groups.

Many of the parent groups that are reported in the literature
combine elements of both education and therapy (Hornby, 1994a,
2000; Seligman & Marshak, 2003). An integrated model is based on
the premise that group formats should be based on the needs of families and that the family's response to the child is multidetermined.
Group goals and content should be based on a careful assessment of
parent needs (see Chapter 12). Families need both knowledge *and*
emotional support in order to cope with the stresses that occur in raising a child with a disability.

Negative emotions are more universal and normal than parents
may think. This is reflected in the following comment made to a group
leader Marsh (1992):

Meeting other mothers with similar experiences was wonderful. As much as we love our handicapped children, it was such an eye-opener to learn that other mothers had intense feelings at times of guilt, anger toward the child, resentment toward an abnormal lifestyle, and other negative feelings. I thought I was the only one that still felt this way after so many years. I left the meetings uplifted that my feelings were quite typical and really normal considering what our family has gone through. (p. 195)

Parent-to-parent models have become popular in the United States and elsewhere. Such groups have increased to over 600 active local and statewide programs, with at least one in every state (Turnbull et al., 2006). Parent-to-parent programs consist of one-to-one meetings between one parent with experience as a parent of a child with a disability and another with a recently diagnosed child. They are round-the-clock services as opposed to the more restricted hours of professional availability (Santelli, Payadue, & Young, 2001).

Hornby (1994a), who pioneered parent-to-parent programs in New Zealand and Great Britain, stated that parents who are accepted as leaders in the programs are closely monitored to be sure that they are performing without major problems. This scrutiny is based on the belief that parents are often under enough stress without the additional burden of coping with another parent who is also under stress. He noted that, on occasion, a parent who was initially accepted into the program is terminated due to inadequate interpersonal skills or unresolved emotional problems. Hornby added that the trained parents come together periodically for additional training and to discuss dilemmas they encounter in their contact with other parents. A full discussion of recruitment, retention, and training is included in Hornby (1994a) and Santelli et al. (2001).

Siblings sometimes do not receive the parenting accorded to their seemingly needier brother or sister with a disability. Some siblings fare well, whereas others do not (Ufner, 2004). Some group models for siblings have emerged out of the recognition that some cope poorly. However, there is a full spectrum of responses to having a brother or sister with a disability. Whether a sibling struggles with his or her special circumstances depends on the factors mentioned in Chaper 9.

These groups have goals similar to those of groups that exist for other family members. Siblings gain an understanding of their brother or sister's condition, its etiology and prognosis, and the knowledge that others who have siblings with disabilities struggle with similar issues. Siblings explore feelings of love, hate, and ambivalence; talk about their fear of developing the same condition; and discuss their concerns about how to handle awkward social situations and how to cope with major anxieties about what the future holds for them. Siblings need a safe environment in which to discuss their feelings of guilt and anger, how they feel their unique situation has affected family life, and how being a sibling of a brother or sister with a disability may influence their choice of a career (Meyer & Vadasy, 1994).

In developing support groups for siblings, the following issues should be carefully considered:

- Whether the group will be heterogeneous or homogeneous regarding age: This issue requires careful thought in that children and adolescents vary considerably over 2- to 3-year spans.
- Whether the group will be heterogeneous or homogeneous in regard to the type of impairment or severity of the disability: There is little lost and perhaps a great deal to gain from more heterogeneous groups.
- What activities will reflect the group's goals and purposes: Some view sibling groups as primarily informational and recreational, whereas others stress emotional adjustment. There probably is considerable value in both of these goals.
- Practical issues, such as the length of each session (keeping in mind the children's ages and the activities planned) and the long-term duration of the group: Some groups span a relatively brief period of time, with each session being well planned, whereas others meet for longer periods with more open-ended sessions.
- Whether a follow-up meeting is deemed necessary: Sibling groups may stir up feelings beyond the group's life, and it may be beneficial to have one or two follow-up meetings to help siblings achieve closure.
- Information content: What information would siblings find relevant to their situation?
- Leadership: Leaders should be chosen who have had some experience with disabilities and group process.
- Discussion materials: Before the meeting participants can be asked to read certain books or articles for discussion purposes. Books and articles should be age appropriate.

We want to mention a particularly well-designed sibling group model developed by Reynolds and Zellmer (1985) that illustrates a structured, time-limited group experience. The group was co-led by a social worker and preschool teacher. Six siblings, ages 7–14, participated in the 1-hour per week, six-session experience.

- Session I: Participants brought family pictures to the first session to facilitate a discussion about themselves and their families.
- Session II: "What is a disability?" was the theme of the second meeting. Siblings explored how every person has some kind of disability. Medical problems of their brothers and sisters with disabilities were also discussed.
- Session III: Group members participated in simulating disabilities so that they could empathize with their siblings. (This technique has been criticized by some; see, French, 1996).
- Session IV: This session focused on what it is like to have a brother or sister with a disability. Books and articles or diaries (e.g., Meyer's 2005 book *The Sibling Slam Book*) authored by siblings can be used to stimulate discussion.
- Session V: Siblings discussed ways to deal with their feelings. The notion that all feelings have value and are not bad was stressed. Role playing of key problematic situations was employed.
- Session VI: This wrap-up session was used to discuss unfinished business. The meeting was held in a relaxed social setting with food available.

This and other group models can be applied flexibly. Sibling age, gender, and the brother or sister's disability can suggest the content. Very young children may be more involved when play and activities are included. Age can determine length and duration of the meetings.

DYSFUNCTIONAL FAMILY DYNAMICS

The selection of an approach to help families cope and adapt rests on family systems theory elaborated in Chapter 2. It is not our intent to repeat family systems concepts here, nor is it our goal to speak with authority about specific family interventions. It is assumed that professionals who plan to conduct family therapy with family members or with the entire family are well grounded in the theory and practice of this intervention.

Dysfunctional, tension-filled families are in a poor position to cope with a family member who is disabled (Marshak & Prezant, 2007). These authors noted, "children have a powerful impact on a marriage; children with disabilities often change the structure of a marriage even more because disability typically amplifies aspects of life. If the foundation of a marriage is somewhat 'off kilter' to begin with, the unique pressures of raising children with disabilities may further alter the structure of the marriage" (p. 43). Although there have been reports that some families have become more cohesive as a result of a childhood disability, these families probably had a minimum of preexisting pathology. Troubled families tend to become more dysfunctional in the face of crises and chronic stressors, whereas strong ones adapt, cope, and grow in the wake of crises.

Following are potential problematic family patterns:

1. In families into which a nondisabled infant is born, fathers sometimes feel neglected, or "left behind." This is an especially salient issue when the infant has a disability and requires significant care. Some husbands initially resent losing the attention after the child is born (Goffman, 1963). This may be more problematic if the spouse had been accustomed to a great deal of attention. The mother may feel incapable of nurturing both her child and her husband, as one mother noted: "More attention was taken from him when these problems with our daughter came up. A mature man would have probably handled it. I wasn't married to a mature person. He acted like it was a competition a lot of time, and she was winning" (Marshak & Prezant, 2007, p. 52).

2. A child with a disability can be the recipient of excessive attention because he or she is seen as the neediest family member. Other family members, such as nondisabled siblings, experience their parents' withdrawing from them, and as a result, feel angry toward the parents and the privileged (disabled) child. Siblings may also feel resentful and unloved, and they may act out their anger in an effort to capture some of the attention for which they long. Unfortunately, the methods some nondisabled children use to gain parental attention may further alienate the parents, thus increasing the likelihood of additional disruptive behavior. Professionals can assist families so embroiled by helping them understand that although a child with a disability may appear to be the neediest, in fact, the other children may be the most emotionally deprived. Furthermore, nondisabled siblings can be helped to understand their well-intentioned parents, who

focused on the child they erroneously thought needed the most attention.

3. Grandparents who may be struggling to accept their grandchild's disability add to the parents' burdens. This scenario can create tension within the parental dyad and between the parents and the grandparents. It is easy to see how parents can be torn in their attempts to be effective parents to their child while remaining connected to their parents.

4. Families who experience themselves as stigmatized by their community are in danger of becoming isolated, bitter, and withdrawn. Although the danger comes from outside of the family, the perception of a hostile community can create major tensions within the family. Professionals can help family members to consider alternative explanations for the behaviors they experience and to become more proficient at detecting their misperceptions of others who are actually supportive of them. They may also be referred to a support group where they can share their perceptions and discover from others that some people are actually supportive, helpful, and kind. The point of this perspective, however, is not to minimize the stigmatizing attitudes and behaviors of some members of the general public and those of professionals.

5. Poor relationships with professionals and the absence of important social services can have negative effects on the family. Families feel unsupported and overburdened, which, in turn, creates tension and stress. In these cases, families need to seek out professionals, like social workers, who are experts at exploring alternative service delivery systems and service providers who devote a portion of their practice to the area of childhood disability.

6. As noted earlier, the birth of a child with a disability to a troubled family can exacerbate existing family tension. Fragile families cannot tolerate additional pressures, and the presence of a child with a disability is not only an additional burden of some magnitude, but also a chronic one (Marshak & Prezant, 2007). Some family members find it difficult to be cooperative with and supportive of each other due to conditions of unemployment and poverty. Significantly troubled families can be helped by agencies that provide a full range of services, including in-home help.

7. A common situation is one in which parents, expecting a typical baby, discover that their newborn has an impairment. The potential immediate effects are considerable: shock; the realization that they must make major changes in their life, in their expectations, and

the like. Over time, families learn to cope by altering their values, expectations, and goals, without abandoning important life objectives. For those family members who find it difficult to come to grips with their circumstances, professional psychological help combined with support group membership can prove beneficial.

Another potentially problematic dynamic occurs when parents have difficulty maintaining appropriate boundaries concerning their child's privacy and growing independence. They can find it difficult to support each other, especially in the area of how best to manage a child with a chronic illness (Drotar, Crawford, & Bush, 1984). Although a child's chronic illness can cause family strain, it is not necessarily the cause of marital dysfunction. In this regard, Venter (as cited in Drotar et al., 1984) suggested that the parents' ability to construct meaning from the child's chronic illness experience may help the family to cope. In writing about coping with his son Andrew, who has Down syndrome, Nicholas Kappes (1995) embraced the concept of relativity to help place his son's disability within a broad philosophical context:

> I find peace in relativity. It governs our universe—it also governs our lives. No matter who or where we are we can always look up to greater and down to lower. Presidents and kings have their heroes and their inadequacies. No one is completely happy or has it all figured out to their satisfaction, and even those in tragic, painful circumstances cling to each precious moment of life—so it must be worth it for all. (p. 27)

Another relevant concept is the family's subsystems, such as the parent and sibling subsystems (see Chapter 9 for a fuller discussion; Turnbull et al., 2006). Attention to subsystems allows the professional to evaluate and intervene in the smaller unit within the family that may be problematic, although he or she should lose sight of how the subsystem (e.g., a parent and the child with a disability) can influence the whole family. As already noted, the concept of boundary is especially relevant for those who work with children who have disabilities and their families. The concepts of boundaries and subsystems go hand-in-hand, because families need to negotiate appropriate space between subsystems.

One of the chief contributors to dysfunctional families is the violation of boundaries by the intrusion of family members into functions that are the domains of other family members (Elman, 1991). An example is an overprotective, controlling mother's thwarting of the father's involvement with his son, who has a disability. Another illustration is the parents' violation of the sibling subsystems when they interfere with their children's methods of solving conflicts among themselves.

Boundary violations can occur in relationships between professionals and the family: "Families vary in their comfort about being asked questions. Some families believe that most or all questions challenge their competency, invade their privacy, or both. One African-American parent said she was raised by her parents, and she raised her own children, with the firm belief that, "what happens in this house stays in this house" (Turnbull et al., 2006, p. 191). Professionals need to be respectful of what is private or public information. Generally speaking, if there is not a compelling reason to ask a particular question, don't ask it. Do not ask a question if it is designed just to satisfy your own curiosity.

A professional's contact with a family generally begins at the point of the child's diagnosis. These initial contacts can send unintended, powerful messages to families, of which professionals should be aware. For example, if professionals maintain contact with the mother only, the family may interpret this as an indicator that she should be involved in all subsequent contacts. The message that is communicated is that it is the mother who should be the primary caregiver, rather than having shared caregiving. These early interactions between professional staff members and the mother can isolate the father and other children from the mother–child dyad. A more adaptive model is to involve as many family members as possible, especially at the point of initial diagnosis.

Professionals should explore how the family has dealt with previous stressors. Rolland (2003) contended that it is helpful to track family illnesses and determine how family members have coped with them in the past. Professionals should attempt to understand the roles family members play in handling emotional and practical tasks and explore whether they emerged from coping with disability or illness with a sense of competence or insecurity.

Whether the family tends to catastrophize events may be an important area to explore (Elman, 1991). Relatedly, the professional might inquire about whether the child is capable of some emotional reciprocity with family members and to what extent the disability impairs the child's functioning. The expected level of the child's ongoing dependency and the severity of the disability should be explored, as well as his or her age, gender, and "launchibility."

These factors may interact with other variables, such as a father's emotional difficulty with a son who has a disability; an adolescent's search for a sense of identity, competence, and self-esteem; or a young adult's continued dependence on the family when independent living is possible.

Reframing and normalizing are important intervention strategies when there is a disability (Elman, 1991). Normalizing can help reduce feelings of isolation and stigma by communicating that the emotions and struggle experienced by the family are both normal and expectable. Support groups are an ideal source for normalizing, in that family members experience others who are struggling similarly and who have been able to adopt a normalized life style. The danger with normalizing is that it can be viewed as trivializing the family's problems. When done by a sensitive professional, however, normalizing can help reduce anxiety and the sense of catastrophe that some family members experience.

Reframing is a powerful and effective strategy to help family members change the meaning of disability in their lives. Reframing means reinterpreting behavior by putting it into a new "frame," or by changing your thinking about a situation to emphasize positive aspects instead of negative ones (Hastings & Taunt, 2002). Reframing also allows the family to change its perception of the disabling condition, such as changing the perception of a child from a severely disabled one to a youngster who has abilities and strengths. In the area of family therapy, the most useful reframing is to redefine a behavior as benignly motivated and capable of being changed (Hoffman, 1981). Following is an illustration of a helpful reframe:

> If a mother is defined as overinvolved and intrusive, the family therapist can respond empathically to how much she cares for her child and how hard she has tried to find ways to help the child to grow as successfully as possible. The therapist can further comment on the difficulty of knowing how to change in the face of the child's and family's changing needs. This basically simple reframe of the mother's behavior, from intrusive to caring, concerned and confused about change, alters the perception of and meaning attributed to the experience. The mother probably feels more understood than she has in the past and feels that continuing effort is worthwhile, even if it has not always worked. The rest of the family also views the mother in a different perspective. An underinvolved parent or relative may feel more able to choose alternative responses when the behavior is framed as one that encourages self-care or independence. (Elman, 1991, p. 394)

Family-oriented approaches can alter the counterproductive belief that the child with a disability should be the sole focus of concern. The family should be considered the client, not the child. Professionals must also keep in mind that some children with disabilities live in fragmented and highly chaotic situations that do not provide a nurturing environment. In the case of difficult family environments that are the result of larger, societally induced factors such as poverty, the counselor may at times have to acknowledge that finding family-based intervention will be a challenge.

Finally, we cannot assume that professionals have a right to intervene in families simply because those families happen to have a child with a disability. One parent wrote:

> No one ever seemed to examine professionals' reactions. Parents are turned into patients and are endlessly analyzed, scrutinized, and finally packaged into neat stages as if they were one-celled animals going through mitosis. Although parents and people with disabilities do have obligations and responsibilities, they must not be victimized by their status. (Pieper, in Darling & Darling, 1982, p. viii)

It is our perspective that parents must be active participants in determining what kinds of help they need and how much help is needed. All decisions about assistance should be made by the family alone or by family members with the aid of a competent professional. Those in positions of authority should not prescribe an approach in the absence of family input.

13

Applying a Partnership Approach to Addressing Family Resources, Concerns, and Priorities

Developing Family Service Plans

As noted repeatedly in this volume, the recognition of the importance of the family as a whole in services to children with disabilities is a relatively recent development in the history of the field. In the past, medical, educational, and therapeutic services were designed to meet only the needs of the child. The needs of parents and other family members were neglected or left to mental health professionals who had little direct influence on the child's educational or therapeutic program. In recent years, professionals have come to recognize that child needs and family concerns are not separate and distinct. This recognition achieved legal acknowledgment with the passage of landmark legislation in 1986, the Education of the Handicapped Act amendments—Public Law 99-457 (since amended and renamed the Individuals with Disabilities Education Act). Part H of that law, which applies to infants and toddlers with disabilities, estab-

lished a policy to assist state governments "to develop and imple-
ment a statewide, comprehensive, coordinated, multidisciplinary inter-
agency program of early intervention services for handicapped infants
and toddlers *and their families*" (pp. 1–2, emphasis added). A similar
shift toward family-based services has occurred in the fields of psychology, social work, and other disciplines that serve families of children with disabilities.

In this chapter we provide examples that illustrate the application
of family-centered principles to the provision of services for families
of children with disabilities. Unlike the last chapter, which focused on
changes within the family system, this chapter addresses approaches to
changing the larger social systems within which families reside.

THE PARTNERSHIP MODEL[1]

As noted in Chapter 11, the status inequality perspective characterized
most human service practice in the decades preceding the 1980s.
Sometimes it led to successful treatments and cures. Certainly, the
health status of people around the world has improved dramatically as
a result of various medical and surgical interventions based on this
model. Diagnostic categories are useful when they point the way
toward effective intervention. On the other hand, the status inequality
model has failed miserably in treating some problems. Social workers
have been counseling poor people for years but have not succeeded in
eliminating poverty by this method. Similarly, programs for the rehabilitation of drug addicts, juvenile delinquents, and adult criminals
have experienced frustratingly high rates of recidivism. Even in the
field of medicine, established treatment regimens do not always work.

Failed attempts at intervention are often the result of a poor
understanding of the nature of a problem. Although some pathologies
do rest within individuals, often the source of a problem is external to
the individual and the family. With respect to early education programs for poor children, Bowman (1992, pp. 104–105) wrote:

> Many of us who work in poverty communities believe that we can and
> should be able to change the developmental outcomes of children in
> these profoundly depriving environments. But success is limited and

---

[1] The following sections are adapted from Darling (2000). Copyright 2000 by Kluwer Aca-
demic/Plenum Publishers. Adapted by permission of Springer Science and Business Media.

burnout is rampant. . . . The truth of the matter is that trying to cure sociological problems with treatments aimed at the intrapsychic organizations of individuals is counterproductive at best. It may be immoral.

Mercer (1965), who described the clinical perspective discussed in Chapter 11, argued that the source of the problem often lies within the *social system* rather than the individual. In the case of the families that she studied, a child's label was contingent on the situation in which the child was placed. In the institutional setting, lower-SES children might be regarded as mentally deficient; however, when these same children were removed from the institution and returned to their home communities, they were likely to be regarded as normal. Thus, Mercer suggested that the solution to some problems might involve changing the norms of the social system or, alternatively, relocating the individual to a system that does not regard his or her behavior or condition as pathological.

This social system perspective is in many ways identical to the partnership approach that is becoming the norm in many human service fields today. In the partnership approach, the professional's definition of the situation is not necessarily seen as "right." Rather, the definitions of all parties are accepted as meaningful for the purpose of designing effective interventions. In this approach, the service user and the service provider become partners in the problem-solving endeavor. The professional contributes expertise based on his or her training and past experience, and the client contributes the expertise that comes from intimate familiarity with his or her social world.

After a review of 130 published sources in a variety of disciplines, a group of researchers ("Family-Centered Service Delivery," 1997, p. 1) identified a number of key components of these newer models of practice, including the following:

- Organizing assistance collaboratively (e.g., ensuring mutual respect and teamwork between team workers and clients)
- Organizing assistance in accordance with each individual family's wishes so that the family ultimately directs decision making
- Considering family strengths (versus dwelling on family deficiencies)
- Addressing family needs holistically (rather than focusing on a member with a "problem")
- Normalizing perspectives (i.e., recognizing that much of what those receiving services are experiencing is typical)
- Structuring service delivery to ensure accessibility, minimal disruption of family integrity and routine.

Some examples of the independent movement of a variety of disciplines toward a partnership approach are explored in the next section.

Education

In the field of education, the shift toward a partnership perspective has been especially notable in the area of early intervention. As noted earlier, much of the early literature in this field tended to take a victim-blaming stance toward the families of these children. Service plans generally focused on the child and did not take family concerns into account. When families were included at all, they were typically treated as clients themselves, and treatment centered around improving their ability to cope with and adjust to their children's disabilities.

As recently as 1986, *Topics in Early Childhood Special Education*, a major journal in the early intervention field, published a thematic issue titled "Assessment of Handicapped Children and Their Families: New Directions." The assessment of families was based on a status inequality model that suggested that professionals knew better than parents what was best for their children. However, just 4 years later, the same journal published an issue titled, "Gathering Family Information: Procedures, Products, and Precautions." The change in terminology marked a shift in thinking about families. In a relatively short period of time, the field had moved from talking about "assessing" families to viewing families as equal partners who could provide valuable information.

This newer perspective is reflected especially in the writing of Carl Dunst and his colleagues, who suggested an "enablement and empowerment" perspective:

> A fuller understanding of empowerment requires that we take a broader-based view of the conditions that influence the behavior of people during help-seeker and help-giver exchanges. . . . Empowerment implies that what you see as poor functioning is a result of social structure and lack of resources which make it impossible for the existing competencies to operate. (Dunst, Trivette, & Deal, 1987, p. 3)

They described how a social system perspective views a family as a social unit embedded within other formal and informal social units and networks. They proposed a "social systems definition of intervention": "the provision of support (i.e., resources provided by others) by members of a family's informal and formal social network that either directly or indirectly influences child, parent, and family functioning" (p. 3).

In a similar vein, as noted in the last chapter, Donald Bailey and his colleagues have developed a curriculum and materials for early intervention professionals based on a "family-focused" perspective (e.g., Bailey et al., 1986; Winton & Bailey, 1988). They discussed the need for intervention to fit the individualized needs of families. Among the intervention goals they listed is the following: "To preserve and reinforce the dignity of families by respecting and responding to their desire for services and incorporating them in the assessment, planning, and evaluation process" (Bailey et al., 1986, p. 158). Thus the family's definition of the situation, rather than the professional's, becomes the focus for service provision.

Why has this shift occurred? Several factors seem to have played a role: (1) Probably most important is the role played by families themselves. Increasingly, parents of children with disabilities began to speak out against practices based on status inequality and to demand a larger part in determining the services their children received (for a further discussion of the parent movement of the 1970s–1980s, see Pizzo, 1983; Darling, 1988). (2) Professionals also began to realize the inefficacy of status inequality approaches in their day-to-day work with families. Especially as home visiting became a more popular method in the field, professionals began to acquire a new respect for the family's perspective. This point of view was expressed in this professional's quote that appeared in an earlier chapter: "Before I had Peter I gave out [physical therapy] programs that would have taken all day. I don't know when I expected mothers to change diapers, sort laundry, or buy groceries" (Featherstone, 1980, p. 57). (3) Research with families also led increasingly to an appreciation of their perspective. For example, as cited in previous chapters, one early study of parents of children with disabilities in an Australian city with few services available (Schonell & Watts, 1956) concluded that the parents' concerns were pathological. When the same population was studied following the establishment of new services in the city (Schonell & Rorke, 1960), their "neurotic" symptoms had disappeared. Their "pathology," then, seemed to be an artifact of the lack of resources—their limited structure of opportunities—rather than the manifestation of some inherent, psychological disorder.

Newer, system-based perspectives in the field of early intervention have been reflected in practice. The "Individualized Family Service Plans" mandated by law now tend to be products of a partnership between families and professionals, and services are based on the *family's* resources, concerns, and priorities. Guidelines for practice usually reflect the new approaches, as illustrated by the following "underlying principles" from a seminal document in the field:

- Each family has its own structure, roles, values, beliefs, and coping styles. Respect for and acceptance of this diversity is a cornerstone of family-centered early intervention.
- Respect for family autonomy, independence, and decision making means that families must be able to choose the level and nature of an early intervention program's involvement in their life.
- An enabling approach to working with families requires that professionals re-examine their traditional roles and practices and develop new practices when necessary. (Johnson, McGonigel, & Kaufmann, 1989, p. 3)

This newer perspective does not deny the existence of diagnosable developmental disabilities in children. However, it asserts that the existence of diagnosable disabilities in children does not require that their parents be diagnosed and categorized as well. Rather, parents become respected members of the treatment team.

Social Work

A strand that values the strengths and perspectives of service users has always existed in the field of social work (Simon, 1994). However, for a number of years, that strand seemed to be overshadowed by approaches based more on status inequality. Specht and Courtney (1994) noted, for example, a trend toward the private practice of psychotherapy among social workers during the past 60 years. Recently, however, social system approaches have experienced a resurgence.

Adams and Nelson (1995) suggested that the new movement toward community- and family-centered practice was stimulated by concerns about the "fragmented, bureaucratic, rule-driven, ineffective way" (p. 3) in which human service agencies had been operating. They posed a series of questions suggesting their vision of a more effective, social system model:

What would it be like if services were designed to strengthen rather than substitute for the caring capacity of families and communities? What if services were shaped by and available to all citizens in their communities, so people could get a little help when they needed it, without always having to fit into a narrow category or be formally processed as "clients"? What if services were geared to recognizing and building on the strengths and resources of families and communities, rather than focusing on their deficits? (p. 2)

A major component of newer, social system approaches in social work has been the concept of *empowerment*. Lee (1994) argued that an empowerment approach is based on a number of underlying principles, including the following:

- People empower themselves: social workers should assist.
- Social workers should establish an "I and I" [partnership] relationship with clients.
- Social workers should encourage the client to say her own word [and not use the language of the oppressor].
- The worker should maintain a focus on the person as victor and not victim.
- Social workers should maintain a social change focus. (pp. 27–28)

She argued further that social workers need to develop "fifocal vision," based on historical, ecological, "ethclass," feminist, and critical perspectives.

The family support movement has been growing rapidly in the United States. As Zigler and Black (1989) noted, a number of social trends have increased stresses on families, creating a need for support. The goal of family support programs is "not to provide families with direct services, but to enhance parent empowerment—to enable families to help themselves and their children" (Zigler & Black, 1989, p. 7). The need for agency services can often be avoided when support is provided to families even before problems occur. Such models also suggest that *all* families could use some help from time to time; yet being labeled as a client can be demeaning and may discourage people from seeking the help they need. The Family Support America website (www.familysupportamerica.org) provides information on the extent of the family support movement today.

In the child welfare field, family-centered practice has resulted in the creation of "family preservation programs" (Cameron & Vanderwoerd, 1997; Fraser, Pecora, & Haapala, 1991; Nelson & Allen, 1995; Wells & Biegel, 1991; Whittaker, Kenney, Tracy, & Booth, 1990). Rather than removing children perceived to be at risk from their homes and placing them in foster care, these programs build on family strengths and work to keep families together. The family support and preservation philosophy has guided funding for child protective services in recent years and has given rise to new programs throughout the United States, many of which are based on home visiting or family center models.

Psychology/Mental Health

The field of psychology has been moving toward a partnership model in a number of areas. Social system principles underlie the theoretical literature in the ecological and family systems approaches (discussed in detail in Chapter 2) that have been popular in recent years. These principles can also be seen in several practice models, including behavioral health care delivery and children's mental health care, among others.

In 1997 the National Community Behavioral Healthcare Council proposed a new model for services that is consumer-centered and based on an understanding of the importance of the social system. A series of "principles for consumer-centered care" include, among others:

- The provision of services and support should take place in the consumer's environment and be directed by his or her needs and desires, wherever possible.
- Consumer needs, strengths, and choices should be considered, and the involvement of the individual should be demonstrated, in service planning and implementation, in order to help consumers take charge of their lives through informed decision-making.
- Services should be culturally and linguistically appropriate. Providers should demonstrate responsiveness, understanding, and respect for the consumer's culture and language and should make every effort to provide services in the person's preferred language. (pp. 15–16)

A shift in perspectives in the mental health field is also apparent in professional support for self-help groups. As Wasow (1997) noted, in the past, consumer organizations were seen by professionals as suspect. Today, many professionals recommend such groups to their clients, and the consumer advocacy movement is growing.

One area of mental health practice that seems to have moved almost completely toward a partnership model is that of services to children. In the past, when children were diagnosed with behavioral and emotional disorders, their families were typically seen as the cause of their problem. In characteristic victim-blaming fashion, parents were labeled as "overprotective" or "too permissive," or by some other term suggesting their ineptness. Although some parents certainly do contribute to their children's difficulties, blaming models have not been productive in creating positive outcomes for children and families. More recent models have regarded families as allies and have looked beyond the family for system-based causes of children's behavior.

The federally sponsored Child and Adolescent Service System Program (CASSP) approach noted in Chapter 11 is based on a partnership between service providers and families (Cohen & Lavach, 1995). In this model, parents are acknowledged to be experts about, and advocates for, their children. Parent involvement has been encouraged through mutual support or self-help groups, joint service planning, and increased recognition by professionals of the constraints on families imposed by their social and cultural environments. Greater flexibility in service delivery is also an important feature of the model.

Today, mental health services are delivered in a variety of settings, including schools, child care centers, and family homes, in addition to the offices and clinics that are the "natural habitats" of professionals. Although older, status inequality models still determine eligibility for services in many cases (especially in some of the newer managed care plans), professionals seem to be more aware of the importance of the service user's usual environment and definition of the situation. Thus, like the other helping professions, psychological practice has been moving toward a more partnership-based approach.

Health Care

Family-centered health care was tried in various forms throughout much of the 20th century (Doherty, 1985). Projects such as the Peckham Experiment, the Cornell Project, and the Montefiore Medical Group attempted to apply a holistic perspective, rather than treating patients in isolation from their familial and social milieus. However, the area in the health care field that has moved most closely to a partnership perspective is probably maternal and child health. Perhaps the role of the family was most obvious in the case of infant and child patients.

During the past 20 years or so, the family-centered care movement has been gaining momentum in maternal and child health. This movement recognizes that "families are the primary caregivers and advocates for their children" and encourages parent–professional collaboration rather than professional dominance (Hostler, 1991). "Within this philosophy is the idea that families should be supported in their natural care-giving and decision-making roles by building on their unique strengths as people and families" (Brewer, McPherson, Magrab, & Hutchins, 1989). Family-centered care was incorporated into the 1989 amendments to Title V of the Social Security Act.

The U.S. Bureau of Maternal and Child Health has provided funding for various initiatives, including the Center for Family-Centered Care at the Association for the Care of Children's Health and various "Special Projects of Regional and National Significance" (SPRANS), including physician-training projects in several states. The "Healthy Tomorrows Partnership" between the U.S. Maternal and Child Health Bureau and the American Academy of Pediatrics, which funded various child health initiatives, required that projects be community-based, family-centered, comprehensive and culturally relevant. Further, Ireys and Nelson (1992) suggested that pediatric training programs at all levels need to incorporate the principles of community-based, family-centered care into their curricula.

The Institute for Family-Centered Care lists the following "core principles":

- In family-centered health care, people are treated with dignity and respect.
- In family-centered health care, health care providers communicate and share complete and unbiased information with patients and families in ways that are affirming and useful.
- In family-centered health care, individuals and family members build on their strengths by participating in experiences that enhance control and independence.
- In family-centered health care, collaboration among patients, families, and providers occurs in policy and program development and professional education, as well as in the delivery of care. ("Core Principles of Family-Centered Health Care," 1998, pp. 2–3)

As noted in Chapter 11, physician-training programs based on a partnership model have been especially prevalent in the area of children with special health care needs. Parents of such children are included as faculty in these programs throughout the country, at both the medical school and residency levels, as well as in continuing education programs for practicing physicians. Usually, pediatricians and family physicians are targeted.

One model program at the medical-school level (Lewis & Greenstein, 1994) requires first-year medical students to make six to eight home visits to a family of a child with special health needs over the course of one semester. These students clearly come away with a new appreciation of the family's definition of the situation:

> Above all, no one can really see what this family experiences. I think I see a window into their life: their daily routines, their minor setbacks offset by victories. One of their most fervent desires is to make me understand that I cannot feel their painful experience, but that I should recognize and acknowledge it and incorporate this into my fiber as a professional. Another lesson: chronic illness does not stop when the patient leaves the office; it is a way of life. . . . There is some sort of lesson here, although I don't think I fully understand it yet. It is something about the value of having a relationship that is close enough to be painful. (Lewis & Greenstein, 1994, p. 89)

Similar programs also exist at the residency level (Cooley, 1994). Many of these programs bring families into the classroom. Others require pediatric residents to spend time with families, either as observers or as respite care providers.

Physicians practicing in the community have been targeted by similar training programs. For example, a major SPRANS grant project in Hawaii developed a curriculum for practicing physicians based on the American Pediatric Association's concept of "medical home" (Peter & Sia, 1994). This concept designates physicians as service coordinators for their patients and suggests the integration of medical services with those provided by school and community agencies. The Hawaii curriculum has been adopted in many states. (For a further discussion of this and other projects designed to train physicians in a partnership perspective, see Darling & Peter, 1994.)

Thus the professional dominance of physicians seems to be declining in favor of a newer perspective that takes the patient's (and/or patient's family's) views into account. Newer training programs in the health care field acknowledge that patients seen in medical offices, clinics, or hospitals are impacted by their lives in nonmedical settings and that medical professionals cannot gain a complete understanding of their patients' needs unless they come to recognize the totality of their social worlds.

As the sections above have shown, virtually all of the helping professions are moving toward newer partnership models of practice. However, professionals trained in older approaches may not have the "tools" necessary to empower families to express their wishes or to develop treatment outcomes based on those wishes. The next section illustrates the development of service plans using a family-driven, partnership approach.

THE IDENTIFICATION OF RESOURCES, CONCERNS, AND PRIORITIES

How should professionals working with families of children who have disabilities apply the principles of partnership in their practice? The first step in providing family-centered services involves the identification of a family's resources, concerns, and priorities. This process replaces the professionally dominated "assessment" of "needs" that occurred in older, clinical models of intervention. Because a family-centered partnership model focuses on family-identified issues, the role of the professional becomes one of helping the family to articulate the areas in which professional assistance may be desired. In addition to addressing concerns, the partnership model also focuses on family strengths or resources. Rather than encouraging families to rely on professional expertise, this approach seeks to identify areas in which a family can achieve desired outcomes through more informal means that will be continuously available, even after professional intervention has ended. The following sections describe the areas on which professionals need to focus in helping families identify their resources, concerns, and priorities.

Information

Information or knowledge can be both a resource and a concern. Some families with prior experience in the human service system already know a considerable amount about help-seeking procedures before they encounter a new professional. Others may know very little about where to turn for the kinds of help they need.

The kind of information that families want varies. Most families want to know as much as possible about the issues that concern them, especially if they are in a state of anomie (cf. Chapter 4). Sometimes, because of previously encountered professional dominance or a concern that is new, a family's priority may be to better define what is troubling them. As noted in earlier chapters, a number of studies have indicated that the desire for information is the *most* salient concern among parents of young children with disabilities.

Some parents have good research skills, a resource in the information area. These individuals may have access to good libraries or may be skilled at using the Internet to obtain information. Typically, research skills are commensurate with education, and parents who are college graduates may be better at finding information on their own than those who did not graduate from high school. On the other hand, individuals with considerable experience in using human services, regardless of education level or social class, may be very adept at using the telephone and locating knowledgeable experts in their area of concern.

Once a concern has been defined, families typically seek information about available services. The role of the professional in providing this kind of information varies. Sometimes the agency with which the family is already involved may provide the kinds of services the family wants. Often, though, the professional will need to make a referral to a different agency. For this reason, professionals need to be knowledgeable about all the services located in the community. Many communities maintain directories of human services, and networking through councils and consortia of agencies is also helpful.

Material Support

Like information, material support can be both a resource and a concern. Material support refers to goods or things (as opposed to services) that a family might have or want. Some common examples of material support include money, government benefits, food, clothing, shelter, furnishings, medical equipment, a means of transportation, and toys and leisure items. Clearly, material support is a more common resource among the rich than among the poor and, conversely, a more common concern among the poor. For the poorest families, material support is likely to be the concern of highest priority. Material support may be provided informally, through friends or relatives, or formally, through human service agencies, such as food banks and homeless shelters, or government programs such as subsidized housing or Medicaid.

Because of the priority of material support, service professionals will usually want to identify the nature of a family's resources in this area, even when the family is referred for assistance with a child's disability. If the parents are struggling to make ends meet, they may not be as concerned about their child's disability as they are about their financial situation. On the other hand, asking questions about finances may be regarded as intrusive by a family for whom material support is not a major concern. In fact, in the experience of one of us (R. B. D.) in early intervention, some middle- and upper-class families refused services rather than disclose information about their financial status. Appropriate methods for obtaining information about material support and other sensitive areas are addressed later in this chapter.

Informal Support

Informal support refers to the assistance people receive as a result of their relationships with their primary groups—family, friends, neighbors, fellow churchgoers or clergy, and coworkers. This support may take the form of assistance with material needs, as discussed in the last section, with service needs, such as the need for child care, or with emotional needs, through simply listening or otherwise acknowledging the validity of an individual's concerns.

Some individuals have extensive support networks, whereas others have few people they can rely on for assistance when needed. In a study of one group of single African American mothers in a poor neighborhood (Cook & Fine, 1995), for example, the women "felt bereft of positive social networks. . . . They reported being 'the sickly sister who stayed in the neighborhood,' 'The kid they thought was slow' " (p. 126). These women provided considerable support for children, parents, and neighbors but could not identify anyone who regularly supported them.

Perhaps the people with the least informal support in society are those who are homeless. Numerous studies of homeless individuals (see, e.g., Kozol, 1988; Liebow, 1993) have suggested that many people become homeless when they are rejected by their families. A typical career path of homeless families includes varying periods of time during which the families live with relatives after losing their own homes. Homelessness commonly occurs when these relatives are no longer able or willing to house these families.

Usually, the main source of support is an individual's immediate family. Consequently, professionals need to look most closely at the relationships among these individuals. The literature in the field of family systems theory and methods (see Chapter 2) can be valuable here. In addition, the concerns of other family members are important. For example, a woman who is caring for her chronically ill mother may not have the time or emotional energy to help her child with the disability that brought the family to the attention of an agency. Concerns involving other members of the family can compete with the concerns for which families are referred for help. Also, when other family members have concerns of their own, they are not likely to be able to provide support to the family of a child with a disability.

Cameron and Vanderwoerd (1997, pp. 21–23) suggested the following structural dimensions of support networks:

- *Range of supports available* (the types of available support, such as material, emotional, or service).
- *Levels of support available* (the adequacy of supports in buffering the effects of stressors).
- *Length of commitment.*
- *Reciprocity.*
- *Technical expertise.*
- *Openness to all in need* (availability to stigmatized and other "undesirable" cases).
- *Availability in a crisis.*
- *Motivation and skill requirements* (willingness and ability to help).

Human service professionals can assist their clients by helping to mobilize existing networks of support.

Formal Support

Formal support becomes important when opportunities for informal support are limited. Baxter (1987) found, in a study of parents of children with intellectual disabilities, that those parents experiencing the highest levels of stress expressed the greatest need for professional help. In addition, professionals may, because of their training and experience, be better equipped than laypersons to provide some technical services, such as medical care. *Formal support* refers to services provided by agencies and professionals and includes emotional, technical, and service support.

Emotional support involves the provision of empathy and assurance to individuals who do not have sufficient support within their primary groups. A common mechanism for the provision of such support is support groups. As noted in the last chapter, these are usually professionally organized groups of individuals with similar concerns that meet on a regular basis. Through these groups, individuals come to realize that their concerns are shared. The groups also serve as forums for the exchange of information as well as sources of role models for the members. The counseling literature contains much information on organizing and conducting support groups. Many professionals prefer to gradually turn the control of the group over to the members, and many successful groups have been organized by parents themselves, without any professional intervention at all.

Technical support refers to services such as medical and dental care, education, legal services, therapy, and other specialized forms of treatment. These services are designed to improve the functioning of children with disabilities. Technical support is often provided within a status inequality framework; however, it can also be provided within a partnership perspective when a concern in this area is *family defined* and not merely professionally diagnosed.

Finally, *service support* includes the provision of services such as child care, respite care, organized recreational programs, and other services to meet family-defined needs. As noted in the information section above, professionals may be able to provide needed services directly, or they may have to refer families to other agencies. When needed services are not available or are available on only a limited basis in a community, professionals may need to become advocates for their clients in an attempt to secure additional funding or to otherwise lobby those in positions of power to expand service offerings.

As in the other areas that have been discussed, formal support can be both a resource and a concern for families. Some families are satisfied with the services they are receiving; others may be dissatisfied or even disillusioned with what they have received (or not received) from agencies and professionals.

In identifying their clients' resources and concerns in this area, agency staff need to determine which services families are already using and whether they are satisfied with those services. After this determination has been made, the staff can assist families in exploring concerns that are not currently being met. Finally, they can try to match these concerns with existing services. Sometimes the needed service will be available within the agency; sometimes referral to another agency may be required. When no available agency can meet identified concerns, advocacy or activism may be desirable. The following sections illustrate the process of developing a service plan to address family-identified concerns in the areas of information, and material, informal, and formal support.

DEVELOPING A FAMILY SERVICE PLAN

The program type highlighted in this section is designed to provide early intervention services to young children with disabilities and their families. However, the procedures described could be applied equally well to other kinds of programs serving families of children with disabilities. Although developmental outcomes for the child are also important in services for this population, our discussion focuses on *family outcomes*.

The first step in developing a family service plan involves identifying a family's resources, concerns, and priorities. Various methods can be used in the identification process, including observation, interviewing, and written questionnaires. The following sections discuss three techniques that have been shown to be effective in early intervention programs: the Parent Needs Survey, the family interview, and observation. (For a more in-depth discussion of identification methods, see Darling, 2000.)

The Parent Needs Survey

The Parent Needs Survey (PNS) is a questionnaire-type instrument that exemplifies a tool based on a social system/partnership perspective, in that needs are defined by the family rather than by the professional. The PNS has been used for over 15 years in a program previously directed by one of us (R. B. D.) and was also field tested in other early intervention programs around the country (see Darling & Baxter, 1996, for a discussion of the testing process). Figure 13.1 is a sample survey form. The codes (e.g., I, FS, IS) that follow each statement do not appear on the instrument that parents fill out; they are explained in the following text.

The PNS was developed from an overview of the literature (presented in earlier chapters) on families of young children with disabilities. The literature indicates six major areas of need or concern in this population:

1. *Information* about diagnosis, prognosis, and treatment
2. *Intervention* for the child (medical, therapeutic, and educational)
3. *Formal support* from public and private agencies
4. *Informal support* from relatives, friends, neighbors, coworkers, and other parents

Date: _____

Name of person completing form: _____

Relationship to child: _____

Parents of young children have many different needs. Not all parents need the same kinds of help. For each of the needs listed below, please check (x) the space that best describes your need or desire for help in that area. Although we may not be able to help you with all your needs, your answers will help us improve our program.

		I really need some help in this area.	I would like some help, but my need is not that great.	I don't need any help in this area.
1. More information about my child's disability.	I			
2. Someone who can help me feel better about myself.	FS, IS			
3. Help with child care.	FS, IS			
4. More money/financial help.	MS, CN			
5. Someone who can babysit for a day or evening so I can get away.	CN			
6. Better medical care for my child.	T			
7. More information about child development.	I			
8. More information about behavior problems.	I, T			
9. More information about programs that can help my child.	I, T			
10. Counseling to help me cope with my situation.	FS			
11. Better/more frequent teaching or therapy services for my child.	T			
12. Day care so I can get a job.	FS, CN			
13. A bigger or better house or apartment.	CN			
14. More information about how I can help my child.	I, T			
15. More information about nutrition or feeding.	I, T			

(continued)

FIGURE 13.1. Parent Needs Survey.

		I really need some help in this area.	I would like some help, but my need is not that great.	I don't need any help in this area.
16. Learning how to handle my other children's jealousy of their brother or sister.	CN			
17. Problems with in-laws or other relatives.	IS, CN			
18. Problems with friends or neighbors.	IS, CN			
19. Special equipment to meet my child's needs.	T, MS			
20. More friends who have a child like mine.	IS			
21. Someone to talk to about my problems.	FS, IS			
22. Problems with my husband (wife).	IS, CN			
23. A car or other form of transportation.	MS, CN			
24. Medical care for myself.	CN			
25. More time for myself.	CN			
26. More time to be with my child.	CN			

Please list any needs we have forgotten:

27.				
28.				
29.				
30.				
31.				
32.				
33.				
34.				

FIGURE 13.1. (*continued*)

5. *Material support*, including financial support and access to resources
6. Elimination of *competing family needs*, that is, needs of other family members (parents, siblings) that may affect the family's ability to attend to the needs of the child with a disability

The PNS contains items that relate to each of these categories of need, as follows:

1. I: Information—items 1, 7, 8, 9, 14, 15
2. T: Intervention (a form of technical formal support)—items 6, 8, 9, 11, 14, 15, 19
3. FS: Formal support (other than treatment for the child)—items 2, 3, 10, 12, 21
4. IS: Informal support—items 2, 3, 17, 18, 20, 21, 22
5. MS: Material support—items 4, 19, 23
6. CN: Competing needs (an area affecting the availability of informal support)—items 4, 5, 12, 13, 16, 17, 18, 22, 23, 24, 25, 26

Field-test studies of the PNS (reported in Darling & Baxter, 1996) have indicated that information is by far the greatest area of need expressed by parents of very young children with disabilities, followed by concerns relating to intervention for the child. Needs for material support also tend to be relatively high among families of lower SES. In general, needs relating to both formal and informal support are expressed by only a small minority of families, probably because most families already receive some support from family, friends, and community agencies. Needs in all areas tend to decrease over time among families involved in early intervention programs. No doubt these programs provide much of the information, intervention, and support that families need. Information gathered from an instrument such as the PNS, along with information from a family interview and from observation, can be used in the development of a family service plan.

Family Interview

No checklist-type instrument provides qualitative, in-depth information about families. True understanding of a family's situation can only be obtained by talking with family members about their resources and concerns or through long-term observation. (Observation will be discussed more fully in the next section.) Here we suggest that a well-constructed depth interview can provide valuable information.

The following interview schedule is a suggested model excerpted from one used in the early intervention program mentioned in the previous section (see Darling & Baxter, 1996, for an extended discussion of interviewing in this context). The interview should be conducted in a relaxed, conversational style, and follow-up questions should be asked to clarify statements made by parents and other family members. The interviewer must be careful to listen empathically and without personal judgment. The interview may be used separately with mothers and fathers or with other family members, or with both parents or the whole family present together.

> I'd like to ask you some questions about your family to help us understand how we can best meet your needs and help you help your child. If I ask you anything you'd rather not answer, just tell me, and we'll skip that question. Please tell me, too, if there's anything you'd like to talk about that I may forget to ask.
>
> First, it would help me to know a little about your (and your husband's or wife's) background.
>
> Where are you from originally?
>
> Was your family large?
>
> Where did you go to school? What was the last grade in school you completed?
>
> While you were growing up, did you know any children or adults with any kind of disability?
>
> Had you ever heard of (child's disability) before _____ was born?
>
> Do you remember the kinds of things you were thinking before _____ was born? Did you ever think he (or she) might have a problem of any kind?
>
> Is _____ your first child?
>
> When did you first learn that _____ had a problem? How did you feel when you first heard (or suspected) this?
>
> What kinds of things have you worried about since you first learned about _____'s disability?
>
> Have you told other people—siblings, grandparents, friends, minister/priest/rabbi, neighbors, coworkers? How have they reacted to the news? How have they reacted to the baby?
>
> Do you know any other parents of children with special needs? Would you like to talk to other parents?
>
> How did you learn about this program?
>
> Has it been hard to get information about available services?
>
> Have you been satisfied with your child's medical treatment so far?

How about your health; has it been good?

Has anyone else in the family had any medical problems?

Do you work? (If not) Have you worked in the past? What kind of work do you do?

(If not working) Would you work if you had someone to take care of _____?

Does your husband (or wife or partner) help with child care?

Do family members live nearby? Do they help you with anything?

Do any of your other children have any special needs?

Have you had any problems with the baby—with sleeping, feeding, handling, or other areas of care?

Is there anything you need for the baby—furniture, clothing, equipment, toys?

Do you have a car or other means of transportation?

Would you say that you are coping pretty well with your problems right now, or would you like some help with things that are bothering you?

As part of this program, you will be asked to work on some activities with your baby at home. Do you think you will have any difficulty finding enough time to work on these activities? Do you like the idea of being your baby's teacher? Do you think you might have any special experience, skills, or feelings that will make you a good teacher for your baby?

Can you think of anything else right now that our program might be able to help you with?

Note that the areas covered in the family interview are the same as those covered in the PNS—information, intervention, formal support, informal support, material support, competing needs. The interview provides another way of eliciting and elaborating on this kind of information and, as such, provides a valuable supplement to the checklist.

Interviewing skills should be part of the training that professionals working with families receive. Without such training, they may feel uncomfortable asking personal questions and may not be able to elicit valid responses; they also may make families feel uncomfortable. We would recommend that a course in social research methods, counseling techniques, or a similar subject be included as part of the preprofessional curriculum offered to those planning to enter the disability services field. An alternative for those already working in the field would be appropriate inservice training. The family interview format included here is intended to serve as a guide and should not generally be used by untrained staff.

Regardless of the level of staff training, data from an initial family interview should be regarded with some caution. The interviewer is a stranger to the family and may not be trusted at the beginning of an intervention program. As a relationship develops between a practitioner and a family, the family is likely to reveal additional information about its concerns. Concerns also change over time. Consequently, the identification process should be ongoing, and the practitioner should be sensitive to any changes in family status that occur. Finally, interviews, like other methods of assisting families, should be conducted in a spirit of partnership with family members. In this case, the *family* is the expert, and the professional is the student who needs to learn about the family's resources, concerns, and priorities.

Observation

Professionals acquire information about families simply by being with them. In the course of interaction, they observe how the family dresses, how family members interact with one another, what conversational mannerisms are employed, and how feelings are revealed. Professionals who work with families in their homes also have the privilege of observing furnishings, toys, and other material resources; daily routines; family photos and memorabilia; and more "natural" interactions among family members. Such information may be valuable in developing the family service plan, but the professional should be careful to ask families if they want it to be included; *they* may see such inclusion as intrusive and inappropriate.

Observation may be the most appropriate method to use in the case of some culturally diverse families that are suspicious of questionnaires or uncomfortable revealing personal information in the verbal format of an interview. In general, though, observation should only be used to *supplement* information obtained in other ways. The observer who is not familiar with a family's lifestyle and interaction patterns may draw incorrect inferences about the family's concerns and priorities. Thus, he or she should always *ask* family members about observed behaviors (e.g., "I see that your children are playing very well together; do they always cooperate so nicely?").

Home visits are almost essential for professionals who want to get to know families well. Recommended courses of action that seem to make sense in an office or at a center may not work at all in the home environment. Some homes are very small and cramped, with many people (both related and unrelated) living together. In other cases, the impact of many siblings all needing attention at the same time cannot be fully understood outside the home setting. Only through observation in the home can the professional be reasonably confident that a plan will work for a given child and family.

Writing the Plan

In deciding which methods to use in identifying family concerns and priorities for the plan, the practitioner should try to simplify the identification process as much as possible. Most families resent having to fill out numerous forms or submit to more than one interview; unfortunately, when a professional first meets a family, the family has probably already been asked many questions by intake workers or professionals in other agencies. Intrusion into a family's private life should be kept to a minimum, and only methods that are truly necessary for an understanding of the family's situation should be used.

After the needs identification process has been completed, the professional and the family collaborate to write the service plan. Many or most of the written outcomes in the plan will relate to the child; many guidelines exist in the educational literature for developing such outcomes based on an assessment of the child. We will not concern ourselves here with outcomes that relate specifically to the child (e.g., "Johnny will learn to walk"). Rather, we consider the process of developing outcomes that relate to the *family*.

In order to be sure that all possible areas of family concern have been addressed, the professional should check to see that all of the areas noted above are included: information and formal, informal, and material support. Not all families have concerns in all areas; however, listing a family's *resources* in all areas can be helpful in fostering family empowerment. For example, even if parents express no concerns regarding the technical support (intervention) their child is receiving, a statement such as the following might be included: "The Smiths are satisfied with Johnny's medical care and are pleased with the progress he has made in the early intervention program; they do not have any concerns in this area at the present time."

Examples of action steps based on expressed concerns in each area follow:

Area of concern	*Suggested action*
1. Information (e.g., parent wants more information about child's disability)	1. Provide information or make referral to appropriate professional.
2. Informal support (e.g., parents are concerned because grandparents will not acknowledge child's disability)	2. Provide information to grandparents and provide or make referral to grandparent support group.

3. Formal support (e.g., parent is concerned because child is 3 years old and not yet talking)

3. Provide speech therapy or make appropriate referral.

4. Material support (e.g., parents do not have enough money to meet child's needs)

4. Refer to appropriate community resources (e.g., supplemental security income [SSI])

In some cases, resources may not be readily available in the community to meet identified needs. For example, babysitters trained to care for children who have seizure disorders or who are dependent on highly technical medical equipment may be difficult to locate. In such instances, professionals may wish to explore the possibility of starting new programs or help parents advocate for the creation of such programs. Advocacy involves knowledge of legal parameters and family rights, research skills to identify successful models and funding sources that may exist elsewhere, grant-writing skills, and political skills such as organizing and lobbying. (The role of the professional as an advocate is discussed in Chapter 11. (Further information about advocacy techniques can be found in Alper, Schloss, & Schloss [1996] and Richan [1991], amoing other sources.) The actual service plan also contains (1) time frames within which activities will occur and (2) outcomes that are expected to be achieved as a result of these activities.

The degree to which programs are able to meet all of the needs expressed by families varies considerably. Programs that employ appropriately trained psychologists may be able to provide family counseling in accordance with the model suggested in Chapter 12. Programs without such resources will need to make referrals to other agencies or professionals. Some needs may not be able to be met at all (e.g., the need for a cure, in the case of chronic or terminal illness); in such cases, the professional may only be able to help the family cope.

Other needs are the result of major social problems that cannot be corrected through intervention by helping professionals. For example, many material needs reflect a family's underlying poverty; intervention at the family level cannot change the stratified structure of society or an economy that does not provide enough jobs that pay a living wage for all people. Sociologists refer to concerns such as poverty or racism as *macro-level* or social problems. Human services are generally designed to address *micro-* or *meso-level* concerns that derive from problems in the family itself (micro) or in the service system or community (meso). The interventions that are suggested in this chapter involve changing a family's opportunity structure through the expansion of resources at the meso-level. (Micro-level interventions were discussed in Chapter 12.)

Programs that do have competent psychologists or counselors on staff should not necessarily include clinical treatment outcomes for families. Just as all children do not need physical therapy, all parents do not need counseling. The methods described in this chapter allow the family to define its own needs. In some cases, the professional might not agree with the family's definitions; however, professionals do not have the right to impose their judgments on families. Except in extreme cases such as child abuse, the family's wishes should prevail. As noted earlier, this model of family-centered and family-directed services is supported by recent practice and legislation in the fields of both early intervention and maternal and child health, among others.

The application of the methods of questionnaire administration, interviewing, and observation to service plan development is best illustrated through a case example. The case described below is a fictitious composite of several real families in an early intervention program. (The complete case description also appears in Darling & Baxter, 1996.)

Case Example: The Torres Family

This family consists of 3-month-old Amanda, who was just discharged from a neonatal intensive care unit; her 2-year-old brother, Raymond; her 4-year-old sister, Jennifer; and her 21-year-old mother, Elena. Amanda was born prematurely at 32 weeks' gestation. She had an intraventricular hemorrhage shortly after birth, developed hydrocephalus, and underwent surgery to have a shunt inserted to drain the fluid from her head. She had seizures right after the surgery, but these seem to be under control now. Amanda has been referred to a local early intervention program.

Observation

Elena brings the baby to the early intervention center for a team assessment. Kate (child development specialist), Susan (speech therapist), Paul (physical therapist), and Nancy (occupational therapist) are involved. They notice that Elena seems tired and has a bruise under one eye. Raymond and Jennifer seem quiet. Amanda is wearing a pink dress that looks new and a matching bonnet and booties.

Barbara (social worker) makes a home visit. She sees that the family lives in a cramped, sparsely furnished, two-bedroom apartment in a run-down building. She does not see any toys. The paint on the baby's crib is peeling. The older children are sitting at a kitchen table eating their breakfast—cereal and milk. It is 1 P.M. and they have just awakened. Elena looks as though she has been crying.

Interview

Because the family has just entered the early intervention program, they are assigned a service coordinator, Judy, by the Department of Human Services, which funds the program. Judy meets with the family when they arrive at the center for Amanda's team assessment and asks for some background information, including Amanda's birth history, her hospital course, and how she has been doing since she has been home.

Elena tells her that Amanda seems to be doing all right, although she seems sleepy all the time. Elena is worried about the possibility of another seizure. Judy also asks Elena for some additional information about the family, including household composition and who cares for the baby. She learns that Elena lives alone with the children; she is the only caregiver.

Barbara conducts a more in-depth interview during her home visit but does not repeat questions Judy has already asked. The format Barbara follows is the one suggested earlier in this chapter. As a result of this interview, Barbara learns that Elena comes from a large family. One of her sisters lives a few blocks away from her, but the rest of the family lives in another state.

Elena dropped out of high school in her senior year while she was pregnant with Jennifer. She lived with Jennifer's father, Joe, for a while and planned to marry him, but while she was pregnant with Raymond, Joe started seeing other women. They had arguments, which were sometimes violent. Elena says that her mother was not supportive because "they didn't want me to live with Joe in the first place." As a result, Elena reports that she moved to the state where she currently resides to be near her sister, who paid her moving expenses.

Elena met Amanda's father, Mike, shortly after moving here. He was very nice to her at first and brought presents for her and the children. He was employed and, until recently when he lost his job, contributed toward the family's support. After that, Elena and Mike began to argue frequently. He would drink and become abusive toward her. Elena says that she does not see Mike very often now and that he has no interest in Amanda; however, he made one of his infrequent visits the previous night.

When Barbara asks Elena how she feels about Amanda's medical problems, Elena says, "Scared." She says she is afraid that the baby will have a seizure or that the shunt will malfunction and she will not know what to do. She explains that she has no experience with problems of this kind—her other children were "normal." Barbara asks Elena about her resources. She learns that the family receives public assistance (Temporary Assistance to Needy Families, or TANF) and that Elena's sister, Maria, who has a clerical job, helps them some, but "we still don't have enough to pay the bills." Maria also helps a little with babysitting, but she works full time and has two school-age children of her own, including one who is "hyperactive." Elena says she has no close friends. Her neighbors are "nice, but they have enough of their own problems." Barbara notes that the family applied for TANF only after Mike stopped supporting them. Elena has some time before she will need to look for work; TANF time limits will need to be addressed in the future, though.

Elena reports that her other two children are healthy. Jennifer goes to Head Start and really likes it. She says that Mike has never hurt, or threatened to hurt, any of her children.

As for her own health, Elena notes that she has had intermittent bleeding since Amanda was born and that she always feels tired. When asked, she says she has no regular doctor for herself but has recently found a pediatrician she likes for the children, and he accepts the medical (assistance) card. Barbara asks if she has any difficulty getting to medical or early intervention appointments. Elena says she usually takes the bus, but that taking three young children on the bus is not easy.

Barbara asks if Elena needs anything for herself or the children. Elena says she could use a new crib; the one she got from a neighbor is not in good condition. She says she gets food stamps and help from the Women, Infants, and Children Program (WIC) and usually has enough food in the house, "but we can't afford anything extra that the kids want." She says she does not need clothes for the baby—she has "hand-me-downs" from Jennifer and her sister's children. She does not have enough money to buy the children the nice toys they should have, however. Throughout the interview Elena says often that she wants the best for her children.

Questionnaires

Barbara asks Elena if she would like to fill out the PNS "in case there's something I forgot to ask you about," but Elena declines. Judy has told

Barbara that Elena seemed to have difficulty with the intake forms at the early intervention center, so Barbara does not try to encourage her to complete the form.

Because she does not see any toys in the home, Barbara asks Elena to complete the toy checklist from the HOME Screening Questionnaire (JFK Child Development Center, 1981). She offers to read it to her, and Elena accepts her offer. The results indicate that the family does not have most of the items on the list. The only age-appropriate toys that Elena has for Amanda are a few rattles.

Developing Family Outcomes

In reviewing all the information that has been gathered, Elena and the team list the family's resources and concerns, as illustrated in Table 13.1. They note the following priorities:

1. Help with medical concerns about the baby.
2. Not having to take the children on the bus for Amanda's physical therapy appointment, scheduled for later this week.

TABLE 13.1. The Torres Family's Resources and Concerns

Area	Resources	Concerns
Information	Elena knows about child development in general, because she has two older children.	Elena would like more information about hydrocephalus and seizure management.
Formal support	Elena is satisfied with Amanda's medical care. Jennifer is enrolled in Head Start. Elena is interested in learning more about agencies that can help her family.	Elena is concerned about getting to the early intervention center by bus. Elena could use more help with child care. Elena would like medical care for herself.
Informal support	Jennifer and Raymond are healthy. Elena's sister helps with babysitting when she can.	Although she does not desire assistance at present, Elena is interested in learning more about dealing with Mike's violence.
Material support	The family receives support from TANF, food stamps, and WIC and some help from Elena's sister and from neighbors. Amanda has enough clothes; she has some toys.	Elena would like a crib and more toys for Amanda. Elena would like more help with meeting household expenses.

Based on this prioritized list, the following service plan outcomes are written:

INFORMATION

Outcome: Elena will have the knowledge she desires regarding hydrocephalus and seizure management.

Service activities: Barbara will immediately make a referral to the public health nurse, who will make home visits to provide information and support to Elena regarding hydrocephalus and seizure management.

Rationale: Because of Elena's apparent difficulty with printed material, modeling and discussion appear to be better in this case than booklets, handouts, and library references.

INFORMAL/FORMAL SUPPORT

Outcome: All early intervention services will be home based; Elena will receive the medical care she desires; Elena will receive child care services in addition to those she receives informally from her sister; Elena will have information about resources available for victims of domestic violence.

Service activities:

1. Judy [service coordinator] will make arrangements for all early intervention services to be provided through home visits rather than at the center. These services will begin immediately.
2. Barbara will give Elena a list of family doctors and ob–gyn specialists who accept the medical card and are easily accessible with public transportation.
3. Barbara will make a referral to the free babysitting program offered by the Association for Children with Special Needs.
4. Barbara will give Elena information about the support group for abused women and other services at the Women's Help Center.

Rationale: During their discussion, Elena indicated to Barbara that she was "not ready" for Barbara to make a referral; she wanted the information so she could call and get help "when she needed it." She said she would call if Mike hit her again.

If the children were being abused, Barbara would have an ethical (and probably legal) obligation to report the situation to children's protective services. In the current circumstances, however, she should respect Elena's decision. She will continue to work very closely with her and encourage her to seek help, if necessary. Such situations always involve a delicate balance between respecting a family's privacy and doing what the professional considers to be best for the family.

5. Barbara will give Elena information about the "Moms of Tots" support group that meets monthly at a church near her home.

Rationale: Elena expressed considerable interest in this group when Barbara explained that this church-sponsored group included other young mothers like herself and that babysitting was provided. Elena was not interested in the early intervention program's support group, which included only parents of children with disabilities.

MATERIAL SUPPORT

Outcome: Elena will obtain a new crib and toys for the children; Elena will know about additional sources of financial support.
Service activities:

1. Barbara will assist Elena in locating a crib at the Salvation Army store or another thrift shop.
2. Barbara will assist Elena in applying for Supplemental Security Income (SSI) for Amanda. (She assumes that Elena's TANF caseworker is investigating the possibility of child support from the children's fathers.)
3. Kate [the child development specialist] will review the agency's toy-lending library list with Elena and will bring to the home the toys that Elena selects (both for Amanda and the other children).

The outcomes and activities listed above would not constitute the entire service plan. Typically, the plan would include outcomes for the child, in addition to family outcomes such as those listed above. For a child like Amanda, those outcomes would probably focus on facilitating her achievement of normal developmental milestones in the motor, cognitive, language, and social areas. In the past, service plans included *only* child outcomes; today, plans must include family outcomes as well. In the case of a two-parent family, the interventionist would identify the concerns and priorities of both parents and develop outcomes addressing each of their concerns separately. Similarly, in cases in which grandparents or other relatives are part of the household unit, they would be included in the identification process as well. The resulting plan would reflect the concerns of all family members.

CHILDREN AND FAMILIES: A SUMMARY

Professionals who work with children who have disabilities must recognize the resources and concerns of the family as a whole. Professionals working in medical and educational settings historically developed a kind of tunnel vision—that is, they focused exclusively on the child as patient, student, or client and ignored the world within which the child lived. In recent years, human services have broadened that focus because of the inescapable recognition that children and their families are clinically inseparable.

The process described above for the development of family service plans can be used, to some extent, in any kind of helping relationship between professionals and families. Regardless of professional discipline, all those who work with families need to address the family's location in society. Not all families have equal access to resources and opportunities; families also differ in their priorities for their children. In the case illustration above, the mother was most concerned about her baby's medical needs. A professional evaluating the same case might have listed the father's abuse of the mother as the primary concern. Professionals need to take their lead from families. They need to listen to what family members are saying, especially when their own ideas about appropriate intervention approaches are different from those of the family.

In this book we have tried to show how a child's disability has an impact on mothers, fathers, siblings, grandparents, and all other family members whose lives intersect with the child's life. These family members, in turn, play the most important role in shaping the child's future. Families are circles of interaction, and all of their members affect one another. Professionals who treat children must acknowledge families, the cultural worlds within which those families live, and the right of families to determine their own destiny.

In review, then, we have looked at childhood disability from the broad perspective of both *family systems* and *social systems*. Chapters 1 and 2 reviewed the sociological and psychological literature on social and family systems and showed the relevance of this literature for professionals working with families of children with disabilities. Chapter 3 explored the social system in greater depth and showed the importance of social and cultural diversity in shaping families' opportunities, beliefs, values, and lifestyles. Society and culture shape the effect of a child's disability on the family as a whole, as well as the family's interaction within a social world of friends, relatives, professionals, and strangers. The family's definition of its situation is the product of all of these interactional experiences. If professionals want to understand families, they must come to understand their interactional worlds.

Specifically, as Chapter 4 suggests, families are located in social worlds long before their children are born. These worlds provide families with definitions of children and of disabilities, and these definitions shape family reactions to a child's birth and diagnosis. Preexisting definitions, however, generally prepare families poorly for the birth of a child with a disability. As a result, families strive to overcome their initial reaction of anomie and to reestablish meaning in, and control over, their lives. Children themselves play an important role in this definitional process as they grow and develop and respond to their families' attempts at interacting with them.

As Chapter 5 indicates, the period of acute anomie usually ends with infancy. After their initial needs for information and intervention for their child have been satisfied, most families are able to maintain a normalized lifestyle. As long as the surrounding social system is supportive, families who have children with disabilities can return to the routines of career, household, and recreational pursuits during the years of childhood and adolescence. However, new concerns may emerge during adolescence and early adulthood. For some families, normalization remains elusive through most or all of the childhood period. When formal and informal sources of support are not available or other family members have overwhelming problems, a child's disability can have a continuing, negative impact on a family's lifestyle.

Virtually all parents want their children to become happy, productive adults, and professionals who work with families try to help them attain that goal. Chapter 6 explores the outcomes for children with disabilities by examining the range of identities and orientations toward disability that exists among adults. The chapter shows how adult identities are being shaped by social forces, including the disability rights movement, and suggests some strategies that parents can use to prepare their children for the future.

As Chapters 7 through 10 reveal, childhood disability can have both positive and negative effects on mothers, fathers, siblings, grandparents, and other family members. Each of these family members experiences the child's disability in a different way and is differently positioned to contribute to either positive or negative outcomes for the child and the family. These family experiences are always shaped by the availability of resources in the family's social world.

The first 10 chapters, then, further our understanding of the social and personal worlds of the family. Chapter 11 shows what happens when these worlds intersect with that of the professional. Many professionals have been trained to hold a clinical worldview, which is different from the perspective of the family. The clinical view tends to define children and families narrowly in terms of a disability category or value-based label. The family, on the other hand, tends to define its situation within the broader parameters of its various interactional contexts. The difference in perspectives can result in conflict when families and professionals interact. Recently, a number of professional fields have been moving away from a clinical worldview toward a more system-based perspective.

Finally, Chapters 12 and 13 attempt to apply the systems perspective developed in earlier chapters to actual interventions with families. Sometimes family relationships become inordinately disturbed, and families express a need for professional intervention. Chapter 12 describes a family systems approach to providing counseling in such situations. In this approach, the interactions among family members become the locus of concern. The present chapter suggests a model for applying the social system perspective in developing family service plans. By rejecting a traditional clinical assessment in favor of identifying family-defined concerns and priorities, professionals and families can work together to develop system-based outcomes. Tools such as the PNS do not impose an external interpretation on a family's definition of the situation. We hope that an increasing recognition of, and respect for, the family's point of view will result in the development of similarly based instruments in all professional disciplines in the field.

Since the first edition of this book was published in 1989, a number of professional disciplines have moved closer to a systems model. Examples abound in the fields of education, social work, medicine, and child development, among others, of approaches that take the whole family into account. A growing interest in cultural diversity also reflects increasing awareness of the family's location in a social world. We have tried to record some of these changes throughout the book.

We hope that this edition has not only recorded, but will also contribute to, this trend.

Families are our greatest resource. They provide individuals with their earliest emotional and educational experiences. Children from strong families have the opportunity to become strong adults. Professionals cannot help children without the help of families. Only through a family–professional partnership can effective intervention occur. Professionals, then, must work to understand the world in which a child lives—the world of the family.

Families, in turn, reside within larger social structures. They are parts of systems of beliefs, values, and behaviors that shape their thinking and actions. Reactions to childhood disability are social products resulting from a lifetime of interactional experiences. If we truly want to help families, we must do it on their terms, within the context of *their* system of meaning. Only through such a systems perspective can we hope to improve the quality of life for ordinary families who happen to have children with out-of-the-ordinary needs.

References

Abbott, A. (2004). My mother's warnings. In S. D. Klein & J. D. Kemo (Eds.), *Reflections from a different journey: What adults with disabilities wish all parents knew* (pp. 140–144). New York: McGraw-Hill.

Ablon, J. (1982). The parents' auxiliary of Little People of America: A self-help model for social support for families of short-statured children. In L. D. Borman (Ed.), *Helping people to help themselves* (pp. 31–46). New York: Haworth Press.

Adams, M. (1973). Science, technology, and some dilemmas of advocacy. *Science, 180*, 840–842.

Adams, P. N., & Nelson, K. (Eds.). (1995). *Reinventing human services: Community- and family-centered practice*. New York: Aldine deGruyter.

Adapting research to cultures and countries. (1995–1996, Fall–Winter). *Impact: World Institute on Disability Semi Annual Report, p. 5.*

Agee, L. C., Innocenti, M., & Boyce, G. C. (1995). I'm all stressed out: The impact of parenting stress on the effectiveness of a parent involvement program. *Center for Persons with Disabilities News, 8*, 4–7.

Albrecht, G. L., & Devlieger, P. J. (1999). The disability paradox: High quality of life against all odds. *Social Science and Medicine, 48*, 977–988.

Alper, S. K., Schloss, P. J., & Schloss, C. N. (1994). *Families of students with disabilities: Consultation and advising*. Boston: Allyn & Bacon.

Alper, S. K., Schloss, P. J., & Schloss, C. N. (1996). Families of children with disabilities in elementary and middle school: Advocacy models and strategies. *Exceptional Children, 62*(3), 261–270.

Altman, B. M. (1997). Parents and children, children and parents: The disability context. *Disability Studies Quarterly, 17*(3), 154–156.

Altman, B. M., & Rasch, E. K. (2003). Disability among Native Americans. *Research in Social Science and Disability, 3*, 299–326.

Alvard, M. K., & Grados, J. J. (2005). Enhancing resilience in children: A proactive approach. *Professional Psychology: Research and Practice, 36*, 238–245.

Alvirez, D., & Bean, F. D. (1976). The Mexican-American family. In C. H. Mindel & R.

381

W. Habenstein (Eds.), *Ethnic families in America: Patterns and variations* (pp. 271–292). New York: Elsevier.

Anderegg, M. L., Vergason, G. A., & Smith, M. C. (1992). A visual presentation of the grief cycle for use by teachers with families of children with disabilities. *Remedial and Special Education, 13,* 17–23.

Anderson, P. (1988). *Serving culturally diverse populations of infants and toddlers with disabilities.* Washington, DC: Society for Disability Studies.

Anderton, J. M., Elfert, H., & Lai, M. (1989). Ideology in the clinical context: Chronic illness, ethnicity and the discourse of normalisation. *Sociology of Health and Illness, 11,* 253–258.

Andrew, G. (1968). Determinants of Negro family decisions in management of retardation. *Journal of Marriage and the Family, 30,* 612–617.

Anspach, R. R. (1979). From stigma to identity politics: Political activism among the physically disabled and former mental patients. *Social Science and Medicine, 13A,* 765–773.

Anspach, R. R. (1993). *Deciding who lives: Fateful choices in the intensive-care nursery.* Berkeley: University of California Press.

Appoloni, T. (1987, November/December). Guardianship: New options for parents. *Exceptional Parent,* pp. 24–48.

Arango, G. A. (2001). What can I say? In S. D. Klein & K. Schive (Eds.), *You will dream new dreams: Inspiring stories by parents of children with disabilities.* New York: Kensington Books.

Ariel, C. N., & Naseef, R. A. (2006). *Voices from the spectrum.* London: Jessica Kingsley.

Aswad, B. C. (1997). Arab American families. In M. K. DeGenova (Ed.), *Families in cultural context: Strengths and challenges in diversity* (pp. 213–237). Mountain View, CA: Mayfield.

Attneave, C. (1982). American Indians and Alaska Native families: Emigrants in their own homeland. In M. McGoldrick, J. K. Pearce, & J. Giordano (Eds.), *Ethnicity and family therapy* (pp. 55–83). New York: Guilford Press.

Ayer, S. (1984). Community care: The failure of professionals to meet the family needs. *Child: Health and Development, 10,* 127–140.

Azar, B. (1994). Research plumbs why the "talking cure" works. *APA Monitor,* p. 24.

Azziz, R. (1981). The Hispanic parent. *Pennsylvania Medicine,* pp. 22–25.

Baca Zinn, M., & Pok, A. Y. H. (2002). Tradition and transition in Mexican-origin families. In R. J. Taylor (Ed.), *Minority families in the United States: A multicultural perspective* (3rd ed., pp. 79–100). Upper Saddle River, NJ: Prentice Hall.

Baca Zinn, M., & Wells, B. (2000). Diversity within Latino families: New lessons for family social science. In D. H. Demo, K. R. Allen, & M. A. Fine (Eds.), *Handbook of family diversity* (pp. 252–273). New York: Oxford University Press.

Bach, J. R., & Tilton, M. C. (1994). Life satisfaction and well-being measures in ventilator assisted individuals with traumatic tetraplegia. *Archives of Physical Medicine and Rehabilitation, 75,* 626–632.

Bailey, D. B., Jr., & Simeonsson, R. J. (1984). Critical issues underlying research and intervention with families of young handicapped children. *Journal of the Division for Early Childhood, 9,* 38–48.

Bailey, D. B., Jr., Simeonsson, R. J., Winton, P. J., Huntington, G. S., Comfort, M. I., P., O'Donnell, K. J., et al. (1986). Family-focused intervention: A functional model for planning, implementing, and evaluating individual family services in early intervention. *Journal of the Division for Early Childhood, 10,* 156–171.

Bailey, D. B., Jr., Skinner, D., Rodriguez, P., Gut, D., & Correa, V. (1999). Awareness, use, and satisfaction with services for Latino parents of young children with disabilities. *Exceptional Children, 65*(3), 367–381.

Bailey, D. B., Jr., & Wolery, M. R. (1984). *Teaching infants and preschoolers with handicaps.* Columbus, OH: Merrill.

Baker, B. L. (1989). *Parent training and developmental disabilities.* Washington, DC: American Association on Mental Retardation.

Bank, S. P., & Kahn, M. D. (1997). *The sibling bond* (2nd ed.). New York: Basic Books.

Banks, M. E., & Kaschak, E. (2003). *Women with visible and invisible disabilities.* New York: Haworth Press.

Baranowski, M. D. (1982). Grandparent–adolescent relations: Beyond the nuclear family. *Adolescence, 17,* 574–584.

Baranowski, M. D., & Schilmoeller, G. L. (1999). Grandparents in the lives of grandchildren: Mothers' perceptions. *Education and Treatment of Children, 22,* 427–446.

Barkley, R. A. (2004, July). ADHD and Mom's love. *Monitor on Psychology,* p. 11.

Barnett, W. D. (1995). Effects of children with Down syndrome on parents' activities. *American Journal on Mental Retardation, 100,* 115–127.

Barnwell, D. A., & Day, M. (1996). Providing support to diverse families. In P. J. Beckman (Ed.), *Strategies for working with families of young children with disabilities* (pp. 47–68). Baltimore: Brookes.

Barrera, M., Chung, J. Y. Y., Greenberg, M., & Fleming, C. (2002). Preliminary investigation of a group intervention for siblings of pediatric cancer patients. *Children's Health Care, 3,* 131–142.

Bartz, K. W., & Levine, E. S. (1978). Childbearing by black parents: A description and comparison to Anglo and Chicano parents. *Journal of Marriage and the Family, 40,* 709–719.

Batshaw, M. L. (Ed.). (2002). *Children with disabilities* (5th ed.). Baltimore: Brookes.

Bauer, A. M., & Shea, T. M. (2003). *Parents and schools: Creating a successful partnership.* Upper Saddle River, NJ: Merrill/Prentice Hall.

Baxter, C. (1986). *Intellectual disability: Parental perceptions and stigma as stress.* Victoria, Australia: Monash University.

Baxter, C. (1987). Professional services as support: Perceptions of parents. *Australia and New Zealand Journal of Developmental Disabilities, 13,* 243–253.

Beach Center on Families and Disability. (1997, Spring). Families make transition happen. *Families and Disability Newsletter,* p. 4.

Beatty, L. A. (2003). Substance abuse, disabilities, and black women. In M. E. Banks & E. Kashak (Eds.), *Women with visible and invisible disabilities* (pp. 223–236). New York: Haworth Press.

Beckman, P. J. (1983). Influence of selected child characteristics on stress in families of handicapped infants. *American Journal on Mental Deficiency, 88,* 150–156.

Beckman, P. J. (2002). Providing family-centered care. In M. L. Batshaw (Ed.), *Children with disabilities* (5th ed., pp. 683–691). Baltimore: Brookes.

Beckman, P. J., & Porkorni, J. L. (1988). A longitudinal study of families of preterm infants: Change in stress and support over the first two years. *Journal of Special Education, 22,* 66–75.

Beinart, P. (1997, August 9). Jews, Latinos and the US political landscape. *The [Toronto] Globe and Mail,* p. 21.

Benson, B. A., & Gross, A. M. (1989). The effect of a congenitally handicapped child upon the marital dyad. *Clinical Psychology Review, 9,* 747–758.

Berg, J. M., Gilderdale, S., & Way, J. (1969). On telling parents of the diagnosis of Mongolism. *British Journal of Psychiatry, 115,* 1195–1196.

Berg, R. C., Landreth, G. L., & Fall, K. A. (2006). *Group counseling: Concepts and procedures*. New York: Routledge.

Berger, M., & Foster, M. (1986). Applications of family therapy theory to research and interventions with families with mentally retarded children. In J. J. Gallagher & P. M. Vietze (Eds.), *Families of handicapped persons* (pp. 251–260). Baltimore: Brookes.

Bernard, A. W. (1974). A comparative study of marital integration and sibling role tension differences between families who have a severely mentally retarded child and families of non-handicapped. *Dissertation Abstracts International, 35*(5), 2800A–2801A.

Bernheim, K. F., & Lehman, A. (1985). *Working with families of the mentally ill*. New York: Norton.

Berry, J. O., & Hardman, M. L. (1998). *Lifespan perspectives on the family and disability*. Boston: Allyn & Bacon.

Berube, M. (1996). *Life as we know it: A father, a family, and an exceptional child*. New York: Vintage Books.

Betz, M., & O'Connell, L. (1983). Changing doctor–patient relationships and the rise in concern for accountability. *Social Problems, 31*, 84–95.

Beveridge, C. J. (2001). I am a father. In S. D. Klein & K. Schieve (Eds.), *You will dream new dreams: Inspiring personal stories by parents of children with disabilities* (pp. 81–84). New York: Kensington Books.

Beyer, H. A. (1986). Estate planning: Providing for your child's future. *Exceptional Parent*, pp. 12–18.

Biegel, D. E., Sales, E., & Schulz, R. (1991). *Family care giving in chronic illness*. Newbury Park, CA: Sage.

Biklen, D. (1974). *Let our children go: An organizing manual for advocates and parents*. Syracuse, NY: Human Policy Press.

Biller, H. B., & Kimpton, J. L. (1997). The father and the school aged child. In M. E. Lamb (Ed.), *The role of the father in child development* (3rd ed., pp. 143–161). New York: Wiley.

Birenbaum, A. (1970). On managing a courtesy stigma. *Journal of Health and Social Behavior, 11*, 196–206.

Birenbaum, A. (1971). The mentally retarded child in the home and the family cycle. *Journal of Health and Social Behavior, 12*, 55–65.

Blacher, J. (1984a). A dynamic perspective on the impact of a severely handicapped child on the family. In J. Blacher (Ed.), *Severely handicapped young children and their families: Research in review* (pp. 196–228). Orlando, FL: Academic Press.

Blacher, J. (1984b). Sequential stages of parental adjustment to the birth of a child with handicaps: Fact or artifact? *Mental Retardation, 22*, 55–68.

Blacher, J. (Ed.). (1984c). *Severely handicapped young children and their families: Research in review*. Orlando, FL: Academic Press.

Blacher, J. (2003). The sunny side of the street: Multi-national family research. *Exceptional Parent Magazine*, pp. 77–79.

Blacher, J., Nihira, K., & Meyers, C. E. (1987). Characteristics of home environments of families with mentally retarded children: Comparison across levels of retardation. *American Journal on Mental Deficiency, 91*, 313–320.

Blackard, M. K., & Barsch, E. T. (1982). Parents' and professionals' perceptions of the handicapped child's impact on the family. *TASH Journal, 7*, 62–70.

Blue-Banning, M., Summers, J. A., Frankland, H. C., Nelson, L. L., & Beegle, G. (2004). Dimensions of family and professional partnerships: Constructive guidelines for collaboration. *Exceptional Children, 70*(2), 167–184.

Blumberg, B. D., Lewis, M. J., & Susman, E. J. (1984). Adolescence: A time of transition. In M. G. Eisenberg, L. C. Sutkin, & M. A. Jansen (Eds.), *Chronic illness and disability through the life span: Effects on self and family* (pp. 133–149). New York: Springer.

Blumberg, L. (2004). The virtues of "ballpark normalcy." In S. D. Klein & J. D. Kemp (Eds.), *Reflections from a different journey: What adults with disabilities wish all parents knew* (pp. 23–26). New York: McGraw-Hill.

Boles, G. (1959). Personality factors in mothers of cerebral palsied children. *Genetic Psychology Monographs, 59*, 160–218.

Bonilla-Santiago, G. (1996). Latino battered women: Barriers to service delivery and cultural considerations. In A. R. Roberts (Ed.), *Helping battered women: New perspectives and remedies* (pp. 229–234). New York: Oxford University Press.

Bowen, M. (1978). *Family therapy in clinical practice*. New York: Aronson.

Bowlby, J. (1951). *Maternal care and mental health*. Geneva: World Health Organization.

Bowman, B. T. (1992). Who is at risk for what and why? *Journal of Early Intervention, 16*(2), 101–108.

Boyd, B. A. (2002). Examining the relationship between stress and lack of support in mothers of children with autism. *Focus on Autism and Other Developmental Disabilities, 17*, 208–215.

Boyce, G. C., & Barnett, S. W. (1991). *Siblings of persons with mental retardation: A historical perspective and recent findings*. Unpublished manuscript, Utah State University.

Brewer, E. J., Jr., McPherson, M., Magrab, P. R., & Hutchins, V.L. (1989). Family-centered, community-based, coordinated care for children with special health care needs. *Pediatrics, 83*, 1055–1060.

Brinthaupt, J. (1991). Pediatric chronic illness, cystic fibrosis, and parental adjustment. In M. Seligman (Ed.), *The family with a handicapped child* (2nd ed., pp. 295–336). Boston: Allyn & Bacon.

Bristol, M. M. (1984). Family resources and successful adaptation to autistic children. In E. Schopler & G. B. Mesibov (Eds.), *The effects of autism on the family* (pp. 289–310). New York: Plenum Press.

Bristol, M. M. (1987). Methodological caveats in the assessment of single-parent families of handicapped children. *Journal of the Division for Early Childhood, 11*, 135–143.

Bristol, M. M., & Schopler, E. (1984). A developmental perspective on stress and coping in families of autistic children. In J. Blacher (Ed.), *Severely handicapped young children and their families: Research in review* (pp. 91–141). Orlando, FL: Academic Press.

Bronfenbrenner, U. (1979). *The ecology of human development*. Cambridge, MA: Harvard University Press.

Bronfenbrenner, U. (1990). Discovering what families do. In D. Blankenhorn, S. Bayme, & J. B. Elshtain (Eds.), *Rebuilding the nest: A new commitment to the American family* (pp. 27–38). Milwaukee, WI: Family Service America.

Brotherson, M. J., Backus, L. H., Summers, J. A., & Turnbull, A. P. (1986). Transition to adulthood. In J. A. Summers (Ed.), *The right to grow up: An introduction to adults with developmental disabilities* (pp. 17–44). Baltimore: Brookes.

Brown, I., Anand, S., Fung, W., Isaacs, B., & Baum, N. (2003). Family quality of life: Canadian results from an international study. *Journal of Developmental and Physical Disabilities, 15*, 207–229.

Browner, C. H., Preloran, H.M., & Cox, S.J. (1999). Ethnicity, bioethics, and prenatal diagnosis: The amniocentesis decisions of Mexican-origin women and their partners. *American Journal of Public Health, 89*, 1658–1666.

Bubolz, M. M., & Whiren, A. P. (1984). The family of the handicapped: An ecological model for policy and practice. *Family Relations, 33,* 5–12.

Bumpass, L. L., Sweet, J. A., & Cherlin, A. (1998). The Role of cohabitation in declining rates of marriage. In S. J. Ferguson (Ed.), *Shifting the center: Understanding contemporary families* (pp. 146–160). Mountain View, CA: Mayfield.

Butler, J. A., Rosenbaum, S., & Palfrey, J. S. (1987). Ensuring access to health care for children with disabilities. *New England Journal of Medicine, 317*(3), 162–165.

Byrnes, A. L., Berk, N. W., Cooper, M. F., & Marazita, M. L. (2003). Parental evaluation of informing interviews for cleft lip and/or palate. *Pediatrics, 112*(2), 308–314.

Caldwell, B., & Guze, S. (1960). A study of the adjustment of parents and siblings of institutionalized and noninstitutionalized retarded children. *American Journal of Mental Deficiency, 64,* 839–844.

Cameron, G., & Vanderwoerd, J. (1997). *Protecting children and supporting families: Promising programs and organizational realities* . New York: Aldine de Gruyter.

Camp cares for handicapped kids. (1986, April 18). *Johnstown [PA] Tribune Democrat,* p. 5C.

Cantwell, D. P., & Baker, L. (1984). Research concerning families of children with autism. In E. Schopler & G. B. Mesibov (Eds.), *The effects of autism on the family* (pp. 41–63). New York: Plenum Press.

Capper, C. (1990). Students with low incidence disabilities in disadvantaged, rural settings. *Exceptional Children, 56*(4), 338–344.

Carolan, M. T. (1999). Contemporary Muslim women and the family. In H. P. McAdoo (Ed.), *Family ethnicity: Strength in diversity* (2nd ed., pp. 213–221). Thousand Oaks, CA: Sage.

Carr, E. G., Horner, R. H., Turnbull, A. P., Marquis, J. G., Magito-McLaughlin, D., & McAtee, M. L. (1999). *Positive behavioral support as an approach for dealing with problem behavior in people with developmental disabilities: A research synthesis.* Washington, DC: American Association on Mental Retardation Monograph Series.

Carr, J. (1970). Mongolism: Telling the parents. *Developmental Medicine and Child Neurology, 12,* 213.

Carr, J. (1988). Six-weeks to twenty-one years old: A longitudinal study of children with Down syndrome and their families. *Journal of Child Psychology and Psychiatry, 29,* 407–431.

Carrasquillo, H. (2002). The Puerto Rican Family. In R. J. Taylor (Ed.), *Minority families in the United States: A multicultural perspective* (3rd ed., pp. 101–113). Upper Saddle River, NJ: Prentice Hall.

Carter, B., & McGoldrick, M. (1999). Overview: The expanded family life cycle: Individual, family and social perspectives. In B. Carter & M. McGoldrick (Eds.), *The expanded family life cycle: Individual, family and social perspectives* (3rd ed., pp. 135–148). Boston: Allyn & Bacon.

Carter, B., & McGoldrick, M. (2003). *The expanded family life cycle: Individual, family, and child social perspectives* . Boston: Allyn & Bacon.

Case, S. (2000). Refocusing on the parent: What are the social issues of concern for parents of disabled children? *Disability and Society, 15*(2), 271–292.

Case, S. (2001). Learning to partner, disabling conflict: Early indications of an improving relationship between parents and professionals with regard to service provision for children with learning disabilities. *Disability and Society, 16*(6), 837–854.

Chan, S. (1998). Families with Asian roots. In E. W. Lynch & M. J. Hanson (Eds.), *Developing cross-cultural competence: A guide for working with young children and their families* (2nd ed., pp. 251–354). Baltimore: Brookes.

Chan, S., & Lee, E. (2004). Families with Asian roots. In E. W. Lynch & M. J. Hanson

(Eds.), *Developing cross-cultural competence* (3rd ed., pp. 219–298). Baltimore: Brookes.

Charlton, J. I. (1998). *Nothing about us without us: Disability oppression and empowerment* Berkeley: University of California Press.

Chesler, M. (1965). Ethnocentrism and attitudes toward the physically disabled. *Journal of Personality and Social Psychology, 2,* 877–892.

Chesler, M. A., & Barbarin, G. A. (1987). *Childhood cancer and the family.* New York: Brunner/Mazel.

Chigier, E. (1972). *Down's syndrome.* Lexington, MA: Heath.

Children with special health care needs listserv. (1994–1998). Retrieved on various dates (see text) from CHSCN-L@lists.ufl.edu

Cho, S.-J., Singer, G. H. S., & Brenner, M. (2000). Adaptation and accommodation to young children with disabilities: A comparison of Korean and Korean American parents. *Topics in Early Childhood Special Education, 20*(4), 236–250.

Cicirelli, V. G. (1995). *Sibling relationships across the life span.* New York: Plenum Press.

Cigno, K., & Burke, P. (1997). Single mothers of children with learning disabilities: An undervalued group. *Journal of Interprofessional Care, 11,* 177–186.

Clark, M. J., Kendrick, M., Coffin, K., Conway, A., et al. (1996). *"They just don't get it": What families want professionals to know about their children.* Orono: Center for Community Inclusion, University of Maine.

Clemens, A. W., & Axelson, L. J. (1985). The not so empty nest: The return of the fledgling adult. *Family Relations, 34,* 259–264.

Clemens, S. L. (1963). What is man? In C. Neider (Ed.), *The complete essays of Mark Twain* (pp. 132–144). Garden City, NY: Doubleday.

Cleveland, D. W., & Miller, N. (1977). Attitudes and life commitments of older siblings of mentally retarded adults. *Mental Retardation, 15,* 38–41.

Click, J. (1986). Grandparent concerns: Learning to be special. *Sibling Information Network Newsletter, 5,* 3–4.

Cobb, S. (1976). Social support as a moderator of life stress. *Psychosomatic Medicine, 38,* 300–314.

Cohen, R., & Lavach, C. (1995). Strengthening partnerships between families and service providers. In P. Adams & K. Nelson (Eds.), *Reinventing human services: Community- and family-centered practice* (pp. 261–277). New York: Aldine de Gruyter.

Collins-Moore, M. S. (1984). Birth and diagnosis: A family crisis. In M. G. Eisenberg, L. C. Sutkin, & M. A. Jansen (Eds.), *Chronic illness and disability through the life span: Effects on self and family* (pp. 39–46). New York: Springer.

Coltrane, S. (1998). Changing patterns of family work: Chicano men and housework. In S. J. Ferguson (Ed.), *Shifting the center: Understanding contemporary families* (pp. 547–562). Mountain View, CA: Mayfield.

Cook, D. A., & Fine, M. (1995). "Motherwit": Childrearing lessons from African American mothers of low income. In B. B. S. Wadener & S. Lubeck (Eds.), *Children and families "at promise": Deconstructing the discourse of risk* (pp. 118–142). Albany: State University of New York Press.

Cook, R. E., Klein, D. M., & Tessier, A. (2004). *Adapting early childhood curricula for children in inclusive settings* (6th ed.). Upper Saddle River, NJ: Pearson/Merrill/Prentice Hall.

Cooley, C. H. (1964). *Human nature and the social order.* New York: Schocken Books.

Cooley, W. C. (1994). Graduate medical education in pediatrics: Preparing reliable allies for parents of children with special health care needs. In R. B. Darling & M. I. Peter (Eds.), *Families, physicians, and children with social health care needs: Collaborative medical education models* (pp. 109–120). Westport, CT: Auburn House.

Core principles of family-centered health care. (1998, Summer). *Advances*, pp. 2–3.

Coulter, A. (1997). Partnerships with patients: The pros and cons of shared clinical decision-making. *Journal of Health Services Research and Policy, 2,* 112–121.

Council for Exceptional Children. (1981). Editor's note. *Exceptional Children, 47,* 492–493.

Cox, C. B. (2003). Designing interventions for grandparent caregivers: The need for an ecological perspective for practice. *Families in Society, 84*(1), 127–134.

Cox, F. D. (1996). *Human intimacy.* Minneapolis, MN: West.

Crnic, K. A., Friedrich, N. W., & Greenberg, M. T. (1983). Adaptation of families with mentally retarded children: A model of stress, coping, and family ecology. *American Journal on Mental Deficiency, 88,* 125–138.

Crnic, K. A., Greenberg, M. T., Ragozin, A. S., Robinson, N. M., & Basham, R. B. (1983). Effects of stress and social support on mothers and premature and full-term infants. *Child Development, 54,* 209–217.

Crocker, J., Major, B., & Steele, C. (1998). Social stigma. In D. Gilbert, S. T. Fiske, & G. Lindzey (Eds.), *Handbook of social psychology* (4th ed., pp. 504–553). Boston: McGraw-Hill.

Cromwell, V. L., & Cromwell, R. E. (1978). Perceived dominance in decision making and conflict resolution among Anglo, black, and Chicano couples. *Journal of Marriage and the Family, 19,* 749–759.

Crowley, S. L., & Taylor, J. M. (1994). Mothers' and fathers' perceptions of family functioning in families having children with disabilities. *Early Education and Development, 5,* 213–225.

Cummings, S. T. (1976). The impact of the child's deficiency on the father: A study of fathers of mentally retarded and of chronically-ill children. *American Journal of Orthopsychiatry, 46,* 246–255.

Cuskelly, M., & Gunn, P. (2003). Sibling relationships of children with Down syndrome. *American Journal on Mental Retardation, 108,* 234–244.

Danielson, P. (2004). Disability does not equal liability. In S. D. Klein & J. D. Kemp (Eds.), *Reflections from a different journey: What adults with disabilities wish all parents knew* (pp. 8–12). New York: McGraw-Hill.

D'Arcy, E. (1968). Congenital defects: Mothers' reactions to children with birth defects. *British Medical Journal, iii,* 796–798.

Darling, R. B. (1979). *Families against society: A study of reactions to children with birth defects.* Beverly Hills, CA: Sage.

Darling, R. B. (1987). The economic and psycho-social consequences of disability: Family–society relationships. In M. Ferrari & M. B. Sussman (Eds.), *Childhood disability and family systems* (pp. 45–61). New York: Haworth Press.

Darling, R. B. (1988). Parental entrepreneurship: A consumerist response to professional dominance. *Journal of Social Issues, 44,* 141–158.

Darling, R. B. (1989). Using the social system perspective in early intervention: The value of a sociological approach. *Journal of Early Intervention, 13,* 24–35.

Darling, R. B. (1991). Initial and continuing adaptation to the birth of a disabled child. In M. Seligman (Ed.), *The family with a handicapped child* (2nd ed., pp. 55–89). Boston: Allyn & Bacon.

Darling, R. B. (1994). Overcoming obstacles to early intervention referral: The development of a video-based training model for community physicians. In R. B. Darling & Peter, M. I. (Eds.), *Families, physicians, and children with special health needs: Collaborative medical education models* (pp. 135–148). Westport, CT: Auburn House.

Darling, R. B. (2000). *The partnership model in human services: Sociological foundations and practices.* New York: Kluwer/Plenum.

Darling, R. B. (2003). Toward a model of changing disability identities: A proposed typology and research agenda. *Disability and Society, 18*, 881–895.

Darling, R. B., & Baxter, C. (1996). *Families in focus: Sociological methods in early intervention.* Austin, TX: PRO-ED.

Darling, R. B., & Darling, J. (1982). *Children who are different: Meeting the challenges of birth defects in society.* St. Louis, MO: Mosby.

Darling, R. B., & Darling, J. (1992). Early intervention: A field moving toward a sociological approach. *Sociological Studies in Child Development, 5*, 9–22.

Darling, R. B., Hager, M. A., Stockdale, J. M., & Heckert, D. A. (2002). Divergent views of clients and professionals: A comparison of responses to a needs assessment instrument. *Journal of Social Service Research, 28*(3), 41–63.

Darling, R. B., & Heckert, D. A. (2004, August). *Disability and opportunity: A preliminary test of a typology of orientations toward disability.* Paper presented at the annual meetings of the American Sociological Association, San Francisco.

Darling, R. B., & Peter, M. I. (Eds.). (1994). *Families, physicians and children with special health needs: Collaborative medical evaluation modes .* Westport, CT: Auburn House.

Davidoff, A. J. (2004). Insurance for children with special health care needs: Patterns of coverage and burden on families to provide adequate insurance. *Pediatrics, 114,* 394–403.

Davis, F. (1960). Uncertainty in medical prognosis: Clinical and functional. *American Journal of Sociology, 66,* 41–47.

Davis, F. (1961). Deviance disavowal: The management of strained interaction by the visibly handicapped. *Social Problems, 9,* 120–132.

Deaux, K., Reid, A., Mizrahi, K., & Ethier, A. (1995). Parameters of social identity. *Journal of Personality and Social Psychology, 68,* 280–292.

Dembo, T. (1984). Sensitivity of one person to another. *Rehabilitation Literature, 45,* 90–95.

Dembo, T., Leviton, G. L., & Wright, B. A. (1956). Adjustment to misfortune: A problem of social-psychological rehabilitation. *Artificial Limbs, 3,* 1–62.

DeMyer, M., & Goldberg, P. (1983). Family needs of the autistic adolescent. In E. Schopler & G. Mesibov (Eds.), *Autism in adolescents and adults* (pp. 228–237). New York: Plenum Press.

Developing systems of support with American Indian families of youth with disabilities. (1998, Summer). *Health Issues,* pp. 9–10.

Devlieger, P., & Albrecht, G. (2000). Your experience is not my experience: The concept and experience of disability on Chicago's Near West Side. *Journal of Disability and Policy Studies, 11,* 51–60.

Devore, W., & London, H. (1999). And how are the children?: Diversity in childhood experiences. In H. P. McAdoo (Ed.), *Family ethnicity: Strength in diversity* (2nd ed., pp. 301–320). Thousand Oaks, CA: Sage.

Dickman, I., & Gordon, S. (1985). *One miracle at a time: How to get help for your disabled child–from the experience of other parents.* New York: Simon & Schuster.

Dinsmore, J. (2004). The hand that you're dealt. In S. D. Klein & J. D. Kemp (Eds.), *Reflections from a different journey: What adults with disabilities wish all parents knew* (pp. 113–116). New York: McGraw-Hill.

Disability-research discussion listserv. (1999–2003). Retrieved on various dates (see text) from disability-research@mailbase.ac.uk

DiVenere, N. J. (1994). Parents as educators of medical students. In R. B. Darling & M. I. Peter (Eds.), *Families, physicians, and children with special needs: Collaborative medical education models* (pp. 101–108). Westport, CT: Auburn House.

DoAmaral, R. (2003). How do children with disabilities impact their parents' parental satisfaction, self-esteem, symptoms of stress, ways of coping, marital satisfaction, and family support? *Dissertation Abstracts International, 64*(4), A.

Dobson, B., & Middleton, S. (1998). *Paying to care: The costs of childhood disability.* York, UK: Joseph Rowntree Foundation.

Dodson, J. (1981). Conceptualizations of black families. In H. P. McAdoo (Ed.), *Black families* (pp. 23–36). Beverly Hills, CA: Sage.

Doering, S. G., Entwisle, D. R., & Quinlan, D. (1980). Modeling the quality of women's birth experience. *Journal of Health and Social Behavior, 21*, 12–21.

Doherty, W. J. (1985). Family intervention in health care. *Family Relations, 34*, 129–137.

Dominguez, S., & Watkins, C. (2003). Creating networks for survival and mobility: Social capital among African-American and Latin-American low-income mothers. *Social Problems, 50*(1), 111–135.

Dorner, S. (1975). The relationship of physical handicap to stress in families with an adolescent with spina bifida. *Developmental Medicine and Child Neurology, 17*, 765–776.

Dovidio, J. F., Major, B., & Crocker, J. (2000). Stigma: Introduction and overview. In T. F. Heatherton, R. E. Kleck, M. R. Hebl, & J. G. Hull (Eds.), *The social psychology of stigma* (pp. 1–28). New York: Guilford Press.

Dow, T. E., Jr. (1966). Optimism, physique, and social class in reaction to disability. *Journal of Health and Social Behavior, 7*, 14–19.

Down syndrome, difficult behavior. (1991, January/February). *Exceptional Parent*, pp. 12–13.

Downey, D. B. (1995). When bigger is not better: Family size, parental resources, and children's educational performance. *American Sociological Review, 60*, 746–761.

Downey, K. J. (1963). Parental interest in the institutionalized severely mentally retarded child. *Social Problems, 11*, 186–193.

Drillien, C. M., & Wilkinson, E. M. (1964). Mongolism: When should parents be told? *British Medical Journal, ii*, 1306–1307.

Drotar, D., Crawford, P., & Bush, M. (1984). The family context of childhood chronic illness. In M. G. Eisenberg, L. C. Sutkin, & M. A. Jansen (Eds.), *Chronic illness and disability through the life span* (pp. 103–129). New York: Springer.

Duncan, D. (1977). *The impact of a handicapped child upon the family.* Paper presented at the Pennsylvania Training Model Sessions, Harrisburg.

Dunst, C. J., Trivette, C. M., & Cross, A. H. (1986). Mediating influences of social support. *American Journal of Mental Deficiency, 90*, 403–417.

Dunst, C. J., Trivette, C. M., & Cross, A. H. (1988). Social support networks of Appalachian and non-Appalachian families with handicapped children: Relationship to personal and family well-being. In S. Keefe (Ed.), *Mental health in Appalachia.* Lexington: University of Kentucky Press.

Dunst, C. J., Trivette, C. M., & Deal, A. G. (1987). *Enabling and empowering families: Principles and guidelines for practice.* Cambridge, MA: Brookline Books.

Dushenko, T. (1981). Cystic fibrosis: Medical overview and critique of the psychological literature. *Social Science and Medicine, 15B*, 43–56.

Duvall, E. (1957). *Family development.* Philadelphia: Lippincott.

Duvdevany, I., & Vudinsky, H. (2005). Out-of-home placement of children with intellectual disability: Israeli-born parents vs. new immigrants from the ex-USSR. *International Journal of Rehabilitation Research, 28*(4), 321–330.

Dwight, V. (2001). Aidan's gift. In S. D. Klein & K. Schive (Eds.), *You will dream new dreams: Inspiring personal stories by parents of children with disabilities* (pp. 31–37). New York: Kensington Books.

Dyson, L. L. (1989). Adjustment of siblings of handicapped children: A comparison. *Journal of Pediatric Psychology, 14,* 215–229.

Dyson, L. L., & Fewell, R. R. (1986). Stress and adaptation in parents of young handicapped and nonhandicapped children: A comparative study. *Journal of the Division for Early Childhood, 10,* 25–35.

Edelman, M. W. (1985). The sea is so wide and my boat is so small: Problems facing black children today. In H. P. McAdoo & J. L. McAdoo (Eds.), *Black children: Social, educational and parental environments* (pp. 72–82). Beverly Hills, CA: Sage.

Edgerton, R. B. (1970). Mental retardation in non-Western societies: Toward a cross-cultural perspective on incompetence. In H. C. Haywood (Ed.), *Social-cultural aspects of mental retardation* (pp. 532–559). New York: Appleton-Century-Crofts.

Edin, K., & Harris, K. M. (1997, August). *Getting off and staying off: Race differences in the work route off welfare.* Paper presented at the meeting of the American Sociological Association, Toronto.

Eliades, D. C., & Suitor, C. W. (1994). *Celebrating diversity: Approaching families through their food.* Arlington, VA: National Center for Education in Maternal and Child Health.

Elman, N. S. (1991). Family therapy. In M. Seligman (Ed.), *The family with a handicapped child* (2nd ed., pp. 369–406). Boston: Allyn & Bacon.

Erickson, M. F., & Kurz-Riemer, K. (1999). *Infants, toddlers, and families.* New York: Guilford Press.

Evans, G. W. (2004). The environment of childhood poverty. *American Psychologist, 59,* 77–92.

Fagan, J., & Schor, D. (1993). Mothers of children with spina bifida: Factors related to maternal psychosocial functioning. *American Journal of Orthopsychiatry, 63,* 146–152.

Falicov, C. J. (1982). Mexican families. In M. McGoldrick, J. K. Pearce, & J. Giordano (Eds.), *Ethnicity and family therapy* (pp. 134–163). New York: Guilford Press.

Falicov, C. J., & Karrer, B. M. (1980). Cultural variations in the family life cycle: The Mexican-American family. In E. A. Carter & M. McGoldrick (Eds.), *The family life cycle: A framework for family therapy* (pp. 383–426). New York: Gardner Press.

Family-centered service delivery. (1997, Summer). *Families and Disability Newsletter,* p. 1.

Farber, B. (1959). Effects of a severely mentally retarded child on family integration. *Monographs of the Society for Research in Child Development, 24*(2, Serial No. 71).

Farber, B. (1960a). Family organization and crisis: Maintenance of integration in families with a severely mentally retarded child. *Monographs of the Society for Research in Child Development, 25*(Serial No. 75).

Farber, B. (1960b). Perceptions of crisis and related variables in the impact of a retarded child on the mother. *Journal of Health and Social Behavior, 1,* 108–118.

Farber, B., & Lewis, M. (1975). The symbolic use of parents: A sociological critique of educational practice. *Journal of Research and Development in Education, 8,* 34–41.

Farber, B., & Ryckman, D. B. (1965). Effects of a severely mentally retarded child on family relationships. *Mental Retardation Abstracts, 11,* 1–17.

Featherstone, H. (1980). *A difference in the family: Life with a disabled child.* New York: Basic Books.

Feldman, S. I., & Tegart, G. (2003). Keep moving: Conceptions of illness and disability of middle-aged African American women with arthritis. In M. E. Banks & E. Kashak (Eds.), *Women with visible and invisible disabilities* (pp. 127–143). New York: Haworth Press.

Femminella, F. X., & Quadagno, J. S. (1976). The Italian-American family. In C. H.

Mindel & R. W. Habenstein (Eds.), *Ethnic families in America: Patterns and variations* (pp. 62–88). New York: Elsevier.

Fewell, R. R. (1986). A handicapped child in the family. In R. R. Fewell & P. F. Vadasy (Eds.), *Families of handicapped children* (pp. 3–34). Austin, TX: PRO-ED.

Fewell, R. R. (1991). Parenting moderately handicapped persons. In M. Seligman (Ed.), *The family with a handicapped child* (2nd ed., pp. 203–232). Boston: Allyn & Bacon.

Findler, L. S. (2000). The role of grandparents in the social support systems of mothers of children with a physical disability. *Families in Society, 81,* 370–381.

Findler, L., & Taubman, B. (2003). Social workers' perceptions and practice regarding grandparents in families of children with developmental disabilities. *Families in Society, 84,* 86–94.

Fish, T. (Producer). (1993). *The next step* (videotape). Available from Publications Office, Nisonger Center, UAP, 434 McCampbell Hall, Ohio State University, 1581 Dodd Dr., Columbus, OH 43210.

Fishman, S., Wolf, L., Ellison, D., & Freeman, T. (2000). A longitudinal study of siblings of children with chronic disabilities. *Canadian Journal of Psychiatry, 45,* 369–375.

Fitzpatrick, J. P. (1976). The Puerto Rican family. In C. H. Mindel & R. W. Habenstein (Eds.), *Ethnic families in America: Patterns and variations.* New York: Elsevier.

Flood, R. (2004). Ain't done too bad for a cauliflower. In S. D. Klein & J. D. Kemp (Eds.), *Reflections from a different journey: What adults with disabilities wish all parents knew* (pp. 3–7). New York: McGraw-Hill.

Folkman, S., Lazarus, R., Dunkel-Schelter, C., DeLongis, A., & Gruen, R. (1986). The dynamics of a stressful encounter: Cognitive appraisal, coping and encounter outcomes. *Journal of Personality and Social Psychology, 50,* 992–1003.

Fong, R. (1994). Family preservation: Making it work for Asians. *Child Welfare, 73,* 331–341.

Force, L. T., Botsford, A., Pisano, P. A., & Holbert, A. (2000). Grandparents raising grandchildren with and without a developmental disability. *Journal of Gerontological Social Work, 33,* 5–21.

Forrer, G. R. (1959). The mother of a defective child. *Psychoanalytic Quarterly, 28,* 59–63.

Fox, R. (1959). *Experiment perilous.* Glencoe, IL: Free Press.

Fracasso, M. P. (1994). Studying the social and emotional development of Hispanic children in the United States. *Zero to Three, 15,* 24–27.

Francis, V., Korsch, B. M., & Morris, M. J. (1968). Gaps in doctor–patient communication: Patients' response to medical advice. *New England Journal of Medicine, 280,* 535–540.

Frankland, H. C. (2001). *Professional collaboration and family–professional partnerships.* Unpublished doctoral dissertation, University of Kansas.

Franklin, A. J., & Boyd-Franklin, N. (1985). A psychoeducational perspective on black parenting. In H. P. McAdoo & J. L. McAdoo (Eds.), *Black children: Social, educational, and parental environments* (pp. 194–210). Beverly Hills, CA: Sage.

Franklin, A. J., Franklin, N. B., & Draper, C. V. (2002). A psychological and educational perspective on black parenting. In H. P. McAdoo (Ed.), *Black children: Social, educational, and parental environments* (2nd ed., pp. 119–140). Thousand Oaks, CA: Sage.

Fraser, M. W., Pecora, P. J., & Haapala, D. A. (1991). *Families in crisis: The impact of intensive family preservation services.* New York: Aldine de Gruyter.

Freedman, A. (2001). The future is now. In S. D. Klein & K. Schive (Eds.), *You will dream new dreams: Inspiring personal stories by parents of children with disabilities* (pp. 38–42). New York: Kensington Books.

Freeman, A., Pretzer, J., Fleming, B., & Simon, K. M. (2004). *Clinical applications of cognitive therapy* (2nd ed.). New York: Kluwer/Plenum.

Freidson, E. (1961). *Patients' views of medical practice.* New York: Russell Sage Foundation.

Freidson, E. (1970). *Professional dominance.* Chicago: Aldine.

French, L. A. (1997). *Counseling American Indians.* Lanham, MD: University Press of America.

French, S. (1996). Simulation exercises in disability awareness training: A critique. In G. Hales (Ed.), *Beyond disability: Towards an enabling society* (pp. 114–123). London: Sage.

Freud, S. (1936). *Inhibitions, symptoms and anxiety.* London: Hogarth Press. (Original work published in 1926)

Freund, P. E., & McGuire, M. (1999). *Health, illness and the social body.* Upper Saddle River, NJ: Prentice Hall.

Frey, K. S., Greenberg, M. T., & Fewell, R. R. (1989). Stress and coping among families of handicapped children. *American Journal of Mental Deficiency, 94,* 240–249.

Friedman, B. B., & Berkeley, T. R. (2002). Encouraging fathers to participate in the school experiences of young children: The teacher's role. *Early Childhood Education Journal, 29,* 209–213.

Friedrich, O. (1977). *Going crazy: An inquiry into madness in our time.* New York: Avon Books.

Friedrich, W. N. (1979). Predictors of the coping behaviors of mothers and handicapped children. *Journal of Consulting and Clinical Psychology, 47,* 486–492.

Friedrich, W. N., & Friedrich, W. L. (1981). Psychological aspects of parents of handicapped and nonhandicapped children. *American Journal of Mental Deficiency, 85,* 551–553.

Friend, M., & Cook, L. (2002). *Interactions: Collaboration skills for school professionals.* Boston: Allyn & Bacon.

Fries, K. (1997). *Staring back: The disability experience from the inside out.* New York: Penguin Putnam.

Frisco, J. (2002). *Grandparents with a disabled grandchild.* Unpublished manuscript.

Frith, C. H. (1981). "Advocate" vs. "professional employee": A question of priorities for special educators. *Exceptional Children, 47,* 486–492.

Gabel, H., McDowell, J., & Cerreto, M. C. (1983). Family adaptation to the handicapped infant. In S. G. Garwood & R. R. Fewell (Eds.), *Educating handicapped infants* (pp. 455–493). Rockville, MD: Aspen.

Gaither, R., Bingen, K., & Hopkins, J. (2000). When the bough breaks: The relationship between chronic illness in children and couple functioning. In K. B. Schmaling & S. T. Goldman (Eds.), *The psychology of couples and illness* (pp. 337–365). Washington, DC: American Psychological Association.

Gallimore, R., Weisner, T. S., Bernheimer, L. P., Guthrie, D., & Nihira, K. (1993). Family responses to young children with developmental delays: Accommodation activity in ecological and cultural context. *American Journal of Mental Retardation, 98*(2), 185–206.

Gallo, L. C., Bogart, L. M., Vranceanu, A., & Matthews, K. A. (2005). Socioeconomic status, resources, psychological experiences, and emotional responses: A test of the reserve capacity model. *Journal of Personality and Social Psychology, 88,* 386–399.

Gannotti, M. E., Handwerker, W. P., Groce, N. E., & Cruz, C. (2001). Sociocultural influences on disability status in Puerto Rican children. *Physical Therapy, 81*(9), 1512–1524.

Garbarino, J. (1989). Maltreatment of young children with disabilities. *Infants and Young Children, 2*, 49–57.

Garbarino, J. (1992). *Families and children in the social environment* (2nd ed.). New York: Aldine De Gruyter.

García-Preto, N. (1982). Puerto Rican families. In M. McGoldrick, J. K. Pearce, & J. Giordano (Eds.), *Ethnicity and family therapy* (pp. 164–186). New York: Guilford Press.

Gardner, J. E., Sherman, A., Mobley, D., Brown, P., & Schutter, M. (1994). Grandparents' beliefs regarding their role and relationships with special needs grandchildren. *Education and Treatment of Children, 17*, 185–196.

Gath, A. (1974). Sibling reactions to mental handicap: A comparison of the brothers and sisters of mongol children. *Journal of Child Psychology and Psychiatry, 15*, 187–198.

Gavin-Williams, R. C., & Esterberg, K. C. (2000). Lesbian, gay, and bisexual families. In D. H. Demo, K. R. Allen, & M. A. Fine (Eds.), *Handbook of family diversity* (pp. 197–215). New York: Oxford University Press.

Gayton, W. F., & Walker, L. (1974). Down's syndrome: Informing the parents. *American Journal of Diseases of Children, 127*, 510–512.

George, J. D. (1988). Therapeutic intervention for grandparents and extended family of children with developmental delays. *Mental Retardation, 26*, 369–375.

Gething, L. (1992). Judgements by health professionals of personal characteristics of people with a visible physical disability. *Social Science and Medicine, 34*(7), 809–815.

Ghali, S. B. (1977). Culture sensitivity and the Puerto Rican client. *Social Casework, 58*, 459–474.

Gill, B. (1997). *Changed by a child*. New York: Broadway Books.

Gill, C. J. (1994). Questioning continuum. In B. Shaw (Ed.), *The ragged edge* (pp. 42–49). Louisville, KY: Advocado Press.

Gill, C. J. (1997). Four types of integration in disability identity development. *Journal of Vocational Rehabilitation, 9*, 39–46.

Gill, V. J., & Maynard, D. W. (1995). On "labeling" in actual interaction: Delivering and receiving diagnoses of developmental disabilities. *Social Problems, 42*(1), 11–37.

Gillman, M., Heyman, B., & Swain, J. (2000). What's in a name?: The implications of diagnosis for people with learning difficulties and their family carers. *Disability and Society, 15*(3), 389–409.

Gilson, S. F., & DePoy, E. (2004). Disability, identity, and cultural diversity. *Review of Disability Studies, 1*(1), 16–23.

Gladding, S. T. (2000). *Counseling: A comprehensive profession* (4th ed.). Upper Saddle River, NJ: Prentice Hall.

Glenn, E. N., & Yap, S. G. H. (2002). Chinese American families. In R. J. Taylor (Ed.), *Minority families in the United States: A multicultural perspective* (3rd ed., pp. 134–163). Upper Saddle River, NJ: Prentice Hall.

Glidden, L. M., & Schoolcraft, S. A. (2003). Depression: Its trajectory and correlates in mothers rearing children with intellectual disability. *Journal of Intellectual Disability Research, 47*, 250–263.

Gliedman, J., & Roth, W. (1980). *The unexpected minority: Handicapped children in America*. New York: Harcourt Brace Jovanovich.

Goffman, E. (1959). *The presentation of self in everyday life*. Garden City, NY: Doubleday.

Goffman, E. (1963). *Stigma: Notes on the management of spoiled identity*. Englewood Cliffs, NJ: Prentice Hall.

Gold, S. J. (1999). Continuity and change among Vietnamese families in the United

States. In H. P. McAdoo (Ed.), *Family ethnicity: Strength in diversity* (2nd ed., pp. 225–234). Thousand Oaks, CA: Sage.

Goldenberg, I., & Goldenberg, H. (2003). *Family therapy: An overview* (6th ed.). Pacific Grove, CA: Brooks/Cole.

Goode, D. A. (1984). Presentation practices of a family with a deaf–blind child. *Family Relations, 33,* 173–185.

Goodheart, C. D., & Lansing, M. H. (1997). *Treating people with chronic disease.* Washington, DC: American Psychological Association.

Goodman, C. I. (1980). *A study of alternative therapeutic relationships: Parent groups and their members.* Unpublished doctoral dissertation, Case Western Reserve University.

Goodman, J. F. (1994). "Empowerment" versus "best interests": Client–professional relationships. *Infants and Young Children, 6,* vi–x.

Gould-Martin, K., & Ngin, C. (1981). Chinese Americans. In A. Harwood (Ed.), *Ethnicity and medical care* (pp. 130–171). Cambridge, MA: Harvard University Press.

Gowen, J. W., Christy, D. S., & Sparling, J. (1993). Informational needs of parents of young children with special needs. *American Journal of Mental Deficiency, 66,* 838–843.

Grakliker, B. V., Fishler, K., & Koch, R. (1962). Teenage reactions to a mentally retarded sibling. *American Journal of Mental Deficiency, 66,* 838–843.

Gray, D. E. (1997). High functioning autistic children and the construction of "normal family life." *Social Science and Medicine, 44*(8), 1097–1106.

Green, S. E. (2001). Grandma's hands: Parental perspectives of the importance of grandparents as secondary caregivers in families of children with disabilities. *International Journal of Aging and Human Development, 53,* 11–33.

Greenberg, J. S., Kim, H. W., & Greenley, J. R. (1997). Factors associated with subjective burden in siblings of adults with severe mental illness. *American Journal of Orthopsychiatry, 67,* 231–241.

Greenspan, S. I., & Wieder, S. (2003). *The child with special needs* (2nd ed.). Da Capo Press.

Grisom, M. O., & Borkowski, J. G. (2002). Self-efficacy in adolescents who have siblings with or without disabilities. *American Journal on Mental Retardation, 107,* 79–90.

Groce, N. (1987, Summer). Cross-cultural research, current strengths, future needs. *Disability Studies Quarterly,* pp. 1–3.

Groce, N. (2005). Immigrants, disability, and rehabilitation. In J. H. Stone (Ed.), *Culture and disability: Providing culturally competent services* (pp. 1–14). Thousand Oaks, CA: Sage.

Grossman, F. K. (1972). *Brothers and sisters of retarded children.* Syracuse, NY: Syracuse University Press.

Gundry, M. (1989, November/December). Wanted: A diagnosis for my son. *Exceptional Parent,* pp. 22–24.

Guralnick, M. J., Bennett, F. C., Heiser, K. E., & Richardson, H. B., Jr. (1987). Training future primary care pediatricians to serve handicapped children and their families. *Topics in Early Childhood Special Education, 6,* 1–11.

Guralnick, M. J., Connor, R. T., & Hammond, M. (1995). Parent perspectives on peer relationships and friendships in integrated and specialized settings. *American Journal on Mental Retardation, 99,* 457–476.

Halpern, R. (1984). Physician–parent communication in the Diagnosis of child handicap: A brief review. *Children's Health Care, 12*(4), 170–174.

Hamre-Nietupski, S., Krajewski, L., Nietupski, J., Ostercamp, D., Sensor, K., & Opheim, B. (1988). Parent/professional partnerships in advocacy: Developing integrated options within resistive systems. *Journal of the Association for Persons with Severe Handicaps, 13*(4), 251–259.

Hannah, M. E., & Midlarsky, E. (1999). Competence and adjustment of siblings of children with mental retardation. *American Journal on Mental Retardation, 104*, 22–37.

Hanson, M. J. (1981). A model for early intervention with culturally diverse single and multiparent families. *Topics in Early Childhood Special Education, 1*, 37–44.

Hanson, M. J., & Lynch, E. W. (2004). *Understanding families: Approaches to diversity, disability, and risk.* Baltimore: Brookes.

Harbaugh, G. R. (1984). *Costs and "out of pocket" costs of rearing a handicapped child.* Unpublished manuscript.

Hardman, M. J., Drew, C. J., & Egan, M. W. (2002). *Human exceptionality: Society, school, and family* (7th ed.). Boston: Allyn & Bacon.

Harris, L., & Associates. (1975). *The myth and reality of aging in America.* Washington, DC: National Council on Aging.

Harris, S. L. (1983). *Families of the developmentally disabled: A guide to behavioral intervention.* New York: Pergamon Press.

Harris, S. (1994). *Siblings of children with autism: A guide for families.* Rockville, MD: Woodbine House.

Harris, S. L. (1996). Serving families of children with developmental disabilities: Reaching diverse populations. *Special Services in the Schools, 12*(1–2), 79–86.

Harris, S. L., & Glasberg, B. A. (2003). *Siblings of children with autism* (2nd ed.). Bethesda, MD: Woodbine.

Harrison, A., Serafica, F., & McAdoo, H. (1984). Ethnic families of color. In R. D. Parke (Ed.), *Review of child development research* (Vol. 7, pp. 329–371). Chicago: University of Chicago Press.

Harry, B. (1992a). *Cultural diversity, families, and the special education system: Communication and empowerment.* New York: Teachers College Press.

Harry, B. (1992b). Developing cultural self-awareness: The first step in values clarification for early interventionists. *Topics in Early Childhood Special Education, 12*, 333–350.

Harry, B. (1992c). Making sense of disability: Low-income Puerto Rican parents' theories of the problem. *Exceptional Children, 59*, 27–40.

Harry, B., Allen, N., & McLaughlin, M. (1995). Communication versus compliance: African-American parents' involvement in special education. *Exceptional Children, 61*, 364–376.

Harry, B., Day, M., & Quist, F. (1998). "He can't really play": An ethnographic study of sibling acceptance and interaction. *Journal of the Association for Persons with Severe Handicaps, 23*, 289–299.

Harry, B., & Kalyanpur, M. (1994). Cultural underpinnings of special education: Implications for professional interactions with culturally diverse families. *Disability and Society, 9*, 145–165.

Harry, B., Otgruson, C., Katkavich, J., & Guerrero, M. (1993). Crossing social class and cultural barriers in working with families: Implications for teacher training. *Teaching Exceptional Children, 26*(1), 48–51.

Hastings, R. P., & Taunt, H. M. (2002). Positive perceptions in families of children with developmental disabilities. *American Journal on Mental Retardation, 107*, 116–127.

Hatchett, S. J., & Jackson, J. S. (1999). African American extended kin systems: An empirical assessment in the National Survey of Black Americans. In H. P. McAdoo (Ed.), *Family ethnicity: Strength in diversity* (2nd ed., pp. 171–190). Thousand Oaks, CA: Sage.

Hatton, C., Blacher, J., & Llewellyn, G. (2003). Guest editorial. *Journal of Intellectual Disability Research, 47*, 215.

Haug, M., & Lavin, B. (1983). *Consumerism in medicine: Challenging physician authority.* Beverly Hills, CA: Sage.

Heatherton, T. F., Kleck, R. E., Hebl, M. R., & Hull, J. G. (Eds.). (2000). *The social psychology of stigma.* New York: Guilford Press.

Heimer, C. A. (1999). Competing institutions: Law, medicine, and family in neonatal intensive care. *Law and Society Review, 33*, 17–66.

Heiss, J. (1981). Women's values regarding marriage and the family. In H. P. McAdoo (Ed.), *Black families* (pp. 186–198). Beverly Hills, CA: Sage.

Helge, D. (1984). The state of the art of rural special education. *Exceptional Children, 50*, 294–305.

Heller, P. G., Quesada, G. M., Harvey, D. L., & Wagner, L. G. (1981). Familism in rural and urban America: Critique and reformulation of a construct. *Rural Sociology, 46*, 116–464.

Heller, T., Hsieh, K., & Rowitz, L. (2000). Grandparents as supports to mothers of persons with intellectual disability. *Journal of Gerontological Social Work, 33*, 23–34.

Herman, S. E., & Thompson, L. (1995). Families' perceptions of their resources for caring for children with developmental disabilities. *Mental Retardation, 33*, 73–83.

Herz, F. M., & Rosen, E. J. (1982). Jewish families. In M. McGoldrick, J. K. Pearce, & J. Giordano (Ed.), *Ethnicity and family therapy* (pp. 84–107). New York: Guilford Press.

Hess, R. D. (1970). Social class and ethnic influences upon socialization. In P. H. Mussen (Ed.), *Carmichael's manual of child psychology* (pp. 457–557). New York: Wiley.

Hetherington, E. M., Bridges, M., & Insabella, G. M. (1998). What matters? What does not? Five perspectives on the association between marital transitions and children's adjustments. *American Psychologist, 53*, 167–184.

Hetherington, E. M., & Stanley-Hagan, M. (2000). Diversity among stepfamilies. In D. H. Demo, K. R. Allen, & M. A. Fine (Eds.), *Handbook of family diversity* (pp. 173–196). New York: Oxford University Press.

Hickman, L. (2000). *Living in my skin: The insider's view of Life with a special needs child.* San Antonio, TX: Communication Skill Builders.

Hickson, G. B., Altemeier, W. A., & O'Connor, S. (1983). Concerns of mothers seeking care in private pediatrics offices: Opportunities for expanding services. *Pediatrics, 72*, 619–624.

Higgins, M. (2002). Posting on the *Disability-research discussion list* [Listserv]. Retrieved February 10, 2002, from disability-research@mailbase.ac.uk

Hill, R. (1949). *Families under stress.* New York: Harper & Row.

Hill, R. (1958). Sociology of marriage and family behavior, 1945–1956: A trend report and bibliography. *Current Sociology, 7*, 10–98.

Hill, R. B. (1999). *The strengths of African American families: Twenty-five years later.* Lanham, MD: University Press of America.

Hines, P. M. (1989). The family life cycle of poor black families. In B. Carter & M. McGoldrick (Eds.), *The changing family life cycle* (2nd ed., pp. 513–544). Boston: Allyn & Bacon.

Hines, P. M., & Boyd-Franklin, N. (1982). Black families. In M. McGoldrick, J. K. Pearce, & J. Giordano (Eds.), *Ethnicity and family therapy* (pp. 84–107). New York: Guilford Press.

Ho, M. K., Rasheed, J. M., & Rasheed, M. N. (2004). *Family therapy with ethnic minorities* (2nd ed.). Thousand Oaks, CA: Sage.

Hobbs, N., Perrin, A., & Ireys, S. (1986). *Chronically ill children and their families* . San Francisco: Jossey-Bass.

Hodapp, R. M., & Krasner, D. V. (1994–1995). Families of children with disabilities: Findings from a national sample of eighth-grade students. *Exceptionality, 5*, 71–81.

Hoffman, L. (1981). *Foundations of family therapy*. New York: Basic Books.

Hollingshead, A. B., & Redlich, F. C. (1958). *Social class and mental illness: A community study*. New York: Wiley.

Holt, K. S. (1958b). *The impact of mentally retarded children upon their families*. Unpublished doctoral dissertation, University of Sheffield, UK.

Honeycutt, A. A., Grosse, S. D., Dunlap, L. J., Schendel, D. E., Chen, H., Brann, F., & alHomsi, G. (2003). Economic costs of mental retardation, cerebral palsy, hearing loss, and vision impairment. In B. M. Altman, S. N. Barnartt, G. E. Hendershot, & S. A. Larson (Eds.), *Using survey data to study disability: Results from the National Health Interview Survey* (Vol. 3, pp. 207–228). Amsterdam: Elsevier.

Hornby, G. (1988). *Fathers of handicapped children*. Unpublished manuscript, University of Hull, UK.

Hornby, G. (1994a). *Counseling in child disability: Skills for working with parents*. London: Chapman & Hall.

Hornby, G. (1994b). Effects of children with disabilities on fathers: A review and analysis of the literature. *International Journal of Disability, Development, and Education, 41*, 171–184.

Hornby, G. (1995a). Fathers' views of the effects on their families of children with Down syndrome. *Journal of Child and Family Studies, 4*, 103–177.

Hornby, G. (1995b). *Working with parents of children with special needs*. London: Cassell.

Hornby, G. (2000). *Improving parental involvement*. London: Continuum.

Hornby, G., & Ashworth, T. (1994). Grandparent support for families who have children with disabilities: A survey of parents. *Journal of Child and Family Studies, 3*, 403–412.

Hornby, G., & Murray, R. (1983). Group programmes for parents of children with various handicaps. *Child Health and Development, 9*, 185–198.

Horton, E. (1985). Unfriendly persuasion. *Science Digest, 93*, 214.

Horton, T. V., & Wallender, J. L. (2001). Hope and social support as resilience factors in psychological distress of mothers who care for children with chronic physical conditions. *Rehabilitation Psychology, 46*, 382–399.

Hostler, S. L. (1991). Family-centered care. *Pediatric Clinics of North America, 38*, 1545–1560.

Houser, R., & Seligman, M. (1991). A comparison of stress and coping by fathers of adolescents with mental retardation and fathers of adolescents without mental retardation. *Research in Developmental Disabilities, 12*, 251–260.

Huang, L. J. (1976). The Chinese-American family. In C. H. Mindel & R. W. Habenstein (Eds.), *Ethnic families in America: Patterns and variations* (pp. 124–147). New York: Elsevier.

Hunt, N., & Marshall, K. (1999). *Exceptional children and youth* (2nd ed.). Boston: Houghton Mifflin.

Hunt, N., & Marshall, K. (2005). *Exceptional children and youth* (4th ed.). Boston: Houghton Mifflin.

Hunt, P. C. (2005). An introduction to Vietnamese culture for rehabilitation service providers in the United States. In J. H. Stone (Ed.), *Culture and disability: Providing culturally competent services* (pp. 203–224). Thousand Oaks, CA: Sage.

Huntington, G. E. (1998). The Amish family. In C. H. Mindel, R. W. Habenstein, & R. Wright, Jr. (Eds.), *Ethnic families in America: Patterns and variations* (4th ed., pp. 450–479). Upper Saddle River, NJ: Prentice Hall.

Hurlbutt, K., & Chalmers, L. (2002). Adults with autism speak out: Perceptions of their life experiences. *Focus on Autism and Other Developmental Disabilities, 17*(2), 103–112.

Institute for Health and Disability, University of Minnesota. (1999, Summer). Families teach residents. *The Second 5 Years*, pp. 16–17.

Ireys, H. T., & Nelson, R. P. (1992). New federal policy for children with special health care needs: Implications for pediatricians. *Pediatrics, 90*, 321–327.

Ishii-Kuntz, M. (1997). Japanese American families. In M. K. DeGenova (Ed.), *Families in cultural context: Strengths and challenges in diversity* (pp. 131–153). Mountain View, CA: Mayfield.

Israelite, N. (1985). Sibling reaction to a hearing-impaired child in the family. *Journal of Rehabilitation of the Deaf, 18*, 1–5.

Jackson, J. J. (1981). Urban black Americans. In A. Harwood (Ed.), *Ethnicity and medical care* (pp. 37–129). Cambridge, MA: Harvard University Press.

Jacobson, R. B., & Humphrey, R. A. (1979). Families in crisis: Research and theory in child mental retardation. *Social Casework, 60*, 597–601.

Janicky, P. M., McCallion, P., Grant-Griffin, L., & Kolomer, S. R. (2000). Grandparent caregivers I: Characteristics of the grandparents and the children with disabilities for whom they care. *Journal of Gerontological Social Work, 33*, 35–55.

Jessop, D. J., & Stein, R. E. (1985). Uncertainty and its relation to the psychological and social correlates of chronic illness in children. *Social Science and Medicine, 20*, 939–999.

Jezewski, M. A., & Sotnik, P. (2005). Disability service providers as culture brokers. In J. H. Stone (Ed.), *Culture and disability: Providing culturally competent services* (pp. 31–64). Thousand Oaks, CA: Sage.

JFK Child Development Center. (1981). *HOME Screening Questionnaire*. Denver, CO: LADOCA.

Joe, J. R., & Malach, R. S. (1992). Families with Native American roots. In E. W. Lynch & M. J. Hanson (Eds.), *Developing cross-cultural competence: A guide for working with young children and their families* (pp. 89–119). Baltimore: Brookes.

John, R. (1998). Native American families. In C. H. Mindel, R. W. Habenstein, & R. Wright, Jr. (Eds.), *Ethnic families in America: Patterns and variations* (4th ed., pp. 382–421). Upper Saddle River, NJ: Prentice Hall.

Johnson, B., McGonigel, M., & Kaufmann, R. (1989). *Guidelines and recommended practices for the individualized family service plan* . Washington, DC: Association for the Care of Children's Health.

Johnson, J., Duffett, A., Farkas, S., & Wilson, L. (2002). *when it's your own child: A report on special education from the families who use it*. New York: Public Agenda.

Judge, G. (1987). Knock, knock. . . . It's no joke. *Zero to Three, 8*, 20–21.

Judge, S. L. (1997). Parental perceptions of help-giving practices and control appraisals in early intervention programs. *Topics in Early Childhood Education, 17*(4), 457–477.

Kahana, G., & Kahana, E. (1970). Grandparenthood from the perspective of the developing grandchild. *Developmental Psychology, 3*, 98–105.

Kaiser, A. P., & Fox, J. J. (1986). Behavioral parent training research. In J. J. Gallagher & P. M. Vietze (Eds.), *Families of handicapped persons* (pp. 219–235). Baltimore: Brookes.

Kalins, I. (1983). Cross-illness comparisons of separation and divorce among parents having a child with a life-threatening illness. *Children's Health Care, 12*, 100–102.

Kalyanpur, M., & Harry, B. (1999). *Culture in special education*. Baltimore: Brookes.

Kappes, N. (1995). Matrix. In D. L. Meyer (Ed.), *Uncommon fathers: Reflections on raising a child with a disability* (pp. 13–18). Bethesda, MD: Woodbine.

Katz, A. H. (1993). *Self help in America*. New York: Twayne.

Kavanagh, K. H., & Kennedy, P. H. (1992). *Promoting cultural diversity: Strategies for health care professionals*. Newbury Park, CA: Sage.

Kazak, A. E., & Marvin, R. S. (1984). Differences, difficulties, and adaptation: Stress and social networks in families with a handicapped child. *Family Relations, 33*, 67–77.

Kazak, A. E., & Wilcox, B. (1984). The structure and function of social support networks in families with handicapped children. *American Journal of Community Psychology, 12*, 645–661.

Keefe, S. E., Padilla, A. M., & Carlos, M. L. (1979). The Mexican American extended family as an emotional support system. *Human Organization, 38*, 144–152.

Kelker, K., Garthwait, C., & Seligman, M. (1992). Rural special education options. *Human Services in the Rural Environment, 15*, 14–17.

Kemp, J. D. (2004). Afterword: Disability culture. In S. D. Klein & J. D. Kemp (Eds.), *Reflections from a different journey: What adults with disabilities wish all parents knew* (pp. 195–200). New York: McGraw-Hill.

Kibert, R. P. (1986). *A descriptive study of the perceptions of normal college age siblings in families with a mentally retarded child*. Unpublished doctoral dissertation, University of Pittsburgh.

Kibria, N. (2002). Vietnamese American families. In R. J. Taylor (Ed.), *Minority families in the United States: A multicultural perspective* (3rd ed., pp. 181–192). Upper Saddle River, NJ: Prentice Hall.

Kisor, H. (1990). *What's that pig outdoors?* New York: Hill & Wang.

Kitano, H. H. L., & Kikumura, A. (1976). The Japanese-American family. In C. H. Mindel & R. W. Habenstein (Eds.), *Ethnic families in America: Patterns and variations* (pp. 41–60). New York: Elsevier.

Klein, C. (1977). Coping patterns of parents of deaf–blind children. *American Annals of the Deaf, 122*, 310–312.

Klein, S. D. (1972). Brother to sister: Sister to brother. *Exceptional Parent, 2*, 10–15.

Klein, S. D., & Kemp, J. D. (Eds.). (2004). *Reflections from a different journey: What adults with disabilities wish all parents knew*. New York: McGraw-Hill.

Klein, S. D., & Schive, K. (Eds.). (2001). *You will dream new dreams: Inspiring personal stories by parents of children with disabilities*. New York: Kensington.

Kliman, J., & Madsen, W. (1999). Social class and the family life cycle. In B. Carter & M. McGoldrick (Eds.), *The expanded family life cycle* (3rd ed.). Boston: Allyn & Bacon.

Kline, F., Acosta, F. X., Austin, W., & Johnson, R. G., Jr. (1980). The misunderstood Spanish-speaking patient. *American Journal of Psychiatry, 137*(12), 1530–1533.

Kohn, M. L. (1969). *Class and conformity: A study in values*. Homewood, IL: Dorsey Press.

Konstam, V., Drainoni, M., Mitchell, G., Houser, R., Reddington, D., & Eaton, D. (1993). Career choices and values of siblings with individuals with developmental disabilities. *School Counselor, 40*, 287–292.

Korn, S. J., Chess, S., & Fernandez, P. (1978). The impact of children's physical handicaps on marital quality and family interaction. In R. M. Lerner & G. B. Spanier (Eds.), *Child influences on marital and family interaction: A lifespan perspective* (pp. 299–326). New York: Academic Press.

Kornblatt, E. S., & Heinrich, J. (1985). Needs and coping abilities in families of children with developmental disabilities. *Mental Retardation, 23,* 13–19.

Kornhaber, A. (2002). *The grandparent guide.* Chicago: Contemporary Books.

Kozol, J. (1988). *Rachel and her children: Homeless families in America.* New York: Fawcett Columbine.

Krahn, G. L. (1993). Conceptualizing social support in families of children with special health needs. *Family Process, 32,* 235–248.

Krahn, G. L., Hallum, A., & Kime, C. (1993). Are there good ways to give "bad news"? *Pediatrics, 91*(3), 578–583.

Krauss, M. W., & Seltzer, M. M. (1993). Coping strategies among older mothers of adults with retardation: A life-span developmental perspective. In A. P. Turnbull, J. M. Patterson, S. K. Behr, D. L. Murphy, J. G. Marquis, & M. J. Blue-Banning (Eds.), *Cognitive coping, families, and disabilities* (pp. 173–182). Baltimore: Brookes.

Kriegsman, K. H., Zaslow, E., & D'Zmura-Rechsteiner, J. (1992). *Taking charge: Teenagers talk about life and physical disabilities.* Bethesda, MD: Woodbine.

Kristoffersen, K., Polit, D. R., & Mastard, G. W. (2000). Towards a theory of interrupted feelings. *Scandinavian Journal of Caring Sciences, 14,* 23–28.

Kübler-Ross, E. (1969). *On death and dying.* New York: Macmillan.

Kunitz, S. J., & Levy, J. E. (1981). Navajos. In A. Harwood (Ed.), *Ethnicity and medical care* (pp. 337–396). Cambridge, MA: Harvard University Press.

Kurtz, R. A. (1977). Advocacy for the mentally retarded: The development of a new social role. In M. J. Begab & S. A. Richardson (Eds.), *The mentally retarded and society: A social science perspective* (pp. 377–394). Baltimore: University Park Press.

Kushner, H. (1981). *When bad things happen to good people.* New York: Avon.

Kuusisto, S. (1998). *Planet of the blind: A memoir.* New York: Dial Press.

Laborde, P. R., & Seligman, M. (1991). Counseling parents of children with disabilities. In M. Seligman (Ed.), *The family with a handicapped child* (2nd ed., pp. 337–369). Boston: Allyn & Bacon.

Lake, J. F., & Billingsley, B. S. (2000). An analysis of factors that contribute to parent–school conflict in special education. *remedial and Special Education, 21,* 240–251.

Lamb, M. E. (1983). Fathers of exceptional children. In M. Seligman (Ed.), *The family with a handicapped child: Understanding and treatment* (pp. 125–146). Orlando, FL: Grune & Stratton.

Lamb, M. E., & Meyer, D. J. (1991). Fathers of children with special needs. In M. Seligman (Ed.), *The family with a handicapped child* (2nd ed., pp. 151–179). Boston: Allyn & Bacon.

Lambie, R. (2000). *Family systems within educational contexts* (2nd ed.). Denver, CO: Love.

Lane, H., Hoffmeister, R., & Bahan, B. (1996). *A journey into the deaf world.* San Diego, CA: Dawn Sign Press.

Laosa, L. M. (1974). Child care and the culturally different child. *Child Care Quarterly, 3,* 214–224.

Laosa, L. M. (1978). Maternal teaching strategies in Chicano families of varied socioeconomic levels. *Child Development, 49,* 1129–1135.

Lardieri, L. A., Blacher, J., & Swanson, H. L. (2000). Sibling relationships and parent stress in families of children with and without learning disabilities. *Learning Disability Quarterly, 23,* 105–116.

LaRossa, R. (1977). *Conflict and power in marriage: Expecting the first child.* Beverly Hills, CA: Sage.

Lavin, J. L. (2001). *Special kids need special parents: A resource for parents of children with special needs.* New York: Penguin.

Lawrence-Webb, C., Okundaye, J. N., & Hafner, G. (2003). Education and kinship caregivers: Creating a new vision. *Families in Society: The Journal of Contemporary Human Services, 84,* 135–142.

Lechtenberg, R. (1984). *Epilepsy and the family.* Cambridge, MA: Harvard University Press.

Lee, E. (1982). A social systems approach to assessment and treatment for Chinese American families. In M. McGoldrick, J. K. Pearce, & J. Giordano (Eds.), *Ethnicity and family therapy* (pp. 527–551). New York: Guilford Press.

Lee, J. A. B. (1994). *The empowerment approach to social work practice.* New York: Columbia University Press.

Lee, S. K., Penner, P. I., & Cox, M. (1991). Comparison of the attitudes of health care professionals and parents toward active treatment of very low birth weight infants. *Pediatrics, 88*(1), 110–115.

Leifield, L., & Murray, T. (1995). Advocating for Aric: Strategies for full inclusion. In B. B. Swadener & S. Lubeck (Eds.), *Children and families "at promise": Deconstructing the discourse of risk* (pp. 238–261). Albany: State University of New York Press.

Leiter, V. (2004). Parental activism, professional dominance, and early childhood disability. *Disability Studies Quarterly, 24*(2), 1–16.

Leiter, V., & Krauss, M. W. (in press). Claims, barriers and satisfaction: Parents' experiences requesting additional special education services. *Journal of Disability Policy Studies.*

Levant, R. F., & Pollack, W. S. (1995). *A new psychology of men.* New York: Basic Books.

Lewis, J., & Greenstein, R. M. (1994). A first-year medical student curriculum about family views of chronic and disabling conditions. In R. B. Darling & M. I. Peter (Eds.), *Families, physicians, and children with special health needs: Collaborative medical education models* (pp. 77–100). Westport, CT: Auburn House.

Lewis, O. (1959). *Five families: An intimate and objective revelation of family life in Mexico today–a dramatic study of the culture of poverty.* New York: Basic Books.

Lidz, T. (1983). *The person: His and her development throughout the life cycle.* New York: Basic Books.

Lieberman, A. F. (1990). Infant–parent intervention with recent immigrants: Reflections on a study with Latino families. *Zero to Three, 10,* 8–11.

Liebow, E. (1993). *Tell them who I am: The lives of homeless women.* New York: Penguin.

Lillie, T. (1993). A harder thing than triumph: Roles of fathers of children with disabilities. *Mental Retardation, 31,* 438–443.

Linn, V. (2005, September 5). Parents of children with autism discuss the results of chelation. *Pittsburgh Post-Gazette,* p. 2.

Linton, S. (1998). *Claiming disability: Knowledge and identity.* New York: New York University Press.

Lipscomb, J., Kolimaga, J. T., Sperduto, P. W., Minnich, J. K., & Fontenot, K. J. (1983). *Cost–benefit and cost-effectiveness analyses of screening for neural tube defects in North Carolina.* Unpublished manuscript, Duke University.

Liu, G. Z. (2005). Best practices: Developing cross-cultural competence from a Chinese perspective. In J. H. Stone (Ed.), *Culture and disability: Providing culturally competent services* (pp. 65–86). Thousand Oaks, CA: Sage.

Lobato, D. J. (1983). Siblings of handicapped children: A review. *Journal of Autism and Developmental Disorders, 13,* 347–364.

Lobato, D. J. (1990). *Brothers, sisters, and special needs.* Baltimore: Brookes.

Locust, C. (1998, June). *Integration of American Indian and scientific concepts of disability: Cross-cultural perspectives.* Paper presented at the meeting of the Society for Disability Studies, Washington, DC.

Loprest, P., & Maag, E. (2003). Issues in job search and work accommodations for adults with disabilities. In B. M. Altman, S. N. Barnartt, G. E. Hendershot, & S. A. Larson (Eds.), *Using survey data to study disability: Results from the National Health Interview Survey on Disability* (Vol. 3, pp. 87–103). Amsterdam: Elsevier.

Lorber, J. (1971). Results of treatment of myelomeningocele. *Developmental Medicine and Child Neurology, 13,* 279–303.

Lugaila, T. A. (1998). *Marital status and living arrangements* (Current Population Reports: Population Characteristics). Atlanta, GA: U.S. Department of Commerce, Bureau of the Census.

Lukens, E. P., Thorning, H., & Rohrer, S. (2004). Sibling perspectives on severe mental illness. *American Journal of Orthopsychiatry, 74,* 489–501.

Lundgren, D., & Morrison, J. W. (2003, May). Involving Spanish-speaking families in early education programs. *Young Children,* pp. 88–95.

Lustig, D. C., & Akey, T. (1999a). Adaptation in families with adult children with mental retardation. *Education and Training in Mental Retardation and Developmental Disabilities, 34,* 260–270.

Lustig, D. C., & Akey, T. (1999b). Adaptation in families with children with mental retardation. *American Journal on Mental Retardation, 104,* 466–482.

Luterman, D. J. (1979). *Counseling parents of hearing-impaired children.* Boston: Little, Brown.

Luterman, D. J. (1991). *Counseling the communicatively disordered and their families* (2nd ed.). Boston: Little, Brown.

Lynch, E. W. (1992). Developing cross-cultural competence. In E. W. Lynch & M. J. Hanson (Eds.), *Developing cross-cultural competence: A guide for working with young children and their families* (pp. 33–59). Baltimore: Brookes.

Lyon, S., & Lyon, G. (1991). Collaboration with families of persons with severe disabilities. In M. Seligman (Ed.), *The family with a handicapped child* (2nd ed., pp. 237–264). Boston: Allyn & Bacon.

Lyon, S., & Preis, A. (1983). Working with families of severely handicapped persons. In M. Seligman (Ed.), *The family with a handicapped child: Understanding and treatment* (pp. 203–232). Orlando, FL: Grune & Stratton.

Lyon, S., Knickelbaum, B. A., & Wolf, P. J. (2005). Inclusion of children and youth with severe disabilities. In S. J. Farenga, B. A. Joyce, & D. Ness (Eds.), *The encyclopedia on education and human development* (pp. 913–929). Armonk, NY: M. E. Sharpe.

Maag, E. (2003). Unmet supportive service needs of children with disabilities. In B. M. Altman, S. N. Barnartt, G. E. Hendershot, & S. A. Larson (Eds.), *Using survey data to study disability: Results from the National Health Interview Survey on Disability* (Vol. 3, pp. 157–183). Amsterdam: Elsevier.

MacGregor, P. (1994). Grief: The unrecognized parental response to mental illness in a child. *Social Work, 39,* 160–166.

MacKeith, R. (1973). The feelings and behavior of parents of handicapped children. *Developmental Medicine and Child Neurology, 15,* 524–527.

MacNeal, N. & Leach, P. (1997, Spring). Health care strategies for working with the Amish community. *Pennsylvania Rural Health News, 7,* 3.

Mahalik, J. R., Good, G. E., & Englar-Carlson, M. (2003). Masculinity scripts, presenting concerns, and help seeking. *Professional Psychology: Research and Practice, 34,* 123–131.

Mairs, N. (1996). *Waist-high in the world: A life among the nondisabled.* Boston: Beacon Press.

Malow-Iroff, M., & Johnson, H. (2005). Health and parenting issues in childhood and adolescence. In S. J. Farenga, B. A., Joyce, & D. Ness (Eds.), *The encyclopedia on education and human development* (pp. 867–902). Armonk, NY: M. E. Sharpe.

Manns, W. (1981). Support systems of significant others in black families. In H. P. McAdoo (Ed.), *Black families* (pp. 238–251). Beverly Hills, CA: Sage.

Marcos, L. R. (1979). Effects of interpreters on the evaluation of psychopathology in non-English-speaking patients. *American Journal of Psychiatry, 136*(2), 171–174.

Marion, R. L. (1981). *Educators, parents, and exceptional children.* Rockville, MD: Aspen.

Marsh, D. T. (1992). *Families and mental retardation.* New York: Praeger.

Marsh, D. T. (1998). *Serious mental illness and the family.* New York: Wiley.

Marshak, L. E., & Prezant, F. (2007). *Married with special needs children: A couples guide to keeping connected.* Bethesda, MD: Woodbine House.

Marshak, L. E., & Seligman, M. (1993). *Counseling persons with disabilities: Theoretical and clinical perspectives.* Austin, TX: PRO-ED.

Marshak, L. E., Seligman, M., & Prezant, F. (1999). *Disability and the family life cycle.* New York: Basic Books.

Martin, E. P., & Martin, J. M. (1995). *Social work and the black experience.* Washington, DC: NASW Press.

Martin, P. (1975). Marital breakdown in families of patients with spina bifida cystica. *Developmental Medicine and Child Neurology, 17,* 757–764.

Martinez, E. A. (1999). Mexican American/Chicano families: Parenting as diverse as the families themselves. In H. P. McAdoo (Ed.), *Family ethnicity: Strength in diversity* (2nd ed., pp. 121–134). Thousand Oaks, CA: Sage.

Mary, L. N. (1990). Reactions of black, Hispanic, and white mothers to having a child with handicaps. *Mental Retardation, 28,* 1–5.

Matheny, K. B., Aycock, D. W., Pugh, J. L., Curlette, W. L., & Canella, K. S. (1986). Stress coping: A qualitative and quantitative synthesis with implications for treatment. *Counseling Psychologist, 14,* 499–549.

Matich-Maroney, J. (2003). Mental health implications for sexually abused adults with mental retardation: Some clinical research findings. *Mental Health Aspects of Developmental Disabilities, 6,* 11–20.

Max, L. (1985). Parents' views of provisions, services, and research. In N. N. Singh & K. M. Wilton (Eds.), *Mental retardation in New Zealand* (pp. 250–262). Christchurch, New Zealand: Whitcoulls.

May, J. (1991). *Fathers of children with special needs.* Bethesda, MD: ACCH.

McAnaney, K. (1990, July–August). How did I get this tough?: Fighting for your child's rights. *Exceptional Parent,* pp. 20–22.

McConkey, R., & Smyth, M. (2003). Parental perceptions of risks with older teenagers who have severe learning difficulties contrasted with the young people's views and experiences. *Children and Society, 17*(1), 18–32.

McCracken, M. J. (1984). Cystic fibrosis in adolescence. In R. W. Blum (Ed.), *Chronic illness and disabilities in childhood and adolescence* (pp. 397–411). Orlando, FL: Grune & Stratton.

McCubbin, H. I., & Patterson, J. M. (1981). *Systematic assessment of family stress, resources, and coping: Tools for research, education, and clinical intervention.* St. Paul: University of Minnesota, Department of Family Social Science, Family Stress and Coping Project.

McCubbin, H. I., & Patterson, J. M. (1983). The family stress process: The double ABCX model of adjustment and adaptation. *Marriage and Family Review, 6*(1–2), 7–37.

McDaniel, S. H. (1995). Collaboration between psychologists and family physicians. *Professional Psychology: Research and Practice, 26,* 117–122.

McDaniel, S. H., Hepworth, J., & Doherty, W. J. (1992). *Medical family therapy.* New York: Basic Books.

McDonald, A. C., Carson, K. L., Palmer, D. J., & Slay, T. (1982). Physicians' diagnostic information to parents of handicapped neonates. *Mental Retardation, 20*, 12–14.

McDowell, A. D., Saylor, C. F., Taylor, M. J., & Boyce, G. C. (1995). Ethnicity and parenting stress change during early intervention. *Early Child Development and Care, 111*, 131–140.

McGoldrick, M. (1982). Ethnicity and family therapy: An overview. In M. McGoldrick, J. K. Pearce, & J. Giordano (Eds.), *Ethnicity and family therapy* (pp. 3–30). New York: Guilford Press.

McGoldrick, M., Giordano, J., & Pierce, J. K. (Eds.). (1996). *Ethnicity and family therapy* (2nd ed.). New York: Guilford Press.

McHale, S. M., & Gamble, W. C. (1987). Sibling relationships and adjustment of children with disabled brothers and sisters. *Journal of Children in Contemporary Society, 19*, 131–158.

McHale, S. M., Sloan, J., & Simeonsson, R. J. (1986). Sibling relationships with autistic, mentally retarded, and non-handicapped brothers and sisters. *Journal of Autism and Developmental Disorders, 16*, 399–414.

McHugh, M. (1999). *Special siblings: Growing up with someone with a disability*. New York: Hyperion.

McHugh, M. (2003). *Special siblings: Growing up with someone with a disability* (rev. ed.). Baltimore: Brookes.

McHugh, P. (1968). *Defining the situation*. Indianapolis, IN: Bobbs-Merrill.

McKay, M., & Hensey, O. (1990). From the other side: Parents' views of their early contacts with health professionals. *Child: Care, Health, and Development, 16*, 23–28.

McLanahan, S., & Sandefur, G. (1994). *Growing up with a single parent: What hurts, what helps*. Cambridge, MA: Harvard University Press.

McMichael, J. K. (1971). *Handicap: A study of physically handicapped children and their families*. Pittsburgh, PA: University of Pittsburgh Press.

McPhee, N. (1982, June). A very special magic: A grandmother's delight. *Exceptional Parent*, pp. 13–16.

McWilliam, R. A., Lang, L., Vandiviers, P., Angell, R., Collins, L., & Underdown, G. (1995). Satisfaction and struggles: Family perceptions of early intervention. *Journal of Early Intervention, 19*, 3–60.

Mead, G. H. (1934). *Mind, self, and society*. Chicago: University of Chicago Press.

Mennuti, R., Freeman, A., & Christner, R. W. (2005). *Cognitive behavioral interventions in educational settings: A handbook for practice*. New York: Routledge.

Mercer, J. R. (1965). Social system perspective and clinical perspective: Frames of reference for understanding career patterns of persons labeled as mentally retarded. *Social Problems, 13*, 18–34.

Meyer, D. (2005). *The sibling slam book*. Bethesda, MD: Woodbine.

Meyer, D. J. (1995). *Uncommon fathers: Reflections on raising a child with a disability*. Bethesda, MD: Woodbine.

Meyer, D. J., & Vadasy, P. F. (1986). *Grandparent workshops: How to organize workshops for grandparents of children with handicaps*. Seattle: University of Washington Press.

Meyer, D. J., & Vadasy, P. F. (1994). *Sibshops: Workshops for siblings of children with special needs*. Baltimore: Brookes.

Meyer, D. J., Vadasy, P. F., Fewell, R. R., & Schell, G. (1985). *A handbook for the Fathers Program*. Seattle: University of Washington Press.

Meyer, J. Y. (1978). One of the family. In S. L. Brown & M. S. Moersch (Eds.), *Parents on the team* (pp. 103–111). Ann Arbor: University of Michigan Press.

Michaelis, C. T. (1980). *Home and school partnerships in exceptional children*. Rockville, MD: Aspen.

Middleton, L. (1999). *Disabled children: Challenging social exclusion*. Oxford: Blackwell Science.

Midence, K., & O'Neill, M. (1999). The experience of parents in the diagnosis of autism: A pilot study. *Autism, 3,* 273–285.

Miller, C. T., & Major, B. (2000). Coping with stigma and prejudice. In T. F. Heatherton, R. E. Kleck, M. R. Hebl, & J. G. Hull (Eds.), *The social psychology of stigma* (4th ed., pp. 504–553). New York: Guilford Press.

Min, P. G. (2002). Korean American families. In R. J. Taylor (Ed.), *Minority families in the United States: A multicultural perspective* (3rd ed., pp. 193–211). Upper Saddle River, NJ: Prentice Hall.

Minkler, M., & Roe, K. M. (1993). *Grandmothers as caregivers: Raising the children of the crack cocaine epidemic*. Thousand Oaks, CA: Sage.

Minnesota Governor's Council on Developmental Disabilities. (2003). *Partners in policymaking* Retrieved February 21, 2005, from http://www.partnersinpolicymaking.com

Minuchin, S. (1974). *Families and family therapy*. Cambridge, MA: Harvard University Press.

Minuchin, S., & Fishman, H. C. (1981). *Family therapy techniques*. Cambridge, MA: Harvard University Press.

Minuchin, S., & Nichols, M. P. (1993). *Family healing: Tales of hope and renewal from family therapy*. New York: Free Press.

Minuchin, S., Rosman, B. L., & Baker, L. (1978). *Psychosomatic families*. Cambridge, MA: Harvard University Press.

Misio, E. (1974). Impact of external systems on the Puerto Rican family. *Social Casework, 55,* 76–83.

Mitchell, D. (1983). Guidance needs and counseling of parents of mentally retarded persons. In N. N. Singh & K. M. Wilton (Eds.), *Mental retardation: Research and services in New Zealand* (pp. 136–156). Christchurch, New Zealand: Whitcoulls.

Moeller, C. J. (1986). The effect of professionals on the family of a handicapped child. In R. R. Fewell & P. F. Vadasy (Eds.), *Families of handicapped children* (pp. 149–166). Austin, TX: PRO-ED.

Moen, P., & Wethington, E. (1999). Midlife development in a life course context. In S. L. Willis & J. D. Ried (Eds.), *Life in the middle: Psychological and social development in middle age* (pp. 3–23). San Diego, CA: Academic Press.

Mondimore, F. M. (2002). *Adolescent depression: A guide for parents*. Baltimore: Johns Hopkins University Press.

Montalvo, B. (1974). Home–school conflict in the Puerto Rican child. *Social Casework, 55,* 76–83.

Moore, K. A., Jekielek, M. A., & Emig, C. (2002). *Marriage from a child's perspective: How does family structure affect children, and what can We do about it?* Child Trends.

Moores, D. (2006). *Education of the deaf: Psychology, principles, and practices*. Boston: Houghton Mifflin.

Moorman, M. (1992a, January–February). My sister's keeper. *Family Therapy Networker,* pp. 41–47.

Moorman, M. (1992b). *My sister's keeper: Learning to cope with a sister's mental illness*. New York: Norton.

Morgan, S. (1987). *Abuse and neglect of handicapped children*. Boston: College-Hill Press.

Mori, A. A. (1983). *Families of children with special needs: Early intervention*. Rockville, MD: Aspen.

Morris, M. M. (1987, March). Health care: Who pays the bills? *Exceptional Parent,* pp. 38–42.

Murphy, A., Paeschel, S., Duffy, T., & Brady, E. (1976). Meeting with brothers and sisters of Down's syndrome children. *Children Today, 5,* 20–23.

Naseef, R. A. (1999). *Big boys don't cry: At least on the outside* [Electronic version]. Retrieved from http://www.fsma.org/bigboys.shtml

Naseef, R. A. (2001a). The rudest awakening. In S. D. Klein & K. Schive (Eds.), *You will dream new dreams: Inspiring personal stories by parents of children with disabilities* (pp. 206–210). New York: Kensington Books.

Naseef, R. A. (2001b). *Special children, challenged parents: The struggles and rewards of raising a child with a disability.* Baltimore: Brookes.

National Clearinghouse on Child Abuse and Neglect (NCCAN). (2004). Child maltreatment 2002: Summary of key findings. Retrieved from http://nccanch.acf.hhs.gov/pubs/factsheets/canstats.cen

National Community Behavioral Healthcare Council. (1997). *Principles for behavioral healthcare delivery.* Rockville, MD: Author.

National Organization on Disability/Harris Survey of Americans with Disabilities. (2000). New York: Harris Interactive.

NCHS studies health insurance and chronically ill children. (1992). *Nation's Health,* p. 13.

Nelson, K., & Allen, M. (1995). Family-centered social services: Moving toward system change. In P. N. Adams & K. Nelson (Eds.), *Reinventing human services: Community-and family-centered practice* (pp. 109–125). New York: Aldine de Gruyter.

Nelson, N. D. (1991, June). Meet my daughter, Annie. *Exceptional Parent,* pp. 22–23.

Neugeboren, J. (1997). *Imagining Robert: My brother, madness, and survival.* New York: Morrow.

Newman, J. (1991). Handicapped persons and their families: Philosophical, historical, and legislative perspectives. In M. Seligman (Ed.), *The family with a handicapped child* (2nd ed., pp. 1–26). Boston: Allyn & Bacon.

Nissenbaum, M. S., Tollefson, N., & Reese, M. R. (2002). The interpretive conference: Sharing a diagnosis of autism with families. *Focus on Autism and Other Developmental Disabilities, 17,* 30–43.

Northy, S., Griffin, W. A., & Krainz, S. (1998). A partial test of the psychosomatic family model: Marital interaction patterns in asthma and nonasthma families. *Journal of Family Psychology, 12,* 220–233.

Offer, D., Ostrov, E., & Howard, K. L. (1984). Body image, self-perception, and chronic illness in adolescence. In R. W. Blum (Ed.), *Chronic illness and disabilities in childhood and adolescence* (pp. 59–73). Orlando, FL: Grune & Stratton.

Oliver, M. (1996). *Understanding disability: From theory to practice.* New York: St. Martin's Press.

Olkin, R. (1999). *What psychotherapists should know about disability.* New York: Guilford Press.

Olshansky, S. (1962). Chronic sorrow: A response to having a mentally defective child. *Social Casework, 43,* 190–193.

Olson, D. H. (1993). Circumplex model of marital and family systems. In F. Walsh (Ed.), *Normal family processes* (2nd ed., pp. 253–268). New York: Guilford Press.

Olson, D. H., McCubbin, H. I., Barnes, H., Larsen, A., Muxen, M., & Wilson, M. (1984). *One thousand families: A national survey.* Beverly Hills, CA: Sage.

Olson, D. H., Russell, C. S., & Sprenkle, D. H. (1980). Circumplex model of marital and family systems II: Empirical studies and clinical intervention. In J. P. Vincent (Ed.), *Advances in family intervention assessment and theory* (Vol. 1, pp. 129–179). Greenwich, CT: JAI Press.

Olsson, M. B., & Hwang, P. C. (2003). Influence of macrostructure of society on the life situation of families with a child with intellectual disability: Sweden as an example. *Journal of Intellectual Disability Research, 47,* 328–341.

Opirhory, G., & Peters, G. A. (1982). Counseling intervention strategies for families with the less than perfect newborn. *Personnel and Guidance Journal, 60,* 451–455.

Orsmond, G. I., & Seltzer, M. M. (2000). Brothers and sisters of adults with mental retardation: Gendered nature of the sibling relationship. *American Journal on Mental Retardation, 105,* 486–508.

Ortiz, V. (1995). Diversity of Latino families. In R. E. Zambrana (Ed.), *Understanding Latino families: Scholarship, policy, and practice* (pp. 18–39). Thousand Oaks, CA: Sage.

Pais, S. (1997). Asian Indian families in America. In M. K. DeGenova (Ed.), *Families in cultural context: Strengths and challenges in diversity* (pp. 173–190). Mountain View, CA: Mayfield.

Paniagua, F. A. (1998). *Assessing and treating culturally diverse clients: A practical guide* (2nd ed.). Thousand Oaks, CA: Sage.

Parham, T. A. (2002). Counseling models for African Americans. In T. A. Parham (Ed.), *Counseling persons of African descent: Raising the bar of practitioner competence* (pp. 100–118). Thousand Oaks, CA: Sage.

Park, J., Turnbull, A. P., & Turnbull, H. R. I. (2002). Impacts of poverty on quality of life in families of children with disabilities. *Exceptional Children, 68*(2), 151–170.

Parke, R. D. (1981). *Fathers.* Cambridge, MA: Harvard University Press.

Parsons, T. (1951). *The social system.* Glencoe, IL: Free Press.

Patterson, J. M. (1985). Critical factors affecting family compliance with home treatment for children with cystic fibrosis. *Family Relations, 34,* 79–89.

Patterson, J. M. (1991). A family systems perspective for working with youth with disability. *Pediatrics, 18,* 129–141.

Paun, M. V. (2006). *A constant burden* (2nd ed.). London: Ashgate.

Peck, J. R., & Stephens, W. B. (1960). A study of the relationship between the attitudes and behavior of parents and that of their mentally defective child. *American Journal of Mental Deficiency, 64,* 839–844.

Peck-Peterson, S. M., Derby, K. M., Berg, W. K., & Horner, R. H. (2002). Collaboration with families in the functional behavior assessment of and intervention for severe behavior problems. *Education and Treatment of Children, 25,* 5–25.

Pelchat, D., Bisson, J., Ricard, N., Perreault, M., & Bouchard, M. (1999). Longitudinal effects of an early family intervention programme on the adaptation of parents of children with a disability. *International Journal of Nursing Studies, 36,* 465–477.

Pelham, T. (2001). Looking toward the future unafraid. In S. D. Klein & K. Schive (Eds.), *You will dream new dreams: Inspiring stories by parents of children with disabilities* (pp. 23–25). New York: Kensington Books.

Pepper, F. C. (1976). Teaching the American Indian child in mainstream settings. In R. L. Jones (Ed.), *Mainstreaming and the minority child* (pp. 108–122). Reston, VA: Council for Exceptional Children.

Perrin, J. M., & MacLean, W. E. (1988). Biomedical and psychosocial dimensions of chronic illness in children. In P. Kardy (Ed.), *Handbook of child health assessment* (pp. 11–29). New York: Wiley.

Perske, R. (1972). The dignity of risk. In W. Wolfensberger (Ed.), *Normalization: The principle of normalization in human services* (pp. 194–200). Toronto: National Institute on Mental Retardation.

Pescosolido, B. A., Tuch, S. A., & Martin, J. K. (2001). The profession of medicine and the public: Examining Americans' changing confidence in physician authority from the beginning of the "health care crisis" to the era of health care reform. *Journal of Health and Social Behavior, 42*(1), 1–16.

Peter, M. I., & Sia, C. C. J. (1994). Preparing physicians through continuing medical education. In R. B. Darling & M. I. Peter (Eds.), *Families, physicians, and children with special health needs: Collaborative medical education models* (pp. 124–134). Westport, CT: Auburn House.

Pilisuk, M., & Parks, S. H. (1986). *The healing web: Social networks and human survival*. Hanover, NH: University Press of New England.

Pizzo, P. (1983). *Parent to parent: Working together for ourselves and our children* Boston: Beacon Press.

Polk, C. (1994). Therapeutic work with African-American families. *Zero to Three, 15*, 9–11.

Pollin, I. (1995). *Medical crisis counseling*. New York: Norton.

Poston, D. J., & Turnbull, A. P. (2004). Role of spirituality and religion in family quality of life for families of children with disabilities. *Education and Training in Developmental Disabilities, 39*, 95–108.

Powell, D. R. (1995). Including Latino fathers in parent education and support programs: Development of a program model. In R. E. Zambrana (Ed.), *Understanding Latino families: Scholarship, policy, and practice* (pp. 85–106). Thousand Oaks, CA: Sage.

Powell, J. D. (1975). *Theory of coping systems: Changes in supportive health organizations*. Cambridge, MA: Schenkman.

Powell, T. H., & Gallagher, P. E. (1993). *Brothers and sisters: A special part of exceptional families* (2nd ed.). Baltimore: Brookes.

Powell, T., & Ogle, P. A. (1993). *Brothers and sisters: A special part of exceptional families*. Baltimore: Brookes.

Power, T. J., DuPaul, G. J., Shapiro, E. S., & Kazak, A. F. (2003). *Promoting children's health*. New York: Guilford Press.

Poznanski, E. (1969). Psychiatric difficulties in siblings of handicapped children. *Pediatrics, 8*, 232–234.

Pratt, J. H. (1907). The class method of treating consumption in the homes of the poor. *Journal of the American Medical Association, 49*, 755–759.

Presley, D. (1995, March). Where are they? *National Fathers' Network Newsletter*.

Price, J. A. (1976). North American Indian families. In C. H. Mindel & R. W. Habenstein (Eds.), *Ethnic families in America: Patterns and variations* (pp. 248–270). New York: Elsevier.

Protection of handicapped newborns. (1986, June 26–27). Hearing held in Washington, DC. Washington, DC: U.S. Commission on Civil Rights.

Pruett, K. D. (1987). *The nurturing father*. New York: Warner.

Purkayastha, B. (2002). Rules, roles, and realities: Indo-American families in the United States. In R. J. Taylor (Ed.), *Minority families in the United States: A multicultural perspective* (3rd ed., pp. 212–224). Upper Saddle River, NJ: Prentice Hall.

Quesada, G. M. (1976). Language and communication barriers for health delivery to a minority group. *Social Science and Medicine, 10*, 323–327.

Quine, L. C., & Pahl, J. (1986). First diagnosis of severe mental handicap: Characteristics of unsatisfactory encounters between doctors and parents. *Social Science and Medicine, 22*, 53–62.

Quine, L. C., & Rutter, D. R. (1994). First diagnosis of severe mental and physical disability: A study of doctor–patient communication. *Journal of Child Psychology and Psychiatry, 35*(7), 1273–1288.

Quinn, D. M. (1999). *Protestant ethic and judgments of stigmatized groups*. Unpublished manuscript, University of Michigan.

Rak, C. F., & Patterson, L. E. (1996). Promoting resilience in at-risk children. *Journal of Counseling and Development, 74*, 368–373.

Ramsey, C. N. (Ed.). (1989). *Family systems in medicine*. New York: Guilford Press.

Rank, M. R. (2000). Poverty and economic hardship in families. In D. H. Demo, K. R. Allen, & M. A. Fine (Eds.), *Handbook of family diversity* (pp. 293–315). New York: Oxford University Press.

Readers' forum. (1985). *Exceptional Parent*, p. 7.

Related services and the Supreme Court: A family's story. (1984, October). *Exceptional Parent*, pp. 36–41.

Resnick, M. D. (1984). The social construction of disability. In R. W. Blum (Ed.), *Chronic illness and disabilities in childhood and adolescence* (pp. 29–46). Orlando, FL: Grune & Stratton.

Reynolds, T., & Zellmer, D. D. (1985). Group for siblings of preschool age children with handicaps. *Sibling Information Network Newsletter*, p. 2.

Ricci, L. A., & Hodapp, R. M. (2003). Fathers of children with Down syndrome versus other types of intellectual disabilities. *Journal of Intellectual Disability Research, 47*, 273–284.

Richan, W. C. (1991). *Lobbying for social change*. New York: Haworth Press.

Richardson, S. A. (1972). People with cerebral palsy talk for themselves. *Developmental Medicine and Child Neurology, 14*, 521–535.

Robert Wood Johnson Foundation. (2004). IPhysician perspectives on communication barriers. Princeton, NJ: Author.

Robson, K. S., & Moss, H. A. (1970). Patterns and determinants of maternal attachment. *Journal of Pediatrics, 77*, 976–985.

Rodwin, M. A. (1994). Patient accountability and quality of care: Lessons from medical consumerism and the patients' rights, women's health and disability rights movements. *American Journal of Law and Medicine, 20*, 147–167.

Rogers, M. L., & Hogan, D. P. (2003). Family life with children with disabilities: The key role of rehabilitation. *Journal of Marriage and the Family, 65*, 818–833.

Rogers-Dulan, J., & Blacher, J. (1995). African American families, religion and disability: A conceptual framework. *Mental Retardation, 33*, 226–238.

Rolland, J. S. (1994). *Families, illness, and disability: An integrative treatment model*. New York: Basic Books.

Rolland, J. S. (2003). Mastering family challenges in serious illness and disability. In F. Walsh (Ed.), *Normal family processes* (3rd ed., pp. 460–489). New York: Guilford Press.

Romaine, M. E. (1982). Clinical management of the Spanish-speaking patient: Pleasures and pitfalls. *Clinical Management in Physical Therapy, 2*, 9–10.

Rosen, E. J., & Weltman, S. F. (1996). Jewish families: An overview. In M. McGoldrick, J. Giordano, & J. K. Pierce (Eds.), *Ethnicity and family therapy* (2nd ed., pp. 611–630). New York: Guilford Press.

Ross, A. O. (1964). *The exceptional child in the family*. New York: Grune & Stratton.

Rousso, H. (1985). Fostering healthy self-esteem. *Exceptional Parent*, pp. 209–214.

Rubin, S., & Quinn-Curran, N. (1983). Lost, then found: Parents' journey through the community service maze. In M. Seligman (Ed.), *The family with a handicapped child: Understanding and treatment* (pp. 63–94). Orlando, FL: Grune & Stratton.

Ruef, M. B., & Turnbull, A. P. (2001). Stakeholder opinions on accessible, informational products helpful in building positive, practical solutions for behavioral challenges of individuals with mental retardation and autism. *Education and Training in Mental Retardation and Developmental Disabilities, 36,* 441–456.

Rump, M. L. (2002). Involving fathers of young children with special needs. *Young Children, 57,* 18–20.

Russell, M. (1994). Malcolm teaches us too. In B. Shaw (Ed.), *The ragged edge: The disability experience from the pages of the first fifteen years of the Disability Rag* (pp. 11–14). Louisville, KY: Advocado Press.

Sabbeth, B. F., & Leventhal, J. M. (1984). Marital adjustment to chronic childhood illness. *Pediatrics, 73,* 762–768.

Safer, J. (2002). *The normal one: Life with a difficult or damaged sibling.* New York: Free Press.

Safilios-Rothschild, C. (1970). *The sociology and social psychology of disability and rehabilitation.* New York: Random House.

San Martino, M., & Newman, M. B. (1974). Siblings of retarded children: A population at risk. *Child Psychiatry and Human Development, 4,* 168–177.

Sanchez, Y. M. (1997). Families of Mexican origin. In M. K. DeGenova (Ed.), *Families in cultural context: Strengths and challenges in diversity* (pp. 61–83). Mountain View, CA: Mayfield.

Santana-Martin, S., & Santana, F. (2005). An introduction to Mexican culture for service providers. In J. H. Stone (Ed.), *Culture and disability: Providing culturally competent services* (pp. 161–186). Thousand Oaks, CA: Sage.

Santelli, B., Poyadue, F. S., & Young, J. L. (2001). *The parent to parent handbook.* Baltimore: Brookes.

Santelli, B., Turnbull, A., Sergeant, J., Lerner, E., & Marquis, J. (1996). Parent to parent programs: Parent preferences for support. *Infants and Young Children, 9,* 53–62.

Santiago-Rivera, A. L., Arrendondo, P., & Gallardo-Cooper, M. (2002). *Counseling Latinos and la familia: A practical guide.* Thousand Oaks, CA: Sage.

Scanlon, C. A., Arick, J., & Phelps, N. (1981). Participation in the development of the IEP: Parents' perspective. *Exceptional Children, 47,* 373–374.

Scanzoni, J. (1985). Black parental values and expectations of children's occupational and educational success: Theoretical implications. In H. P. McAdoo & J. L. McAdoo (Eds.), *Black children: Social, educational, and parental environments* (pp. 113–122). Beverly Hills, CA: Sage.

Schiele, J. H. (2000). *Human services and the Afrocentric paradigm.* New York: Haworth Press.

Schilling, R. F., Gilchrist, L. D., & Schinke, S. P. (1984). Coping and social support in families of developmentally disabled children. *Family Relations, 33,* 47–54.

Schonberg, R. J., & Tifft, C. J. (2002). Birth defects, prenatal diagnoses, and fetal therapy. In M. L. Batshaw (Ed.), *Children with disabilities* (5th ed., pp. 27–41). Baltimore: Brookes.

Schonell, F. J., & Rorke, M. (1960). A second survey of the effects of a subnormal child on the family unit. *American Journal of Mental Deficiency, 64,* 862–868.

Schonell, F. J., & Watts, B. H. (1956). A first survey of the effects of a subnormal child on the family unit. *American Journal of Mental Deficiency, 61,* 210–219.

Schopler, E., & Mesibov, G. (Eds.). (1984). *The effects of autism on the family.* New York: Plenum Press.

Schreiber, J. M., & Feeley, M. (1965). A guided group experience. *Children, 12,* 221–225.

Schreiber, J. M., & Homiak, J. P. (1981). Mexican Americans. In A. Harwood (Ed.), *Ethnicity and medical care* (pp. 264–336). Cambridge, MA: Harvard University Press.

Schulz, J. B. (1987). *Parents and professionals in special education.* Boston: Allyn & Bacon.

Schwab, L. O. (1989). Strengths of families having a member with a disability. *Journal of the Multihandicapped Person, 2,* 105–117.

Scorgie, K., Wilgosh, H., & McDonald, L. (1998). Stress and coping in families of children with disabilities: An examination of recent literature. *Developmental Disabilities Bulletin, 26,* 24–42.

Searle, S. J. (1978). Stages of parents' reaction. *Exceptional Parent, 8,* 27–29.

Segal, U. A. (1998). The Asian Indian-American family. In C. H. Mindel, R. W. Habenstein, & R. Wright, Jr. (Eds.), *Ethnic families in America* (4th ed., pp. 284–314). Upper Saddle River, NJ: Prentice Hall.

Seligman, M. (1979). *Strategies for helping parents of exceptional children: A guide for teachers.* New York: Free Press.

Seligman, M. (Ed.). (1991a). *The family with a handicapped child* (2nd ed.). Boston: Allyn & Bacon.

Seligman, M. (1991b). Grandparents of disabled grandchildren: Hopes, fears, and adaptation. *Families in Society, 72,* 147–152.

Seligman, M. (1993). Group work with parents of children with disabilities. *Journal for Specialists in Group Work, 18,* 115–126.

Seligman, M. (1995). Confessions of a professional/father. In D. Meyer (Ed.), *Uncommon fathers* (pp. 169–183). Bethesda, MD: Woodbine.

Seligman, M. (2000). *Conducting effective conferences with parents of children with disabilities.* New York: Guilford Press.

Seligman, M., & Marshak, L. E. (2003). Group approaches for persons with disabilities. In J. L. Delucia-Waack, D. A. Gerrity, C. R. Kalodner, & M. Riva (Eds.), *Handbook of group counseling and psychotherapy* (pp. 239–252). Thousand Oaks, CA: Sage.

Seltzer, M. M., & Krauss, M. W. (1984). Placement alternatives for mentally retarded children and their families. In J. Blacher (Ed.), *Severely handicapped young children and their families: Research in review* (pp. 143–175). Orlando, FL: Academic Press.

Senator, S. (2004, August 1). Home alone: A mother's mission: That her autistic son become an independent adult. *The New York Times,* p. 34.

Shapiro, J. (1994). *No pity: People with disabilities forging a new civil rights movement.* New York: Times Books.

Shapiro, J., & Tittle, K. (1986). Psychosocial adjustment of poor Mexican mothers of disabled and nondisabled children. *American Journal of Orthopsychiatry, 56,* 289–302.

Shapiro, J., Monzo, L. D., Rueda, R., Gomez, J. A., & Blacher, J. (2004). Alienated advocacy: Perspectives of Latina mothers of young adults with developmental disabilities on service systems. *Mental Retardation, 42,* 37–54.

Sharpe, D., & Rossiter, L. (2002). Siblings of children with a chronic illness: A meta-analysis. *Journal of Pediatric Psychology, 27,* 699–710.

Sherif, B. (1999). Islamic family ideals and their relevance to American Muslim families. In H. P. McAdoo (Ed.), *Family ethnicity: Strength in diversity* (2nd ed., pp. 203–212). Thousand Oaks, CA: Sage.

Shields, M. K., & Behrman, R. E. (2002). Children and welfare reform: Analysis and recommendations. *The Future of Children, 12*(1), 5–25.

Shon, S. P., & Ja, D. Y. (1982). Asian families. In M. McGoldrick, J. K. Pearce, & J. Giordano (Eds.), *Ethnicity and family therapy* (pp. 208–228). New York: Guilford Press.

Siegel, B. (1996). *The world of the autistic child.* New York: Oxford University Press.

Siegel, B. (2003). *Helping children with autism learn.* New York: Oxford University Press.

Siegel, B., & Silverstein, S. (1994). *What about me?: Growing up with a developmentally disabled sibling.* New York: Plenum Press.

Siller, J. (1984). Personality and attitudes toward physical disabilities. In C. J. Golden (Ed.), *Current topics in rehabilitation psychology* (pp. 201–227). New York: Grune and Stratton.

Silverstein, L. B., & Auerbach, C. F. (1999). Deconstructing the essential father. *American Psychologist, 54,* 397–407.

Simeonsson, R. J., & Bailey, D. B. (1986). Siblings of handicapped children. In J. J. Gallagher & W. Vietze (Eds.), *Families of handicapped persons* (pp. 67–77). Baltimore: Brookes.

Simmerman, S., Blacher, J., & Baker, B. (2001). Fathers' and mothers' perceptions of father involvement in families with young children with a disability. *Journal of Intellectual and Developmental Disabilities, 26,* 325–338.

Simon, B. L. (1994). *The empowerment tradition in American social work: A history.* New York: Columbia University Press.

Simon, C. (1997). *Mad house: Growing up in the shadow of mentally ill siblings.* New York: Penguin.

Simons, J. A. (2004, September–October). Thinking about tomorrow: The transition to adult life. *Disability Solutions,* pp. 1, 4–12.

Simos, G. (2002). *Cognitive behavior therapy.* New York: Routledge.

Simpson, R. L. (1990). *Conferencing parents of exceptional children.* Austin, TX: PRO-ED.

Simpson, R. L. (1996). *Working with parents and families of exceptional children and youth.* Austin, TX: Pro-Ed.

Singer, G. H., Marquis, J., Powers, L., Blanchard, L., DiVenere, N., & Santelli, B. (1999). A multi-site evaluation of parent to parent programs for parents of children with disabilities. *Journal of Early Intervention, 22,* 217–219.

Singer, G. H. S., & Powers, L. E. (1993). *Families, disability, and empowerment.* Baltimore: Brookes.

Sivola, S. (2001). Life is good. In S. D. Klein & K. Schive (Eds.), *You will dream new dreams: Inspiring personal stories by parents of children with disabilities* (pp. 11–15). New York: Kensington Books.

Skinner, D. G., Correa, V., Skinner, M., & Bailey, D. B. (2001). Role of religion in the lives of Latino families of young children with developmental delays. *American Journal on Mental Retardation, 106,* 297–313.

Sloman, L. M., Springer, S., & Vachon, M. L. (1993). Disordered communication and grieving in deaf member families. *Family Process, 32,* 171–181.

Sloper, P., Knussen, C., Turner, S., & Cunningham, C. (1991). Factors related to stress and satisfaction with life in families of children with Down's syndrome. *Journal of Child Psychology and Psychiatry, 32,* 655–676.

Sloper, P., & Turner, S. (1991). Parental and professional views of the needs of families with a child with severe physical disability. *Counseling Psychology Quarterly, 4,* 323–330.

Smith, K. (1981). The influence of the male sex role on discussion groups for fathers of exceptional children. *Michigan Personnel and Guidance Journal, 12,* 11–17.

Sommers-Flanagan, J., & Sommers-Flanagan, R. (1993). *Foundations of therapeutic interviewing.* Boston: Allyn & Bacon.

Sonnek, I. M. (1986). Grandparents and the extended family of handicapped children. In R. R. Fewell & P. F. Vadasy (Eds.), *Families of handicapped children* (pp. 99–120). Austin, TX: PRO-ED.

Sontag, J. C., & Schacht, R. (1994). An ethnic comparison of parent participation and information needs in early intervention. *Exceptional Children, 60,* 422–433.

Sosnowitz, B. G. (1984). Managing parents on neonatal intensive care units. *Social Problems, 31,* 390–402.

Sourkes, B. M. (1987). Siblings of a child with a life-threatening illness. *Journal of Children in Contemporary Society, 19*, 159–184.

Spano, S. L. (1994). The miracle of Michael. In R. B. Darling & M. I. Peter (Eds.), *Families, physicians, and children with special health needs: Collaborative medical education models* (pp. 29–50). Westport, CT: Auburn House.

Specht, H., & Courtney, M. E. (1994). *Unfaithful angels: How social work has abandoned its mission.* New York: The Free Press.

Spector, R. E. (1979). *Cultural diversity in health and illness.* New York: Appleton-Century-Crofts.

Spira, J. L. (Ed.). (1997). *Group therapy for medically ill patients.* New York: Guilford Press.

Spruill, L. C. (2004). Affirmation and challenge. In S. D. Klein & J. D. Kemp (Eds.), *Reflections from a different journey: What adults with disabilities wish all parents knew* (pp. 91–95). New York: McGraw-Hill.

Squires, D. A., & Quadagno, J. S. (1998). The Italian-American family. In C. H. Mindel, R. W. Habenstein, & R. Wright, Jr. (Eds.), *Ethnic families in America: Patterns and variations* (4th ed., pp. 102–127). Upper Saddle River, NJ: Prentice Hall.

Stacey, J. (1998). Gay and Lesbian families: Queer like us. In M. A. Mason, A. Skolnick, & S. D. Sugarman (Eds.), *All our families: New policies for a new century* (pp. 117–143). New York: Oxford University Press.

Stein, R. C. (1983). Hispanic parents' perspectives and participation in their children's special education program: Comparisons by program and race. *Learning Disability Quarterly, 6*, 432–439.

Stein, R. E., & Jessop, D. J. (1984). General issues in the care of children with chronic physical condition. *Pediatric Clinics of North America, 31*, 189–198.

Stoneman, Z., & Berman, P. W. (1993). *The effects of mental retardation, disability, and illness on sibling relationships.* Baltimore: Brookes.

Stoneman Z., Brody, G. H., Davis, C. H., Crapps, J. M., & Malone, D. M. (1991). Ascribed role relations between children with mental retardation and their younger siblings. *American Journal of Mental Retardation, 95*, 537–550.

Stotland, J. (1984, February). Relationship of parents to professionals: A challenge to professionals. *Journal of Visual Impairment and Blindness*, pp. 69–74.

Strax, T. E. (1991). Psychological issues faced by adolescents and young adults with disabilities. *Pediatric Annals, 20*, 507–511.

Streiner, D. L., Saigal, S., Burrows, E., Stoskopf, B., & Rosenbaum, P. (2001). Attitudes of parents and health care professionals toward active treatment of extremely premature infants. *Pediatrics, 108*(1), 152–158.

Strohm, K. (2005). *Being the other one: Growing up with a brother or sister who has special needs.* Boston: Shambhala.

Stroman, D. F. (2003). *The disability rights movement: From deinstitutionalization to self-determination.* Lanham, MD: University Press of America.

Stromme, P. (2000). Correlations between socioeconomic status, IQ and aetiology in mental retardation: A population-based study of Norwegian children. *Social Psychiatry and Psychiatric Epidemiology, 35*, 12–18.

Strong, P. M. (1979). *The ceremonial order of the clinic: Parents, doctors, and medical bureaucracies.* London: Routledge & Kegan Paul.

Suelzle, M., & Keenan, V. (1981). Changes in family support networks over the life cycle of mentally retarded persons. *American Journal of Mental Deficiency, 86*, 267–274.

Sullivan, P. M., & Knudson, J. E. (2000). Maltreatment and disabilities: A population-based epidemiological study. *Child Abuse and Neglect: The International Journal, 24*, 1257–1273.

Summers, J. A., Boller, K., & Raikes, H. H. (2004). Preferences and perceptions about getting support expressed by low-income fathers. *Fathering: A Journal of Theory, Research, and Practice about Men as Fathers, 2,* 61–82.

Svarstad, B. L., & Lipton, H. L. (1977). Informing parents about mental retardation: A study of professional communication and parent acceptance. *Social Science and Medicine, 11,* 645–651.

Swados, E. (1991). *The four of us: A family memoir.* New York: Farrar, Strauss, & Giroux.

Swain, J., & French, S. (2000). Towards an affirmation model of Disability. *Disability and Society, 15,* 569–582.

Swain, J., & Walker, C. (2003). Parent–professional power relations: Parent and professional perspectives. *Disability and Society, 18*(5), 547–560.

Szish, J. (2004, Summer). There she is. *Pitt Magazine,* pp. 13–15.

Tallman, I. (1965). Spousal role differentiation and the socialization of severely retarded children. *Journal of Marriage and the Family, 27,* 37–42.

Tartar, S. B. (1987). *Traumatic head injury: Parental stress, coping style and emotional adjustment.* Unpublished doctoral dissertation, University of Pittsburgh.

Taylor, R. J. (2002). Black American families. In R. J. Taylor (Ed.), *Minority families in the United States: A multicultural perspective* (3rd ed., pp. 19–47). Upper Saddle River, NJ: Prentice Hall.

Telford, C. W., & Sawrey, J. M. (1977). *The exceptional individual* (3rd ed.). Englewood Cliffs, NJ: Prentice-Hall.

Tew, B., & Lawrence, K. M. (1975). Mothers, brothers and sisters of patients with spina bifida. *Developmental Medicine and Child Neurology, 15*(Suppl. 29), 69–76.

Tew, B., Lawrence, K. M., Payne, H., & Rawnsley, K. (1977). Marital stability following the birth of a child with spina bifida. *British Journal of Psychiatry, 131,* 79–82.

Teyber, E. (1992). *Helping children cope with divorce.* New York: Lexington Books.

Thibodeau, S. M. (1988). Sibling response to chronic illness: The role of the clinical nurse specialist. *Issues in Comprehensive Pediatric Nursing, 11,* 17–28.

Thompson, R. J., & Gustafson, K. E. (1996). *Adaptation to chronic childhood illness.* Washington, DC: American Psychological Association.

Tillman, F. (2001). Unconditionally yours. In S. D. Klein & K. Schive (Eds.), *You will dream new dreams: Inspiring personal stories by parents of children with disabilities* (pp. 153–155). New York: Kensington Books.

Tolson, T. F. J., & Wilson, M. N. (1990). The impact of two- and three-generational black family structure on perceived family climate. *Child Development, 61,* 416–428.

Trainer, M. (1991). *Differences in common: Straight talk on mental retardation, Down syndrome and life.* Rockville, MD: Woodbine.

Tran, T. V. (1998). The Vietnamese-American family. In C. H. Mindel, R. W. Habenstein, & R. Wright, Jr. (Eds.), *Ethnic families in America: Patterns and variations* (4th ed., pp. 254–283). Upper Saddle River, NJ: Prentice Hall.

Travis, C. (1976). *Chronic illness in children.* Palo Alto, CA: Stanford University Press.

Trevino, F. (1979). Siblings of handicapped children. *Social Casework, 60,* 488–493.

Trimble, J. E., & Thurman, P. J. (2002). Ethnocultural considerations and strategies for providing counseling services to Native American Indians. In P. B. Pedersen, J. G. Draguns, W. J. Lonner, & J. Trimble (Eds.), *Counseling across cultures* (5th ed., pp. 53–91). Thousand Oaks, CA: Sage.

Tripp, J. M., & McGregor, D. (2006). Withholding and withdrawing of life sustaining treatment in the newborn. *Archives of Disease in Childhood, 91,* F67–F71.

Tritt, S. G., & Esses, L. M. (1988). Psychological adaptation of siblings of children with chronic medical illness. *American Journal of Orthopsychiatry, 58,* 211–220.

Trivette, C. M., & Dunst, C. J. (1982). *Proactive influences of social support in families of handicapped children.* Unpublished manuscript.

Trute, B. (1995). Gender differences in the psychological adjustment of parents of young, developmentally disabled children. *Journal of Child Psychology and Psychiatry, 36,* 1225–1242.

Trute, B. (2003). Grandparents of children with developmental disabilities: Intergenerational support and family well-being. *Families in Society, 84,* 119–126.

Turbiville, V. P. (1994). *Fathers, their children, and disability.* Unpublished doctoral dissertation, University of Kansas.

Turk, D. C., & Kerns, R. D. (1985). *Health, illness and families: A life-span perspective.* New York: Wiley.

Turnbull, A. P., Brotherson, M. J., & Summers, J. A. (1985). The impact of deinstitutionalization on families: A family systems approach. In R. H. Bruininks (Ed.), *Living and learning in the least restrictive environment* (pp. 115–152). Baltimore: Brookes.

Turnbull, A. P., Patterson, J. M., Behr, S. R., Murphy, D. L., Marquis, J. G., & Blue-Banning, M. J. (Eds.). (1993). *Cognitive coping, families, and disability.* Baltimore: Brookes.

Turnbull, A. P., Summers, J. A., & Brotherson, M. J. (1986). Family life cycle: Theoretical and empirical implications and future directions for families with mentally retarded members. In J. J. Gallagher & P. M. Vietze (Eds.), *Families of handicapped persons* (pp. 45–65). Baltimore: Brookes.

Turnbull, A. P., & Turnbull, H. R. (1986). *Families, professionals, and exceptionality.* Columbus, OH: Merrill.

Turnbull, A. P., & Turnbull, H. R. (1990). *Families, professionals, and exceptionality* (2nd ed.). Columbus, OH: Merrill.

Turnbull, A. P., & Turnbull, H. R. (1993). Enhancing beneficial linkages across the life span. *Disability Studies Quarterly, 13*(4), 34–36.

Turnbull, A. P., & Turnbull, H. R. (1996). An analysis of self-determination within a culturally responsive family systems perspective: Balancing the family mobile. In L. E. Powers, G. H. S. Singer, & J. Sowers (Ed.), *On the road to autonomy: Promoting self-competence among children and youth with disabilities* (pp. 195–220). Baltimore: Brookes.

Turnbull, A. P., & Turnbull, H. R. (2001). *Families, professionals, and exceptionality* (4th ed.). Upper Saddle River, NJ: Merrill/Prentice Hall.

Turnbull, A. P., Turnbull, H. R., Erwin, E. J., & Soodak, L. C. (2006). *Families, professionals, and exceptionality* (5th ed.). Upper Saddle River, NJ: Pearson/Merrill-Prentice Hall.

Turnbull, A. P., Turnbull, H. R., Shank, M., & Leal, D. (1999). *Exceptional lives: Special education in today's schools* (2nd ed.). Upper Saddle River, NJ: Merrill/Prentice Hall.

Turnbull, H. R., & Turnbull, A. P. (Eds.). (1985). *Parents speak out: Then and now.* Columbus, OH: Merrill.

Ufner, M. J. (2004). *Lifespan effects of having a sibling with schizophrenia.* Unpublished doctoral dissertation, University of Pittsburgh.

U.S. Bureau of the Census. (2003a). *Disability status: 2000–Census 2000 brief.* Washington, DC: Author.

U.S. Bureau of the Census. (2003b). *National population estimates.* Washington, DC: Author.

U.S. Department of Education. (1996). *Eighteenth annual report to congress on the implementation of the Individuals with Disabilities Act.* Washington, DC: Author.

U.S. Department of Education. (2002). *National assessment of educational progress.* Washington, DC: National Center for Education Statistics.

Upshur, C. C. (1982). Respite care for mentally retarded and other disabled populations: Program models and family needs. *Mental Retardation, 20,* 2-6.

Upshur, C. C. (1991). Families and the community service maze. In M. Seligman (Ed.), *The family with a handicapped child* (pp. 91-118). Boston: Allyn & Bacon.

Vadasy, P. F. (1986). Single mothers: A social phenomenon and population in need. In R. R. Fewell & P. F. Vadasy (Eds.), *Families of handicapped children* (pp. 221-249). Austin, TX: PRO-ED.

Vadasy, P. F., & Fewell, R. R. (1986). Mothers of deaf-blind children. In R. R. Fewell & P. F. Vadasy (Eds.), *Families of handicapped children* (pp. 121-148). Austin, TX: PRO-ED.

Vadasy, P. F., Fewell, R. R., Greenberg, M. T., Desmond, N. L., & Meyer, D. J. (1986). Follow-up evaluation of the effects of involvement in the Fathers Program. *Topics in Early Childhood Education, 6,* 16-31.

Vadasy, P. F., Fewell, R. R., & Meyer, D. J. (1986). Grandparents of children with special needs. *Journal of the Division for Early Childhood, 10,* 36-44.

VanDenBerg, J., & Grealish, E. M. (1997). Finding family strengths: A multiple-choice test. *Reaching Today's Youth: The Community Circle of Caring Journal, 1.* Retrieved December 1, 1997, from http://www.air.org/cecp/wraparound/articles.html

Vannatta, K., & Gerhardt, C. A. (2003). Pediatric oncology: Psychological outcomes for children and families. In M. C. Roberts (Ed.), *Handbook of pediatric psychology* (3rd ed., pp. 243-258). New York: Guilford Press.

Van Riper, M. (2000). Family variables associated with well-being in siblings of children with Down syndrome. *Journal of Family Nursing, 6,* 267-286.

Varekamp, M. A., Suurmeijer, P., Rosendaal, F. R., Dijck, H., Uriends, A., & Briet, E. (1990). Family burden in families with a hemophilic child. *Family Systems Medicine, 8,* 291-301.

Vega, W. A. (1995). The study of Latino families: A point of departure. In R. E. Zambrana (Ed.), *Understanding Latino families: Scholarship, policy, and practice* (pp. 3-17). Thousand Oaks, CA: Sage.

Visher, E. B., & Visher, J. S. (1996). *Therapy with stepfamilies.* New York: Brunner/Mazel.

von Bertalanffy, L. (1968). *General systems theory.* New York: Braziller.

Voysey, M. (1972). Impression management by parents with disabled children. *Journal of Health and Social Behavior, 13,* 80-89.

Waechter, E. H. (1977). Bonding problems of infants with congenital anomalies. *Nursing Forum, 16,* 229-318.

Waisbren, E. (1980). Parents' reactions after the birth of a developmentally disabled child. *American Journal of Mental Deficiency, 84,* 345-351.

Waitzkin, H. (1985). Information giving in medical care. *Journal of Health and Social Behavior, 26,* 81-101.

Waitzman, N. J., Scheffler, R. M., & Romano, P. S. (1996). *The cost of birth defects: Estimates of the value of prevention.* Lanham, MD: University Press of America.

Walker, J. H. (1971). Spina bifida—and the parents. *Developmental Medicine and Child Neurology, 13,* 462-476.

Walsh, F. (1989). The family in later life. In B. Carter & M. McGoldrick (Eds.), *The changing family life cycle* (2nd ed., pp. 311-322). Boston: Allyn & Bacon.

Walsh, F. (2003a). Family resilience: A framework for clinical practice. *Family Process, 42,* 1-18.

Walsh, F. (Ed.). (2003b). *Normal family processes* (3rd ed.). New York: Guilford Press.

Wasow, M. (1997). Outcomes measurement and the mental health consumer advocacy movement. In E. J. Mullen & J. L. Magnabosco (Eds.), *Outcomes measurement in the human services* (pp. 160-169). Washington, DC: NASW Press.

Wasow, M., & Wikler, L. (1983). Reflections on professionals' attitudes toward the severely mentally retarded and the chronically ill: Implications for parents. *Family Therapy, 10,* 299–308.

Wasserman, R. (1983). Identifying the counseling needs of the siblings of mentally retarded children. *Personnel and Guidance Journal, 61,* 622–627.

Wayman, K. I., Lynch, E. W., & Hanson, M. J. (1991). Home-based early intervention services: Cultural sensitivity in a family systems approach. *Topics in Early Childhood Special Education, 10,* 56–75.

Weisbren, S. E. (1980). Parents' reactions after the birth of a developmentally disabled child. *American Journal of Mental Deficiency, 84,* 345–351.

Wells, K., & Biegel, D. E. (1991). *Family preservation services: research and evaluation.* Newbury Park, CA: Sage.

Wells, T. P. E., Byron, M. A., McMullen, S. H. P., & Birchall, M. A. (2002). Disability teaching for medical students: Disabled people contribute to curriculum development. *Medical Education, 36*(8), 788–791.

Wendeborn, J. D. (1982). Administrative considerations in treating the Hispanic patient. *Clinical Management in Physical Therapy, 2,* 6–7.

Werner, E. E. & Smith, R. S. (1992). *Overcoming the odds: High-risk children from birth to adulthood.* Ithaca, NY: Cornell University Press.

Wesley, P. W., Buysse, V., & Tyndall, S. (1997). Family and professional perspectives on early intervention: An exploration using focus groups. *Topics in Early Childhood Education, 17*(4), 435–457.

Western Psychiatric Institute and Clinic. (1980). *An intruder in the family: Families with cancer.* Pittsburgh: University of Pittsburgh.

Whitaker, B. (1996, October 13). A plan for parents of disabled children. *The New York Times,* p. 1, 27.

White, C. J. (1995). Native Americans at promise: Travel in Borderlands. In B. B. Swadener & S. Lubeck (Eds.), *Children and families "at promise": Deconstructing the discourse of risk* (pp. 163–184). Albany: State University of New York Press.

White, R., Benedict, M. I., Wulff, L., & Kelley, M. (1987). Physical disabilities as risk factors for child maltreatment: A selected review. *American Journal of Orthopsychiatry, 57,* 93–101.

Whittaker, J. K., Kenney, J., Tracy, E. M., & Booth, C. (1990). *Reaching high-risk families: Intensive family preservation in human services.* New York: Aldine de Gruyter.

Wikler, L. (1981). Chronic stresses of families of mentally retarded children. *Family Relations, 30,* 281–288.

Wilcoxon, A. S. (1987). Grandparents and grandchildren: An often neglected relationship between significant others. *Journal of Counseling and Development, 65,* 289–290.

Wilkinson, D. Y. (1997). American Families of African Descent. In M. K. DeGenova (Ed.), *Families in cultural context: Strengths and challenges in diversity* (pp. 35–59). Mountain View, CA: Mayfield.

Williams, H. B., & Williams, E. (1979). Some aspects of childrearing practices in three minority subcultures in the United States. *Journal of Negro Education, 48,* 408–418.

Willie, C. V., & Reddick, R. J. (2003). *A new look at black families* (5th ed.). Walnut Creek, CA: Altamira Press.

Willoughby, J. C., & Glidden, L. M. (1995). Fathers helping out: Shaped child care and marital satisfaction of parents of children with disabilities. *American Journal of Mental Retardation, 99,* 399–406.

Wilton, K., & Barbour, A. (1978). Mother–child interaction in high-risk and contrast preschoolers of low socioeconomic status. *Child Development, 49,* 1136–1145.

Winton, P. J., & Bailey, D. B., Jr. (1988). The family-focused interview: A collaborative mechanism for family assessment and goal setting. *Journal of the Division for Early Childhood, 12,* 195–207.

Wolfensberger, W. (Ed.). (1972). *Normalization: The principle of normalization in human services.* Toronto: National Institute on Mental Retardation.

Wolin, S., & Wolin, S. (1993). *The resilient self: How survivors of troubled families rise above adversity.* New York: Villard Books.

World Health Organization. (1999). *International classification of functioning, disability, and health.* Geneva: Author.

Wortis, H. Z., & Margolies, J. A. (1955). Parents of children with cerebral palsy. *Medical Social Work, 4,* 110–120.

Wright, B. A. (1983). *Physical disability: A psychosocial approach* (2nd ed.). New York: Harper and Row.

Yalom, I., & Lesczcz, M. (2005). *The theory and practice of group psychotherapy* (5th ed.). New York: Basic Books.

Yedidia, M. J., Gillespie, C. C., Kachur, E., Schwartz, M. D., Ockene, J., Chepaitis, A. E., et al. (2003). Effect of communications training on medical student performance. *Journal of the American Medical Association, 290*(9), 1157–1165.

Yee, L. Y. (1988). Asian children. *Teaching Exceptional Children, 20*(4), 49–50.

Yellowbird, M., & Snipp, C. M. (2002). American Indian families. In R. J. Taylor (Ed.), *Minority families in the United States: A multicultural perspective* (3rd ed., pp. 227–249). Upper Saddle River, NJ: Prentice Hall.

Young, V. H. (1970). Family and childhood in a southern Negro community. *American Anthropologist, 40,* 269–288.

Zambrana, R. E., Dorrington, C., & Hayes-Bautista, D. (1995). Family and child health: A neglected vision. In R. E. Zambrana (Ed.), *Understanding Latino families: Scholarship, policy, and practice* (pp. 157–176). Thousand Oaks, CA: Sage.

Zigler, E., & Black, K. B. (1989). America's family support movement: Strengths and limitations. *American Journal of Orthopsychiatry, 59,* 6–19.

Zinn, M. B., & Eitzen, D. S. (1993). *Diversity in families.* New York: HarperCollins.

Zoints, L. T., Zoints, P., Harrison, S., & Bellinger, O. (2003). Urban African American families' perspective of cultural sensitivity within the special education system. *Focus on Autism and Other Developmental Disabilities, 18,* 41–50.

Zuckoff, M. (2002). *Choosing Naia: A family's journey.* Boston: Beacon Press.

Zuk, G. H. (1959). The religious factor and the role of guilt in parental acceptance of the retarded child. *American Journal of Mental Deficiency, 64,* 139–147.

Zuk, G. H., Miller, R. I., Batrum, J. B., & Kling, F. (1961). Maternal acceptance of retarded children: A questionnaire study of attitudes and religious background. *Child Development, 32,* 525–540.

Zuniga, M. E. (2004). Families with Latino roots. In E. W. Lynch & M. J. Hanson (Eds.), *Developing cross-cultural competence* (pp. 179–217). Baltimore: Brookes.

Index